Principles and Practice of

MANUAL
THERAPEUTICS

MEDICAL GUIDES TO
Complementary & Alternative Medicine

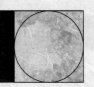

Principles and Practice of
MANUAL THERAPEUTICS

PATRICK COUGHLIN, PhD

Professor
Department of Anatomy
Philadelphia College of Osteopathic Medicine
Philadelphia, Pennsylvania

Series Editor **MARC S. MICOZZI**, MD, PhD

Executive Director
The College of Physicians of Philadelphia
Adjunct Professor of Medicine and of Rehabilitation Medicine
University of Pennsylvania
Bethesda, Maryland, and Philadelphia, Pennsylvania

with 55 illustrations

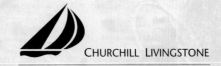

CHURCHILL LIVINGSTONE

An Imprint of Elsevier Science
New York   Edinburgh   London   Philadelphia

CHURCHILL LIVINGSTONE

An Imprint of Elsevier Science

The Curtis Center
Independence Square West
Philadelphia, Pennsylvania 19106

Library of Congress Cataloging in Publication Data

Coughlin, Patrick.
    Principles and practice of manual therapeutics / Patrick Coughlin.
      p. cm.
    Includes bibliographical references and index.
    ISBN 0-443-06559-4
     1. Manipulation (Therapeutics) I. Title.

  RM724 .C68 2002
  615.8'2—dc21

                                       2001058419

Publishing Director: Linda L. Duncan
Associate Editor: Kellie F. Conklin
Associate Developmental Editor: Jennifer L. Watrous
Editorial Assistant: Amanda Carrico
Publishing Services Manager: Deborah L. Vogel
Project Manager: Deon Lee
Design Manager: Bill Drone

About the Cover

The cover image is a color slide of a quilt entitled "Lifelines: Bosnia" made by Judith Tomlinson Trager. "Lifelines: Bosnia" was displayed in the U.S. Embassy in Bosnia from 1999 to 2001. Judith Trager has lived for the past 16 years in Boulder, Colorado, where she is a studio artist. She has made more than 200 quilts in the past 30 years, and her quilts hang in many corporate, public, and private collections, including the Kaiser Permanente Collection, Pikes Peak Community College, and Duke University Children's Hospital. This quilt image is copyrighted by Judith Trager.

PRINCIPLES AND PRACTICE OF MANUAL THERAPEUTICS   ISBN 0-443-06559-4

Contributors

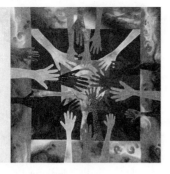

IRIS BURMAN, LMT
Founder and Director
Educating Hands School of Massage
Miami, Florida

LEON CHAITOW, ND, DO
Senior Lecturer
School of Integrated Health
University of Westminster
London, United Kingdom

JUDITH DELANY, LMT
NeuroMuscular Therapy Center
St. Petersburg, Florida

KEVIN V. ERGIL, MA, MS, LAc
Director, Graduate Program in Oriental Medicine
Associate Professor, School of Health Sciences
Touro College
New York, New York

FELICIA FOSTER, DAy, RN
Cardiology Nurse
Fletcher Allan Health Care
Ayurvedic Practitioner and Educator
President
Vermont State Nurse Association
Burlington, Vermont

SANDY FRIEDLAND, LMT
Teacher
Educating Hands School of Massage
Miami, Florida

EARLENE GLEISNER, RN
Reiki Master
Author
Laytonville, California

JOHN M. JONES III, DO
Immediate Past President of the American Academy of
    Osteopathy
Former Chair of the Department of Osteopathic
    Manipulative Medicine
Western University of Health Sciences/College of
    Osteopathic Medicine of the Pacific
Former Chair of the American Association of Colleges of
    Osteopathic Medicine's Educational Council on
    Osteopathic Principles
Dothan, Alabama

JEFFERY MAITLAND, PhD
Advanced Rolfing Instructor
Advanced Rolfer
Philosophical Counselor
Director of Academic Affairs
Rolf Institute
Boulder, Colorado

JOHN M. MCPARTLAND
Assistant Clinical Professor
Michigan State University
Programme Leader
School of Osteopathy, Faculty Health & Environmental
    Science
UNITEC
Auckland, New Zealand

MARC S. MICOZZI, MD, PhD
Executive Director
The College of Physicians of Philadelphia
Adjunct Professor of Medicine and Rehabilitation
    Medicine
University of Pennsylvania
Bethesda, Maryland, and Philadelphia, Pennsylvania

KERRY PALANJIAN, MBA, CMT
Nationally Certified Massage Therapist
Shiatsu Therapy and Owner, Shiatsu On-Site
More than just Massage-in-a-Chair
Hatboro/Greater Philadelphia, Pennsylvania

DANIEL REDWOOD, DC
Redwood Chiropractic and Wellness
Virginia Beach, Virginia

CARLA OSWALD REED, PT
Guild Certified Feldenkrais Practitioner
Physical Therapist
Movement to Wholeness
Sterling, Virginia

JAMES STEPHENS, PT, PhD
Guild Certified Feldenkrais Practitioner
Assistant Professor
Physical Therapy Department
Temple University
Philadelphia, Pennsylvania

ADRIENNE R. STONE
Physical Therapist
Certified Trager Practitioner and Tutor
Instructor of Trager Reflex-Response
Practitioner of Rosen Method Bodywork and Movement
Katonah, New York
Private Practice
Westchester County and Manhattan, New York

DAVID S. WALTHER, DC
Diplomate, International College of Applied Kinesiology
Certified Applied Kinesiology Instructor
Private Practice
Pueblo, Colorado

DIANE WIND WARDELL, PhD, RNC, HNC, CHTP/I
Associate Professor of Nursing
Department of Target Populations
The University of Texas Houston Health Science Center
Director of Research
Healing Touch International, Inc
Houston, Texas

For Liz, David, and Andy

Everything That Rises Must Converge
Flannery O'Connor, Noonday Press, August 1996

Foreword

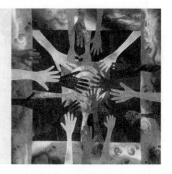

This is a book many of us have wanted and needed for a long time. The methods described in these pages are gaining enormous public acceptance, to the extent that mainstream medicine is finally taking notice.

The dramatic changes taking place in the health care system have been revealed to me by events right here in conservative New England. To my astonishment, in the last few years the local hospitals have begun to offer a growing number of the methods detailed in this book as options for their patients. Those clinical facilities that have not done this are finding themselves at a competitive disadvantage simply because patients appreciate manual therapeutics and prefer to go to facilities that offer them. I never anticipated how rapidly this change could sweep through a health care system that seemed firmly and irrevocably set on a course leading more and more toward breakdown.

Of course, the acceptance of so-called *integrative medicine* varies from city to city, state to state, and country to country. But the overall trend is very clear-cut. People love these therapies and appreciate the personal approach taken by the therapists who provide them. These techniques are enormously cost-effective at a time when the old way is creating debt that will seriously encumber our children and grandchildren. The times are ripe for a change, and it is happening.

Part of the need for this book arises because classically trained physicians are often justifiably bewildered by techniques whose theoretical base is unfamiliar to them. Their patients are asking questions that they are not prepared for. Each of these methods is based on logical premises that anyone can understand, and their practice leads to observations of remarkable phenomena that are open to exploration and verification by scientific methods.

To me, this is the most exciting kind of science—we look at phenomena that are new to the analytical process even though they are old-hat to the therapists who have been doing this work for a long time, seemingly in an intellectual vacuum. In the past, the extraordinary observations therapists make during their day-to-day work have been off-limits to scientific inquiry. This academic "blind spot" has been a huge impediment to the forward progress of biomedicine. Thankfully this primitive outlook is being left behind.

It is for these reasons that there is a need for an organized source of reliable information on manual therapeutics now more than ever, and here it is. Dr. Coughlin is a scholar, and it is therefore no surprise that he has required careful and thoughtful scholarship from his contributors. There is wisdom here that can be used by anyone who uses their hands for the relief of human sufferings.

I believe this is taking us in one direction:

There is this medicine and that medicine, and this method and that method, and then there is how the body really works.

KERRY WEINSTEIN

In spite of their history of effectiveness and acceptance, none of the schools or traditions of manual therapeutics has completed its evolution. All are in development. Each school, from Western biomedicine to the ancient Ayurvedic to Chiropractic to massage to Reiki and so on has a core of insightful and creative individuals who are advancing theory and practice. These visionaries are fascinating to observe because of their eagerness to synthesize and integrate information from modern science as well as from many other sources. Watch them work, and you will see the future of medicine unfolding before your eyes.

A medical and health care revolution is in progress, and it is headed toward a more complete description of what it is to be alive and healthy than we have ever had before. Cross-fertilization between disciplines drives the intellectual side of this revolution. The leaders in every therapeutic school are individuals who can see beyond what they have learned by standing on the shoulders of the giants who have preceded them. They appreciate the accomplishments and insights developed in other therapeutic disciplines and incorporate these lessons into their own unique thinking and hands-on practice.

The medicine that is emerging as you are reading this is increasingly able to treat more and more of the diseases and disorders that conventional medicine is certain are hopeless or incurable. Important for the costly health care crisis and for those who suffer from its inadequacies is that many expensive and dreadfully debilitating chronic problems are being resolved inexpensively by the methods of manual therapeutics.

I would like to single out a chapter in this book for special praise, but I cannot do so. The editor has carefully selected his contributors for their clarity and thoughtfulness. You will find here descriptions that are often more lucid, up-to-date, and insightful than those you have seen elsewhere in the widely scattered literature in these different fields. You will find the rich and fascinating history of each of the disciplines, the life experiences of the founders that led them to their innovations, the clinical trials that have been done, the theoretical underpinnings, and fascinating case studies.

All of those who use their hands to nourish and nurture human beings will derive beneficial insights from each chapter in this book. So regardless of your specialty, I recommend a cover-to-cover reading. You will be rewarded in ways you cannot anticipate and that I cannot predict for you. The publication of this book is a giant step for all of us in the healing arts.

JAMES L. OSCHMAN, PhD
author of *Energy Medicine: The Scientific Basis,*
Churchill Livingstone, 2000

Series Introduction

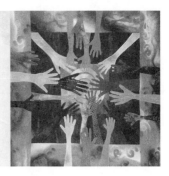

The aim of this series is to provide, for health care professionals and students, clear and rational guides to what is currently known about the following:

- Therapeutic medical systems currently labeled as complementary medicine
- Complementary approaches to specific medical conditions
- Integration of complementary therapy into mainstream medical practice

Each text is written with the needs and questions of a health care audience specifically in mind. Where possible, basic applications in clinical practice are explored.

What is called complementary medicine is being rapidly integrated into mainstream health care largely in response to consumer demand and in recognition of new scientific findings that are expanding our view of health and healing, pushing against the limits of the current biomedical paradigm.

Health care professionals need to know what their patients are doing and what they believe about what has been called *alternative medicine*. In addition, a basic working knowledge of complementary medical therapies is a rapidly growing requirement for primary care, some medical specialties, and throughout the allied health professions. These approaches also expand our view of the art and science of medicine and contribute importantly to the intellectual formation of health professions students.

This series provides a survey of the fundamentals and foundations of complementary medical systems currently available and practiced in North America and Europe. Each topic is presented in ways that are understandable and that provide an important understanding of the intellectual foundations of each system, with translation between the complementary and conventional medical systems when possible. These explanations appropriately draw on the social and scientific foundations of each system of care.

Rapidly growing contemporary research results are included whenever possible. In addition to providing evidence indicating when complementary medicines may be of therapeutic benefit, guidance is provided as to when complementary therapies should not be used.

This field of health is rapidly moving from being considered *alternative* (implying exclusive use of one medical system or another), to *complementary* (used as an adjunct to mainstream medical care), to *integrative medicine* (implying an active, conscious effort by mainstream medicine to incorporate alternatives on the basis of rational clinical and scientific information and judgment).

Likewise, health care professionals and students must move rapidly to learn the fundamentals of complementary medical systems to better serve their patients' needs, protect the public health, and expand their scientific horizons and understandings of health and healing.

MARC S. MICOZZI
Philadelphia, Pennsylvania
1997

Series Editor's Preface

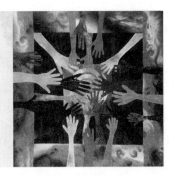

As editor of the textbook *Fundamentals of Complementary and Alternative Medicine,* Second Edition (2001), and series editor for *Medical Guides to Complementary and Alternative Medicine,* I reviewed many contributions on complementary medicine for health care professionals. In my work as a physician and cultural historian, I have made connections between the "new" field of complementary medicine and the ancient history and heritage of healing as a subject common to all human societies in nearly all times and places. Thus we may come to view complementary medicine not as New Age, but as age-old approaches to human healing.

Manual therapies stand at an interesting juncture among healing techniques and traditions. Manual therapies associated with the practice of medicine necessarily involve touch and physical manipulation. When various approaches to manual therapies that have evolved in human societies are surveyed, it is found that the explanations of the therapeutic benefit invoked by these therapies often involve ancient ideas about the manipulation of "vital energy." More recently, science has developed biomechanical models to show how manual therapy works.

However, the human body is not a machine (with apologies to *National Geographic's* popular "incredible machine" metaphor). Human healing involves not only biomechanical manipulation, but also "hands-on" intervention. The benefits of the "laying on of hands" is a well-known and accepted part of the wisdom of clinicians from ancient times to the present in complementary and mainstream medicine.

It has become almost axiomatic that people are often more desirous of "high-touch" than "high-tech" medicine, which can sometimes be seen as impersonal and alienating. People (and practitioners), however, also want medicine that works and are willing to endure a great deal of discomfort to be healed. Increasingly, the high-touch complementary medical modalities are being validated by the standards of contemporary high-tech biomedical science.

Manual therapy has a tremendous opportunity to synthesize the worlds of high-touch and high-tech medicine. Incredibly, I have seen physical therapists who barely touch the patient in favor of biomechanical devices and patient education lectures about stretching and exercise. Patients can get devices and information elsewhere; however, patients turn to manual therapy to be touched therapeutically. That is a role of the healer that cannot be replaced by technology and information.

During the scientific transformation of medical practice in the last century, some manual therapy has become more scientifically based and enfranchised as part of mainstream medical practice. Other manual therapy traditions remain "alternative" or alternatively became mainstreamed, such as the osteopathic medical tradition. In the rush toward scientific validation and integration of complementary therapies into mainstreamed practice, medicine has an interest in reclaiming the general and specific benefits of the laying on of hands in ways that help the body to heal. To the patient, that is what the best manual therapy is about. The twenty-first century should have the opportunity to bring it about.

MARC S. MICOZZI
November 2001
Bethesda, Maryland, and
Philadelphia, Pennsylvania

Preface

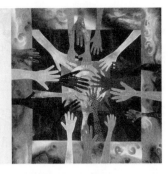

Manipulation as a therapeutic practice has existed for thousands of years. The exact date of origin of the earliest forms of manipulative therapy is unknown. However, because we routinely observe primates in grooming behaviors and giving comfort by means of touch, extrapolating these observations to early hominid behavior indicates that the use of therapeutic touch predates history. In addition, self-treatment by means of stimulus-induced analgesia (e.g., rubbing the site of a traumatic injury or scratching an itch) is a behavior instinctive to a multitude of species. Animals of all stripes touch each other and themselves therapeutically.

It has been recorded that Hippocrates was skilled in the use of manipulation and taught it in his school of medicine more than 2000 years ago. In fact, virtually all of the world's cultures can demonstrate the use of manipulation as a form of therapy. However, much of this information has been passed on as an oral rather than written tradition, so documentation is difficult if not impossible to obtain in many instances (especially in the case of ancient societies such as in India and China, see Chapters 10 and 11).

The late nineteenth century saw a period of great expansion of thought during and immediately following the industrial revolution. It is interesting to note the similarities and differences in the histories of osteopathy and chiropractic. Both began in the midwestern United States during this period. In fact, legend has it that the founders of both professions had contact with one another at one or more points in time (see Chapter 1). Subsequently they diverged philosophically and in practice; the osteopathic profession now much more closely resembles allopathic medicine. Both professions continue to struggle internally with its identity and direction.

There are a number of concepts to bear in mind when considering the principles of manipulation. These concepts are based on physical laws, anatomic principles, and the physiology of the sensorimotor system, and apply to all manipulative practice. Thus association can be made between these concepts and the various forms (styles) of manipulative therapy, resulting in a greater understanding of the rationale for prescribing, applying, or seeking this type of treatment.[3] A conceptual view of manual treatment is the hallmark of the unique presentation of therapeutic massage, found in Chapter 3. These concepts include, but are not limited, to the following:

- The bilateral symmetry of the human neuromusculoskeletal anatomy
- Gravity/tensegrity: the reaction of the human body to the force of gravity and the balance between compressive and tensional forces[2,4]
- Postural maintenance and coordinated movement/orthotropism: the tendency of the human organism toward a vertical posture (see Chapter 5)[5]; this takes place in the body through the interactions of the visual, vestibular, and proprioceptive systems, collectively referred to as the *equilibrial triad,* described in the following:
  - The ubiquitousness of the fascial system and its impact on other body systems
  - Somato-visceral interaction and integration: peripheral and central
  - Pain/muscle spasm/neurologic facilitation: the downward spiral
  - Compensation/decompensation: the adaptive response and its limitations
  - Range of motion/motion barriers and restrictions

- Treatment strategies: active versus passive (i.e., the client as participant in therapy, including the prescription of therapeutic exercise) and direct versus indirect (application of technique toward or away from motion barriers)
- Oscillation: the interplay of body rhythms and the potential harmonic convergence between therapist and client

Based on these defining principles, the practitioner of manual therapy seeks to correct structural and functional imbalances present in the client/patient to optimize the body's ability to self-correct or repair itself, which includes the defense against invasion from foreign substances or organisms. The practitioner is thus a facilitator in a patient/client-centered treatment process, with the client, not the therapist, as the effector of healing. At least three types of balance, which are potential targets of the various styles and techniques employed, follow:

1. The restoration of proper joint range of motion and body symmetry
2. The restoration of balanced nervous system activity
   - Between the sensory and motor systems
   - Between the somatic and autonomic nerves
   - Between the sympathetic and parasympathetic divisions of the autonomic nervous system
3. The restoration of proper arterial flow and venous and lymphatic drainage for proper nutrition of all cells and tissues of the body.

In contrast to biomedical principles prevalent in Western cultures is the Asian model of human anatomy and physiology, which is expressed as energy. In this model, bioenergy (*Qi, Ki, Prana*) flows longitudinally through the body along channels or meridians. Pathology is represented as an improper alteration in energy flow. Consequently, practitioners of Asian manipulation styles treat the channels directly, rather than treating muscle, ligaments, or fascia, for example.

Bioenergy also extends beyond individual bodies and is represented by fields or auras, which can also be manipulated, as found in both eastern and western styles. Qi Gong, Reiki, healing touch, and therapeutic touch all occasionally employ "hands off" techniques to manipulate the energy system.

Even though manipulation can be used symptomatically (using the allopathic disease model), most styles strongly tend toward a holistic view of the patient/client. This viewpoint typically recognizes three parts of the human being: body, mind, and spirit. The recognition of the interaction of these components results in an increased sensitivity of the practitioner to the Reichian concept of body language for the purpose of diagnosis. In addition, manipulative treatment can frequently trigger emotional catharsis in the patient/client, sometimes referred to as somatoemotional release. Occasionally, both practitioners and clients report paranormal (spiritual) experiences as a result of the manipulative experience. Indeed, Feldenkrais and Trager practitioners and others think of the therapist and client as a single unit during treatment.

Until recently, the amount of basic and clinical research on manipulation has been scant. The National Center for Complementary and Alternative Medicine (NCCAM) at the National Institutes of Health was established to fund research on the efficacy of various therapies including manipulation. In each year of its existence the budget for this center has grown exponentially, which has resulted in an ever-growing number of clinical studies. The results of these studies are beginning to find their way into the clinical guidelines published by the Agency for Healthcare Research and Quality.[1] Probably the most confounding question in this research is that of the placebo effect. Constructing appropriate control or sham treatments is very difficult and, when it is considered that any touch may elicit a response, may be impossible.

This book does not purport to be comprehensive. Although not all types of manipulation are covered, the major styles practiced worldwide are represented. Each chapter presents the history, philosophy, technique, and training for and of the practice. The appendix at the end of the book is a compendium of resources from which to obtain additional information.

The prevalence and popularity of manual therapeutics is such that it is rapidly approaching a descriptor of "mainstream" rather than "complementary." Although we have not determined the exact mechanism of action of this treatment modality, what is quite clear is that human beings generally respond favorably to the touch of others and that touch has the potential to affect the outcome of any treatment.

PATRICK COUGHLIN
Philadelphia, Pennsylvania

References

1. Agency for Healthcare Research and Quality: *Clinical practice guidelines.* Available at http://www.ahrq.gov/clinic/cpgsix.htm. [Accessed 12/7/01.]

2. Chen C, Ingber D: Tensegrity and mechanoregulation: from skeleton to cytoskeleton, *Osteoarthritis Cartilage* 7(1):81-94, 1999. Available at http://www.idealibrary.com/links/doi/10.1053/joca.1998.0164. [Accessed on 1/16/02.]

3. Coughlin P: Manual therapies. In Micozzi M, editor: *Fundamentals of complementary medicine,* ed 2, St Louis, 2000, Mosby.

4. Ingber D: The architecture of life, *Sci Am* 2789(1): 48-57, 1998. Available at http://www.sciam.com/1998/0198issue/0198ingber.html. [Accessed on 1/16/02.]

5. Maitland J: Personal communication, January, 2002.

Acknowledgments

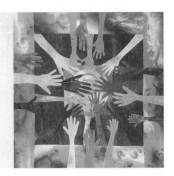

I would like to extend my heartfelt thanks to the individual chapter authors. Their writing skills made my job as compiler an easy one. It should be noted that all of these authors are clinicians, most without an affiliation with an academic institution. The time they spent writing came at considerable personal expense to each of them with no reward other than the satisfaction of a job well done (not even tenure). This was truly a labor of love.

In addition, I would like to thank Jennifer Watrous of Mosby, whose encouragement and cheerleading were a great help to everyone.

Finally, I'd like to thank Marc Micozzi, who had faith in the project from the beginning and who exercised great leadership in the face of seemingly insurmountable difficulty.

Contents

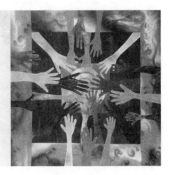

I   EUROPEAN–NORTH AMERICAN MANUAL SYSTEMS, *1*

   1   Osteopathic Medicine, *3*
   JOHN M. JONES III

   2   Chiropractic, *26*
   DANIEL REDWOOD

   3   Massage Therapy: TouchAbilities™, *50*
   IRIS BURMAN AND SANDY FRIEDLAND

   4   Modern Neuromuscular Techniques, *69*
   LEON CHAITOW AND JUDITH DELANY

   5   Cultivating the Vertical: The Rolf Method of Structural Integration, *89*
   JEFFREY MAITLAND

   6   Applied Kinesiology, *100*
   DAVID S. WALTHER

   7   The Trager® Approach, *110*
   ADRIENNE R. STONE

   8   Feldenkrais Method, *119*
   CARLA REED AND JAMES STEPHENS

II   ASIAN MANUAL SYSTEMS, *139*

   9   Shiatsu, *141*
   KERRY PALANJIAN

   10   Ayurvedic Bodywork, *155*
   JOHN M. McPARTLAND AND FELICIA FOSTER

   11   Qi Gong and Tui Na, *165*
   KEVIN V. ERGIL AND MARC S. MICOZZI

III   **MANIPULATION OF BIOENERGY,** *173*

12   Reiki: The Usui System of Natural Healing, *175*
EARLENE GLEISNER

13   Healing Touch and Therapeutic Touch, *184*
DIANE WIND WARDELL

Appendix: Contacts (Professional Organizations/Referral Services), *199*

Index, *217*

Principles and Practice of

MANUAL
THERAPEUTICS

I

EUROPEAN–NORTH AMERICAN MANUAL SYSTEMS

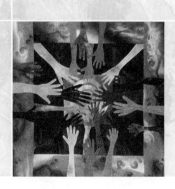

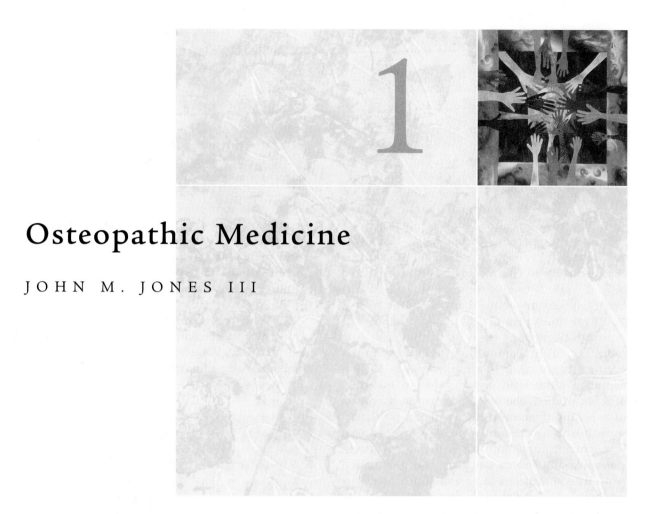

Osteopathic Medicine

JOHN M. JONES III

To find health should be the object of the doctor. Anyone can find disease.

ANDREW TAYLOR STILL, MD, DO, Founder of Osteopathy

HISTORY

Osteopathic medicine began as an offshoot of the standard medical practices of the 1800s when one innovative physician became disenchanted with the inadequate and harmful effects of the medicines being used by the doctors of that era.

Andrew Taylor Still, MD, DO, was born in 1828 in Jonesboro, Virginia. His life experiences and observation led him to question the entire system of medicine that existed in nineteenth century America.

Most medications used in that era were unresearched remedies passed on through tradition. Bleeding and leaching were major components of treatment when Still was trained, as were "purging and puking." One of the most common medications was calomel, a mercuric compound used as a purgative. It was extremely toxic, often causing patients' teeth to fall out and sores to break out in the mouth; calomel undoubtedly contributed to many deaths. Surgery was primitive and performed without antisepsis; anesthetics were just beginning to be used. No antibiotics had been identified, and no microbial cause of infectious illness was proven until 1872. There was no knowledge of the immune system, and heart disease and cancer were not understood. Physicians were capable of diagnosing recognized patterns of illness and in many cases, predicting outcomes. Medical treatment was often more dangerous than doing nothing. In fact, the famous French mathe-

3

matician and philosopher Descartes, developer of the Cartesian system of thought, was reputed to have said, "Before, when I knew I was sick, I thought I might die; now that they are taking me to the chirurgeon, I know I shall."[6]

Still was seeking a philosophy of medicine and system of treatment based on scientific principles as they could be observed in nature. In April 1855, he stated that he began to discuss reasons "for my faith in the laws of life as given to men, worlds, and beings by the God of Nature."[9] He was not alone in his disillusionment with the contemporary state of affairs and quest for a scientifically based philosophy of medicine. The great physician and jurist, Oliver Wendell Holmes, for example, was often quoted as saying that "if the whole of *materia medica* as now used could be sunk to the bottom of the sea, it would be all the better for mankind—and all the worse for the fishes."[4]

By the time of the Civil War, a large number of American physicians were homeopathic or eclectic (nonstandard). In addition, many people on the frontier took care of their own medical needs. Medical education was offered in two ways. At university-affiliated medical schools, students attended a course of 4 months of morning lectures to obtain their degrees. If students voluntarily attended a second year, it was for a repeat of the same lectures. Many American physicians skipped this didactic education and apprenticed themselves to an established physician, reading medical and scientific textbooks and accompanying the physician on his home and office visits. More specialized studies could be undertaken by arranging to work with an established expert, but most doctors did not pursue such studies. These two systems were later combined and evolved into the current system of medical education (2 years of basic science and medical didactics, followed by 2 years during which students continue to read medical books and journals while shadowing and assisting physicians in hospital and ambulatory care settings, after which the graduate physicians do an additional 3 to 7 years of supervised postgraduate hospital residencies).

A.T. Still was the son of Abram Still, a circuit-riding Methodist minister who was also a physician, tending to his flock both spiritually and medically. Shortly after Still was born, the family moved to Missouri so that his father could serve the needs of the church on the western frontier. Abram Still was an ardent abolitionist who sided with the small minority of Methodist ministers in Missouri who were opposed to slavery. When the church split over the issue, he moved the family to Kansas, where they supported the cause of freedom.

Like many pioneer boys, Still grew up contributing to the family food supply by hunting and did much of the butchering of the animals himself. He later stated that his studies of anatomy began this way. In his autobiography, he describes an intense headache that occurred when he was 10 years old. To alleviate his discomfort by taking a nap, he placed his jacket over a rope swing to construct a pillow and then lay down with the base of his skull over the other side of the rope. He fell asleep and a short time later awoke to find his headache gone. This phenomenon impressed him and afterward, as a physician, the memory of it led him to think about the relationship between the body's anatomy and the disease process.

Still obtained his medical education through a process of apprenticeship under an established physician (in Still's case, his father, whom he assisted), combined with reading the medical texts of that time.

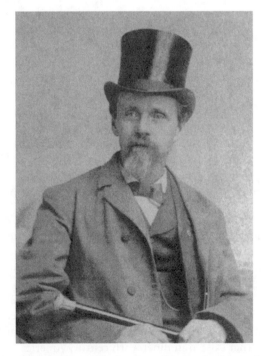

Figure 1-1 A portrait of A.T. Still, the founder of osteopathy, circa 1900. (Courtesy Kirksville College of Osteopathy, A.T. Still Memorial Library, Archives Department, Kirksville, Missouri.)

He later attended a medical school in Kansas City, but he did not complete a degree, finding that the school had little to teach him that he did not already know.

Andrew Taylor Still (Figure 1-1), began his medical career by serving the local community and the Shawnee Indians. Ironically, his maternal grandmother had been kidnapped by that tribe, who had also killed numerous members of that generation of her family. Still had a standard general medical practice, employing the usual medications and involving the full range of available treatment, including obstetrics and minor surgery.

Dr. Still became a battalion surgeon in the Kansas militia during the Civil War; he also served as an officer and led men into battle. He returned to his family in 1864 at the end of the western campaigns, when the Kansas militia was disbanded after Union victory.

Believing that his family was safe because the war was over in that part of the country, he was stunned when three of his children died in an epidemic of spinal meningitis. There were no effective medications to treat such an illness. He called other physicians to attend to his family, rather than manage their cases himself, and called ministers to pray for the children as well. Nothing availed, and the children died. This event caused him to question the entire foundation of medical care in his era. He wrote, "It was when I gazed at three members of my own family —two of my own children and one adopted child— all dead from the disease, spinal meningitis, that I propounded to myself the serious questions 'In sickness has God left man in a world of guessing? Guess what is the matter? What to give, and guess the result? And when dead, guess where he goes?'"[7]

Seeking a more enlightened practice of medicine, Still based his reasoning on the Methodist philosophy of working to attain perfection, which seemed to have something in common with the new idea of natural evolution. The early evolutionists suggested a natural process of working toward perfection of the organism, and that the human being was the highest naturally evolved life form. Still felt that the human being was perfectly constructed by the one he later referred to in his writings as the God of Nature, the Great Architect, the Great Engineer, and the Great Mechanic. If the human body was perfectly constructed as the highest form of machine, he felt it should simply need fuel and, if something went wrong, adjustment.

Like the general population of the nineteenth century, he had a tremendous admiration for engineering and all things mechanical. Still was also an inventor; he had invented a thresher and had obtained patents for a new type of churn and stove. After founding a school of medicine, the American School of Osteopathy (ASO), he would eventually tell his students that they were to become human engineers who knew every part and function of the body.

In 1897 Still wrote in his autobiography that on June 22, 1874, he "flung to the breeze the banner of osteopathy."[7] He was now able to define the principles on which his philosophy and practice of medical care would be based. His new methods involved hands-on treatment adjusting the positions of joints and level of muscle tone; enhancing the circulation of blood, lymphatic, and cerebrospinal fluids; improving the efficiency of respiration; and therefore improving host response to disease.

Still was ostracized in Kansas for leaving the medical fold and denied the opportunity to teach his new ideas at Baker University in Baldwin, Kansas, which his family had helped to build. He moved to Kirksville, Missouri, where he said he found a few people who were willing to listen to reason. He set up a circuit practice of medicine in outlying communities; after being in practice for a while so many people began coming to Kirksville looking for him that he was able to stay in one office. He was not sure what to call his clinical practice; at first he thought his new methods, being hands-on, might have something in common with magnetic healing, and so for a short time he called himself a magnetic healer. Later, he used a business card on which he called himself a lightning bonesetter. The use of this term implies that he had heard of the folk healers who called themselves by that name, although there is no evidence that he ever studied with anyone who had learned this art in the usual way (i.e., it was passed from father to son).

In 1892, shortly before he founded the ASO in Kirksville, he coined the term *osteopathy* (from the Greek roots *osteon* and *pathos*), following the tradition of others who had named their medical approaches after what they thought was the central issue in pathology. In the case of osteopathy, Still reasoned that malpositioned bones and joints, especially in the spine, affected both circulation and nerve function, which, when disturbed, provided the opportunity for the development of disease in the tissues. Starting with about 10 students the first year, the school expanded rapidly, and it became impossible for Still to personally instruct all the students in his methods; thus his first students became the new professors.

To further disseminate his ideas, Still wrote four books: *The Autobiography of Andrew Taylor Still* (1897) describes his life and how he developed osteopathy. *The Philosophy of Osteopathy* (1899) and *The Philosophy and Mechanical Principles of Osteopathy* (copyrighted 1892 but published 1902) describe his philosophical ideas and contain a great deal of speculation about physiology, which was poorly understood at the time. In *Osteopathy: Research and Practice* (1910), Still describes some of his treatment techniques.

These books reveal that he still, on occasion, used some medications—although extremely rarely. He was opposed to the use of opiates and alcohol, having seen much abuse (especially in Civil War victims), and specifically stated that it was foolish for physicians to dissolve most medications in alcohol, because this could lead to addiction. Throughout his books he recommended the use of manipulation to relieve anatomic and therefore physiologic stress on the system, returning the body to a state in which it could cure itself through normal physiologic processes. Still's original philosophical principles are summed up in "Our Platform," which was published in *Osteopathy: Research and Practice,* and adopted by the ASO as the foundation of its educational program.

The allopathic profession, which was becoming successful in establishing a monopoly on medical training and licensure, vigorously fought the new osteopathic profession. Still's followers, however, obtained great success in their treatment of illness in comparison with their MD counterparts, effecting cures in some hopeless cases and treating all types of illnesses. They also had special expertise in neuromusculoskeletal conditions at a time when virtually no physical medicine, rehabilitation, or physical therapy was available to the public. The ASO rapidly expanded, and new schools founded by graduates helped build the osteopathic profession, which attracted supporters such as Teddy Roosevelt, President William Howard Taft, and Mark Twain (who testified in a trial brought against an osteopath). Osteopaths graduated with the title *Doctor of Osteopathy (DO),* which was changed at the end of the twentieth century to *Doctor of Osteopathic Medicine (DO).*

The 1910 Flexner Report, sponsored by the Carnegie Foundation, compared all American medical schools against a standard represented by Johns Hopkins University's School of Medicine. Criticism was so devastating that the majority of American medical schools closed, including many osteopathic medical schools. The surviving osteopathic medical colleges were located in Kirksville, Missouri; Kansas City, Missouri; Des Moines, Iowa; Philadelphia, Pennsylvania; Chicago, Illinois; and Los Angeles, California. Because they were private institutions, none of these schools received public funding at the time. The osteopathic profession was on its own for further development.

Still's central idea was that structural abnormality causes functional abnormality, leading to illness. To regain health, treatments were designed to use the body's own resources. He theorized that manipulation would increase the body's efficiency, promoting appropriate delivery of blood, clearance of blood and lymph, delivery of neurotrophic substances, and transmission of neural impulses. There were relatively few medicines of value for the patient in the preantibiotic era (during the early 1900s). Osteopathic manipulation, on the other hand, was a technique that a physician could use to effect physiologic changes and mount a host defense against illness. In addition, osteopathy directly address a number of needs with which the medical profession had not successfully dealt: musculoskeletal pain, physical rehabilitation, and soft-tissue injuries.

Soon after Still's death in 1917, his new osteopathic physicians were put to the test during the Spanish influenza pandemic of 1919. The results were excellent. The medical profession had little to offer patients other than antitussives and opiates. Osteopathic treatment targeted autonomic changes, blood delivery, lymphatic drainage, and biochemical advantage in respiration. Osteopathic physicians reported dramatically lower morbidity and mortality rates among their influenza patients.

Between the death of Still in 1917 and World War II, osteopathic colleges, like allopathic colleges, gradually improved standards. In the early 1900s, increasing practice of antiseptic procedure helped improve the safety of surgery, as did the development and use of the sulfa antibiotics by the 1930s. Penicillin, although developed in 1927, was not available for practical use until it was prioritized for use with soldiers and sailors during World War II, after the problem of mass production was solved. It was not readily available for the American public until after the war.

Still's students had included MDs who were less opposed to standard medications but integrated his ideas on enhancing the body's own self-healing abilities by treating the structure (anatomy) to enhance the function (physiology) and regain health. By 1928, *materia medica* (the part of medicine concerned with formulation and use of remedies or primitive pharmacologic preparations, taught in allopathic medical schools before the development of modern medications) was taught at all of the osteopathic medical colleges. In addition, the new researched and efficacious antibiotics were discussed as they were developed. Osteopathic physicians, along with their MD peers, increasingly had available medications that actually worked, which they mixed into their general practice of medicine. Early osteopathic physicians had always included surgery in their complete practice of medicine and believed that osteopathic manipulation before and after surgery helped patients tolerate such procedures better and reduced the incidence of complications, such as pneumonia, thereby resulting in a shorter recovery time.

As medical specialties and subspecialties were being developed, most osteopaths were general practitioners. American training programs were not generally open to DOs. A number of osteopathic subspecialists obtained their training in Europe from physicians who did not concern themselves with distinctions between types of American physicians; some of these osteopathic physicians returned and set up training programs in their own profession.

During World War II, osteopaths were not allowed to serve in the armed forces as physicians. A number volunteered and served in other capacities, but many stayed home and took care of patients whose MDs were overseas. In the postwar peroid, as returning soldiers attended universities in record numbers on the GI Bill, osteopathic colleges had record numbers of students.

By 1953 the president of the American Medical Association (AMA) had called for and received a report on the status of osteopathic medicine, indicating that DO training was equivalent to MD training. MDs in general were not concerned with whether their osteopathic colleagues used osteopathic manipulative treatment (OMT) in the care of back pain, sports medicine, and rehabilitation, as long as they also prescribed new medications that were proven to be effective.

Two other events in the middle to late twentieth century helped the osteopathic profession gain acceptance by the allopathic medical profession. One was the merger of the osteopathic profession with the allopathic medical profession in California. A second was the establishment of 10 additional osteopathic medical colleges within a few short years, soon followed by 4 more.

In 1962, California had the largest number of DOs. Voters were convinced to support a plan under which new osteopathic licenses would no longer be issued, with the agreement that any DOs who wished to do so could trade their DO degree and $65 for an MD degree and license. The state osteopathic medical association worked with the California Medical Association to support this merger of professions. At the time, it was difficult for DOs to obtain privileges in most allopathic hospitals. More than 2000 DOs accepted MD degrees and licenses. Benefits to the new MDs included granting of hospital privileges. The largest and arguably most modern school, the College of Osteopathic Physicians and Surgeons at Los Angeles, was transformed into an MD-granting institution, which shortly thereafter affiliated with the University of California at Irvine.

The rest of the osteopathic profession was immediately concerned that the medical establishment, unable to eliminate the osteopathic profession, was attempting to absorb it. Although there was talk of similar offers in other states, there was no continuation of the process. Instead, the developments in California paved the way for further acceptance of the osteopathic medical profession. California MDs had seemingly indicated that the main differences between the two types of physicians were the letters of the degree and $65, and the osteopathic medical profession used this ammunition to approach state legislatures and other authorities in defense of osteopathic medical practice rights. Some state legislatures became convinced that it was in their interest to fund colleges of osteopathic medicine when statistics revealed that most DOs practiced general medicine, with a large proportion doing so in underserved areas (small towns, rural areas, and inner cities).

The osteopathic medical profession rapidly approved the founding of numerous new osteopathic medical colleges, both public and private. Included among the state-funded colleges were schools in Michigan, Texas, Ohio, West Virginia, and Oklahoma. However, this rapid expansion continued the trend toward assimilation into the medical mainstream. In the latter part of the twentieth century there were insufficient numbers of osteopathic physicians to serve as role models, as well as a shortage of postgraduate training positions in osteopathic hospitals, and different interest levels in osteopathic student matriculants. DOs in training therefore began dispersing throughout other hospitals rather than remaining concentrated in osteopathic hospitals. This process increased the number of osteopathic graduates entering allopathic residencies.

In the meantime, the development of the osteopathic profession continued around the world and differed markedly from the American evolution of the profession.

OFFSHOOTS OF THE OSTEOPATHIC PROFESSION

As osteopathic techniques were adapted and used by others who had become convinced of their efficacy, offshoots of the osteopathic profession developed. The first person to investigate osteopathy and found another profession was D.D. Palmer, who founded the chiropractic profession. In his book *The Lengthening Shadow of Dr. Andrew Taylor Still,* Arthur Hildreth, who had been one of the first students at the ASO, mentions that Palmer was a guest of Still's, who often hosted students for dinner.[3] Although the Kirksville College of Osteopathic Medicine does not have records of all matriculated students from the first few years, oral legends persist, passed down from DO parents who had children who became osteopathic physicians. These legends suggest two possibilities. One is that Palmer was a student for a time at the school. A second is that he was not an official student but that he came to town, worked either at the school or in the community, and learned manipulation from the students of Still.

What is clear and indisputable is that Still, a physician, practiced in northern Missouri for almost 20 years before founding his school in 1892. Davenport, Iowa, is not far from Kirksville, Missouri, and Still's reputation was originally regional (although it later became national and international because of national press coverage and outspoken supporters like Mark Twain, Theodore Roosevelt, and other notables).

Still's original students attempted to practice as Still himself had practiced. However, he told his students that they did not have to do exactly as he did if they could achieve the same results. Granted this freedom to explore, they quickly developed high-velocity manipulative techniques that were passed on at the school. By 1915, Edyth Ashmore, DO, who was in charge of teaching manipulative technique at the ASO, recommended in her published manual that the students not be taught the original methods of Still, because they were too hard for the students to learn.

Whether or not Palmer was a student of Still, it would not be surprising if his "serendipitous discovery" of manipulation was based on what he had heard of Still's methods. A number of authorities certainly believe chiropractic to be an offshoot of osteopathy, although founded by a nonphysician, Palmer.

Ida Rolf, the founder of *Rolfing* (see Chapter 5), a method of body work, was clear in her writings that she learned techniques from a blind osteopath and combined them with a knowledge of yoga to create a systematic protocol for whole-body structural integration.

Other adapters of osteopathic technique (and partially of osteopathic philosophy) include John Barnes, a physical therapist who studied myofascial release during postgraduate studies at Michigan State University (MSU) and then taught it to physical therapists, and John Upledger, a DO who mixed cranial and other manipulative techniques taught by Still's student William Garner Sutherland, DO, with light trance work and other techniques to develop what he called *craniosacral therapy,* which is generally practiced by nonphysicians.

In addition, because of the availability of postgraduate programs for physical therapists such as those offered by MSU and courses offered by other osteopathic physicians, physical therapists in the United States began using osteopathic techniques such as muscle energy, mobilization by thrust, myofascial release, and counterstrain. The effect on physical medicine, rehabilitation, sports medicine, and family practice throughout the United States has been considerable, teaching many health care professionals and lay personnel methods of alleviating pain and enhancing physical function.

OSTEOPATHIC PHILOSOPHY

The word *philosophy* often engenders an immediate visceral response in the scientific or technologic mind. The scientific mind is open to processing all new ideas. The technologic mind tends to reject that which has not been statistically demonstrated. Thus the connotation of philosophy as an organization of vague or general thoughts has often been repugnant to the technologic mind of the twentieth century. However, some of our greatest scientists, including Einstein, spoke of the importance of ideas that are not yet statistically evident.

In the last half of the nineteenth century, Still developed a unified philosophy of medicine, which he called *osteopathic philosophy*. This philosophy is best described as a background reference system that identifies the nature of the patient, defines the physician's mission, and establishes the basic premises of the logic of diagnosis and treatment. There remains in the general medical community, which has not been exposed to this organizing system, a poor understanding of exactly what is meant by osteopathic philosophy and why doctors of osteopathic medicine consider it important.

Osteopathic medical philosophy is centered on a profound respect for the inherent ability of the human being, and particularly the body, to heal itself. This philosophy has deep roots through all of recorded history. Over time, all ideas evolve and are integrated with new information. Osteopathic philosophy is no exception: time has produced a distinction between classical osteopathy, which was taught by Still, and contemporary osteopathic medical philosophy, which integrates the basic elements of Still's ideas with subsequent scientific discoveries (Box 1-1).

Classical Osteopathic Philosophy

Classical osteopathic philosophy identifies the human being as a triune being, including body, mind, and spirit. However, Still speaks in his writings very little about how to deal with the spirit or mind, leaving that up to the individual, and confines himself in general to dealing with the body. The osteopathic perspective is that the body is a marvelous machine that will function perfectly if the structure is perfect. If sick, it can be adjusted to the structural ideal to effect a return to physiologic harmony. Surgery and obstetrics are included in this philosophy. Surprisingly, Still believed that the diet of his time was sufficient and that the body (the machine) could handle any fuel as long as the machine was working correctly.

The triune nature of the human being that Still so often mentioned dates back to at least the Greeks and probably the Egyptians. The body is obvious and needs no definition. The mind, however, has been described both as an epiphenomenon of the brain and its biochemistry and as something that is more than the product of chemical interactions. Emotions are generally identified with the mind, but where the mind ends and the spirit begins is open to question. Although many scientists openly question the existence of spirit, it is perhaps easiest to say that throughout history, a possible third factor of human existence has been recognized by all societies. This factor is sometimes regarded as the most potent but the most unpredictable.

Still focused on the relationship between structure (anatomy) and function (physiology). His methods included taking a history, observing and palpating the body, and adjusting the body's constituent parts so that they were in normal positions, with normal motion, thereby promoting normal physiology. At that point, the innate self-healing powers of the body would accomplish what was necessary for healing to take place.

Evolution of the Osteopathic Philosophy

All philosophies that survive must be capable of incorporating newly discovered information. Striking differences from Still's original platform are found in contemporary osteopathic medical philosophy and practice.

Still died in 1917. By 1911 the ASO had incorporated the teaching of vaccines, serum therapy, and antitoxins in the bacteriology course.[11] Also by 1911 the first modern antibiotic, the arsenic compound Salvarsan, which had been developed by Paul Erlich, had been successfully used against syphilis *(Treponema pallidum)*.[7] Following the success of Salvarsan, the sulfa drugs were developed by the 1930s. As new medicines were developed and researched, the faculty and students at the ASO and other osteopathic medical colleges adopted and used them. By the 1930s, the osteopathic philosophy had been expanded to include medicines that had proven their value through research, as illustrated in the following introductory quote from the 1935 edition of the *Sage Sayings of Still:*

Osteopathy is not a drugless therapy in the strict sense of the word. It uses drugs which have specific scientific

BOX 1-1

Traditional Versus Contemporary Osteopathy

Our Platform[9]

It should be known where osteopathy stands and what it stands for. A political party has a platform that all may know its position in regard to matters of public importance, what it stands for and what principles it advocates. The osteopath should make his position just as clear to the public. He should let the public know, in his platform, what he advocates in his campaign against disease. Our position can be tersely stated in the following planks:

First: We believe in sanitation and hygiene.

Second: We are opposed to the use of drugs as remedial agencies.

Third: We are opposed to vaccination.

Fourth: We are opposed to the use of serums in the treatment of disease. Nature furnishes its own serums if we know how to deliver them.

Fifth: We realize that many cases require surgical treatment and therefore advocate it as a last resort. We believe many surgical operations are unnecessarily performed and that many operations can be avoided by osteopathic treatment.

Sixth: The osteopath does not depend on electricity, X-radiance, hydrotherapy or other adjuncts, but relies on osteopathic measures in the treatment of disease.

Seventh: We have a friendly feeling for other non-drug, natural methods of healing, but we do not incorporate any other methods into our system. We are all opposed to drugs; in that respect at least, all nat-

ural, unharmful methods occupy the same ground. The fundamental principles of osteopathy are different from those of any other system and the cause of disease is considered from one standpoint, viz: disease is the result of anatomical abnormalities followed by physiological discord. To cure disease the abnormal parts must be adjusted to the normal; therefore other methods that are entirely different in principle have no place in the osteopathic system.

Eighth: Osteopathy is an independent system and can be applied to all conditions of disease, including purely surgical cases, and in these cases surgery is but a branch of osteopathy.

Ninth: We believe that our therapeutic house is just large enough for osteopathy and that when other methods are brought in just that much osteopathy must move out.

Contemporary Differences with Our Platform

Addressing each of the planks of the platform, today's osteopathic physicians would have the following comments.

1. Hygienic and sanitary measures have, in fact, decreased mortality and morbidity in modern society far more than other medical measures.
2. Much of Still's criticism of the medicine of his day was provoked precisely because it was not researched and therefore, to him, without logic and not scientifically valid. However, there have been

value, such as antiseptics, parasiticides, antidotes, anesthetics or narcotics for the temporary relief of suffering. It is the empirical internal administration of drugs for therapeutic purposes that osteopathy opposes, substituting instead manipulation, mechanical measures and the balancing of the life essentials as more rational and more in keeping with the physiological functions of the body. The osteopathic physician is the skilled engineer of the vital human mechanism, influencing by manipulation and other osteopathic measures the activities of the nerves, cells, glands and organs, the distribution of fluids and the discharge of nerve impulses, thus normalizing tissue, fluid and function.[13]

Antiseptic surgical technique was developed at about the same time as osteopathy and was included in surgical procedures practiced by the new profession. One difference between the allopathic and osteopathic

approaches was that patients received OMT before and after surgery. Postsurgical treatment focused on soft tissue and rib raising, an articulatory treatment designed to increase the efficiency of breathing while calming the sympathetic nervous system.

The development of the sulfa antibiotics (and their increased use in hospitalized patients in the 1930s) and the advent of penicillin (developed in 1927 but not commercially available until after World War II in 1945) significantly changed the practice of all medicine. Except for a very few older DOs who believed manipulation was the only answer, osteopathic physicians adopted these miracle medicines immediately. By accepting the use of thoroughly researched, effective medicines, classical osteopathic philosophy expanded to a more comprehensive contemporary osteopathic medical philosophy.

BOX 1-1

Traditional Versus Contemporary Osteopathy—cont'd

only a very few osteopathic physicians, most of them at the end of the nineteenth or beginning of the twentieth century, who were completely opposed to all medicines. Contemporary medications are often overused; there may be a higher annual number of deaths caused by medication errors and side effects than are caused by highway accidents.

3. Immunization is now achieved with standard purified doses and is better understood. Statistics have demonstrated that the morbidity and mortality rates associated with not using immunizations are considerably worse than those found when immunizations are used. Although it is impossible to predict the outcome of immunization in an individual case, assuming that the patient who succumbs to an idiosyncratic reaction to a vaccine did not have that reaction because of the sensitivity to the medium (e.g., egg protein), that patient may be the one who would have had a similar or worse reaction to the disease in an epidemic if the population were not immunized.

4. Serums or other blood parts in Still's day were much more dangerous than those found today. However, AIDS and other bloodborne diseases have demonstrated that body fluids, cells, and cell parts must be used with appropriate caution.

5. Surgery is necessary but may remain overused in the United States. Twentieth century medicine has improved diagnostic testing and more conservative approaches have decreased the number of unnecessary surgeries. The use of aseptic technique, improved anesthesia, and microscopic and endoscopic surgery has diminished many negative consequences.

6. All therapies that are statistically demonstrated to aid patients are completely acceptable. Still was apparently never opposed to the use of x-rays studies for diagnostic purposes, because the ASO had the second diagnostic x-ray machine west of the Mississippi River. The use of radiation therapy as we know it was unknown in his time, as was the use of lasers for therapeutic purposes.

7. We recognize that disease has multiple causes that were unknown in Still's day (e.g., genetic abnormality, nutritional deficiencies, radiation damage [including sunlight], psychosomatic effects) and that his unifactorial description of the cause of illness is no longer tenable.

8. The therapeutic house of the osteopathic profession, except for a few of its founding members, has always included the latest of research on medications and the expansion in medical knowledge through this past century. However, the incorporation of this expanded knowledge into medical school curricula has resulted in less available instructional time for osteopathic manipulation, leaving some physicians less skilled and neglecting its use in appropriate cases.

"Our Platform" from Korr IM, Olgilvie CD: Health orientation in medical education, U.S. The Texas College of Osteopathic Medicine, *Prev Med* 10:710-718, 1981, Academic Press.

Following the evolution of osteopathic thought, George W. Northup, DO, was quoted in 1996 as saying:

It is now better understood that a given "disease" is not so easily defined as was once believed. The search for a single cause for a single disease has produced disillusionment. Even the "germ theory" is not sufficient to provide a "simple" explanation for infectious diseases. All of us live in a world of potential bacterial invasion, but relatively few become infected. There are multiple causes, even in bacterially induced diseases. Disease is a total body response. It is not merely a stomach ulcer, a broken bone, or a troublesome mother-in-law. It is a disturbance of the structure-function of the body and not an isolated or local insult. Equally important is the recognition that disease is multi-causal. The understanding that multiple causes of disease can arise from remote but interconnected parts of the body will ultimately emerge into a unifying philosophy for all of medicine. When this occurs, it will embrace many of the basic principles of osteopathic medicine.[5]

The shift in osteopathic thought embraced the progress of the scientific development of medicine in the twentieth century but maintained the belief that it is not the physician who heals, but the body itself, which heals through its homeostatic mechanisms. Contemporary osteopathic medical philosophy also maintains a belief in the efficacy of manipulation to decrease physiologic and sometimes psychologic stress, therefore helping the body regain optimal homeostatic levels.

Still's original opposition to the medicine of his time was due to the lack of research on the medicines that were used. One of his better-known quotes is, "Man should study and use the drugs compounded in his own body."[8] This is increasingly the method of study today: finding out how the body works and then using medicines that interact with the body's cellular receptors and that mimic or, in some cases, are identical to the compounds found in the body.

Contemporary Osteopathic Medical Philosophy

As we enter the twenty-first century, we find the following official definition of the term *osteopathic philosophy* in the "Glossary of Osteopathic Terminology" section of the American Osteopathic Association (AOA) Yearbook, 2000:

Osteopathic philosophy: Osteopathic medicine is a philosophy of health care and a distinctive art, supported by expanding scientific knowledge; its philosophy embraces the concept of the unity of the living organism's structure (anatomy) and function (physiology). Its art is the application of the philosophy in the practice of medicine and surgery in all its branches and specialties. Its science includes the behavioral, chemical, physical, spiritual and biological knowledge related to the establishment and maintenance of health as well as the prevention and alleviation of disease.[1]

Osteopathic concepts emphasize the following principles[1]:

1. The human being is a dynamic unit of function.
2. The body possesses self-regulatory mechanisms which are self-healing in nature.
3. Structure and function are interrelated at all levels.
4. Rational treatment is based on these principles.

Contemporary osteopathic medical philosophy begins with classical osteopathy and integrates additional knowledge. Rather than applying the choice *either/or* to manipulation or medicine, *both/and* is often more appropriate. Other evolved changes include recently developed knowledge of nutrition, exercise, environmental factors, genetics, and psychology.

For instance, nutrition is now considered important. Still did not consider it important, and often recommended that the patients just "eat what they want of good plain nutritious food."[8] The importance of nutrition was later added to Still's original philosophy because, although Still commented on not following fad diets, the food Americans ate in his age was very different from the average American diet of our times. During Still's lifetime all crops were grown organically and most of the population of the United States was in a rural environment. Although he mentions good food several times, he assumed that the average diet in those times was sufficient for nourishment.

For exercise, Still occasionally mentioned walking or horseback riding. In the preautomotive society, there was little need to recommend these—everyone in the United States walked or rode horseback to get where they were going. A great many laborsaving devices had not been invented, so normal daily living took care of most of the exercise needs of the population.

Likewise, the dangers of excessive solar radiation to health had not yet become apparent in a society in which tanning was not considered attractive. Farmers often wore long-sleeve shirts and hats, and even swimsuits provided practically full covering of the body and often were paired with a parasol for protection from the sun. Air pollution, water pollution, and noise pollution were not considered as causes of illness, nor were workplace toxins. Radiation damage was undiscovered.

Genetic mutations and deficiencies also were unknown. Physicians were virtually ignorant of the science of genetics at the end of the nineteenth century. Current research promises multiple benefits from our expanding knowledge of molecular biology. This knowledge has great potential for both good and harm. Its application also fits in well with osteopathic philosophy.

Mind/body approaches have shown considerable potential for patient applications. Biofeedback and the relaxation response have been validated by research as ways of manipulating homeostatic values to improve immune system function. Psychologic counseling techniques have advanced the possibilities for patients to address the stresses in their psychosocial milieu.

All of these etiologic factors of illness have therefore been integrated into an expanded contemporary osteopathic philosophy while retaining the profound respect for the body's ability to function in the face of many challenges and its inherent capacity for self-healing when injury or illness is present.

Still thought the body was basically perfect as it was and could process environmental and nutritional input without damage unless there was an injury resulting in structural damage. We now know that the human being is continuous with the environment, and on more than one level (body: physical; mind: thought/emotion; spirit: emotion/beliefs/other subtle factors). Illness is seen by the twenty-first century osteopathic physician as having multiple causes, any one of which can be the initiator or promoter. Nonetheless, all of these factors potentially affect the structure of the body, whether at a gross (neuromusculoskeletal) level or at a microscopic (stereochemical/bioelectrochemical) level.

Wellness therefore lies along a continuum with illness, across the time frame between the points of conception and death. Illness begins as wellness decreases. Wellness indicates that the individual is capable of accepting multiple challenges without homeostasis declining to the point of interference with normal activities. As the system loses optimal homeostatic balance, less of an environmental/mental insult is needed to precipitate a state of illness.

Early in the continuum lie such problems as nutritional deficiency, insufficient exercise or rest, and inappropriate levels of stress. If these problems are addressed while they are simple, the organism recovers and retains adaptability. On an overlapping/interactive continuum lies the problem of gross structural integrity, involving bilateral muscle tone balance and neural activity levels, especially in the autonomic nervous system, particularly as these factors affect the respiratory, circulatory, lymphatic, endocrine, and immune systems.

When nothing is done, our homeostatic mechanisms may effect a recovery from illness without aid. Sometimes the body does not have the ability to recover on its own. In such cases, structural dysfunction at either the gross or the microscopic level can be compounded by the sequelae of inflammation, pain, and tissue congestion. These negative changes in the biochemical environment of the body can cause many variables in the endocrine and immune systems to swing to wider extremes and destabilize one or more of the body's systems, leading to illness. Simple problems can sometimes be solved with manipulation, lifestyle changes (e.g., exercises), or nutrition to reestablish optimal homeostatic set points.

Ideas such as these are not easily understood by a reductionistic approach to the body, in which each variable is analyzed by itself or perhaps in conjunction with one or two other variables (e.g., the balance between insulin and glucagon). Current understanding recognizes much more complexity in the interactions between many more subtle variables, such as eicosanoids, the biochemicals that evolved before homeostatic hormonal control systems and that control many body functions.

Chaos mathematical analysis and fractal analysis have enabled greater understanding of the complexity of dynamic medical systems. Chaos mathematics allows us to understand how affecting a single or even a few variables in one system (e.g., cardiovascular) can affect the function of other systems, and thereby the entire human being. One factor that has been noted is the phenomenon known as *sensitive dependence on initial conditions,* or the *butterfly effect,* which indicates that a simple motion such as that of a butterfly's wings in New York may affect the weather patterns in Moscow 3 months later.[2] Although this is an example that makes us chuckle, the mathematical models following chaos principles appear to be closer to what happens in the natural world than any previous analysis. Mathematicians are working on models of such things as the decompensating cycle of cardiac arrhythmia leading to fatal fibrillation.[2] Understanding new concepts such as point attractors, strange attractors, triviality, nontriviality, and degeneracy leads to a better understanding of the processes of homeostasis and how manipulation of anatomic values and tissue tensions can promote physiologic adaptability.

Each system is understood to be an avenue of access to the entire body, to the whole person. The neuromusculoskeletal system can be considered the largest single system in the body; it reflects the state of health of the other systems, thereby yielding diagnostic clues for systemic or organic function or dysfunction. It can also be used as an access for treatment, through the use of manipulation to change the set points of muscle tone, thereby affecting vascular and lymphatic flow and neural (particularly autonomic) tone.

CURRENT STATUS

Osteopathic Principles

To an osteopathic physician, osteopathic principles are commonsense ideas that serve as a milieu in which to diagnose and treat a patient. Here we consider a series of ideas on how to approach a patient.

At some level, the physician should always be aware of the following considerations:

- Who is the patient? The patient is a human being like ourselves, a functional unity of body (a genetically constructed grouping of cells and systems), mind (thoughts and emotions), and a third factor (identified by some as spirit), which is interactive with the environment at physical, psychosocial, and energetic levels. The human being functions by transforming thought into action through the musculoskeletal system.
- Where does health arise? Health comes from within.
- What is the goal of the osteopathic physician? Seek health in the patient. Wellness and illness exist on a continuum, or on an interactive multidimensional group of continua. Seek the highest possible level of homeostatic balance and performance within the limitations of the individual patient and the current circumstances.
- How do we seek health in the patient? Prevention is the best medicine; we encourage and teach patients to follow healthful practices (e.g., appropriate rest, nutrition, exercise, breathing exercises, positive thoughts and emotions, relaxation, social interaction), and to avoid that which is self-destructive (e.g., tobacco, radiation, toxins, excessive alcohol, drugs).

If the patient has entered the illness end of the continuum, we must take a careful history, perform a physical examination, and formulate a differential diagnosis, including all standard diagnostic medical practices. As we do so, the musculoskeletal system is included as an access point for diagnostic signs that may indicate systemic problems (and later, an access for imparting information to the other systems). Tests may be needed. After arriving at a diagnosis, we decide on necessary treatment, bearing in mind all factors that affect the physiology and performance of the patient.

What factors affect the physiology of the patient? Physiology can be affected by air, water, and food; nutritional supplements; prescription and over-the-counter medications; physical forces and impacts on the system (ranging from the effects of any movement, including exercise, to trauma); thoughts, emotions, stress, or relaxation; and energy (from gravity to sunlight to magnetic field to energies of which we may not yet be aware). All of the body's systems are integrative, but five are more easily seen as unifying systems of global body communication (cardiovascular and lymphatic, respiratory, neurologic, endocrine, and immune systems).

The host has control of vulnerability to illness through the immune system and homeostatic mechanisms (vis medicatrix naturae). When host control decreases and the system downgrades into illness, intervention is necessary. Intervention is designed to support a system that is no longer functioning at an appropriately high level of homeostasis.

How do we intervene? Just as wellness, injury, and illness exist along a continuum, so do treatment approaches. When physical or emotional force has deranged anatomic or physiologic performance, we address the problems with physical approaches ranging from manipulation to surgery. When genetic limitations or illness make it impossible for the body to perform appropriate functions on its own or with the speed required, we use exogenous substances such as nutritional supplementation, medication, or appropriate genetic therapy. (From the point of view of chaos mathematics and dynamical systems, we seek to reverse abnormal trivial point attractors to strange attractor status.) We do this in a conservative manner, bearing in mind the body's innate intelligence and the wisdom of using the least possible intervention (least invasive) for the greatest possible results.

Osteopathic Techniques

Osteopathy is not a system of techniques, but a philosophy that is often applied through techniques of osteopathic manipulative medicine, which were developed by osteopathic physicians. Because of interest in what these techniques may be, several of the more commonly recognized osteopathic diagnosis and treatment systems are described here. There are, of course, many others. These techniques exist along a continuum of effect, one logically leading to another, depending on the problem of the patient and the perception and skill of the osteopathic physician.

It has been said that there are only two types of techniques, direct and indirect. *Direct Treatment* is treatment that confronts restriction of motion, in which the body part is taken in the direction of restriction. *Indirect Treatment* is treatment in which the body part is taken in the direction of ease of motion. Once the body part is appropriately positioned, activating forces are applied to induce changes in muscle tone; central, peripheral, or autonomic nervous system tone (level of activation); and vascular/lymphatic response. The goals of treatment include tissue relaxation, increased physiologic motion, decrease in pain, and optimization of homeostasis. The following are some of the more common systems of OMT. It should be stated that manipulation of any form has both indications and contraindications; these are not discussed here because they are well outlined in other texts.

Soft-Tissue and Lymphatic Treatments

Soft-tissue treatment, generally a direct treatment, was developed by Still and his early students and is sometimes confused with massage. The techniques focus on altering the tone of muscle and connective tissue. Soft-tissue treatment increases arterial delivery, relaxes muscles and connective tissue, and alters the tone of the autonomic nervous system. Whereas soft-tissue treatment definitely affects the lymphatics, specific lymphatic techniques focus on increasing lymphatic and venous drainage.

High-Velocity, Low-Amplitude Thrust

In the direct method of treatment referred to as *high-velocity, low-amplitude (HVLA) thrust,* the restrictive barrier is engaged by precise positioning of the body. The thrust when the body part is at the restrictive barrier is very rapid (high velocity) but operates over a very short distance (low amplitude), gapping the articulation by approximately ⅛ inch or less. This allows a reset of both joint position and muscle tension levels, which causes related neural and vascular readjustment.

Articulatory Technique

The original general articulatory technique, developed by Still and his students, takes the body part being treated to the end portion of its restricted range of motion in a gentle, repetitive fashion. The repeated articulation directly diminishes the restrictive barrier. Movements within one or more planes of motion are treated at a time. This treatment can be used to treat individual joints or regions (e.g., shoulder, cervical spine).

Still also used specific articulation techniques that began with diagnosis, placing the body parts in the direction of ease of motion and rotating them into the direction of restriction. These specific articulation techniques have been called the *Still Technique.*[12]

Facilitated Positional Release[6] is also a variation of the type of work Still himself did.

Muscle Energy

Muscle energy treatment was developed by Fred Mitchell, Sr., DO. It is most commonly used as a direct treatment, and the term *muscle energy* means that the patient uses his or her own energy through directed muscular cooperation with the physician. Reflexive changes in muscle tension are used in a variety of ways to allow dysfunctional, shortened muscles to lengthen; abnormally lengthened muscles to shorten; weakened muscles to strengthen; and hypertonic muscles to relax. Commonly, voluntary isometric contraction of a patient's muscles is followed by a gentle stretch of the dysfunctional, contracted muscles, decreasing abnormal restriction of motion. Other muscle energy techniques use traction on the muscle to pull an articulation back into the appropriate position.

Counterstrain Technique

Counterstrain is a passive positional technique that places the patient's dysfunctional joint (spinal or other) or tissue in a position of ease. This position arrests the inappropriate proprioceptive activity that maintains the somatic dysfunction. Marked shortening of the involved muscle or connective tissue is maintained for 90 seconds. An inappropriate strain reflex (a result of injury) is therefore inhibited by applying counterstrain. Diagnosis is primarily by palpation of areas of tenderness mapped by the originator of this system, Lawrence Jones, DO. This form of diagnosis can also be integrated with positional, movement, or tissue texture abnormalities. The tender point is indicative of inappropriate neurologic balance. This system is ideal for the patient who does not respond well to articulatory techniques, such as the postsurgical patient.

Myofascial Release

Myofascial release is actually a renaming of original osteopathic techniques developed by Still, which were called fascial techniques by the early osteopathic physicians. Anthony Chila, Robert Ward, and John Peckham developed a course in these techniques at MSU, in which they also acknowledged the importance of the muscle tissue to the treatment. This technique may be performed in a direct or indirect manner and involves either shortening the contracted tissue (indirect) or lengthening it (direct) and allowing the nervous and respiratory systems to direct changes. Two physiologic biomechanical tissue processes, creep and hysteresis, also play a role. Compression, traction, respiratory cooperation, or a combination thereof may be included to facilitate treatment.

Osteopathy in the Cranial Field

Osteopathy in the cranial field, also referred to as *OCF, Cranial Osteopathy,* and *Craniosacral Osteopathy,* was developed by William G. Sutherland, DO. It is usually done as a mixture of indirect and direct procedures that work with the body's inherent rhythmic motions. It is commonly used in adults as a treatment for headaches or temporomandibular joint dysfunction syndrome and in infants (whose skulls are more flexible) for treatment of symptoms related to cranial nerve compression (e.g., vomiting, poor sleep, poor feeding). Although OCF techniques often focus on the skull and the sacrum, where the dura mater attaches, they can be and are commonly used throughout the body.

Visceral Techniques

A variety of techniques have been developed from the beginning of the profession to address imbalance in the viscera. These include stretching and balancing techniques related to ligamentous attachments, as originated by Still, and may involve use of inherent visceral motion. More recently, Jean-Pierre Barral, a nonphysician DO from France, has developed and taught an entire system of visceral techniques.

EXAMPLES OF DIAGNOSIS AND TREATMENT IN OSTEOPATHIC MEDICINE

Osteopathic diagnosis and treatment are determined by the osteopathic philosophy, making the practice of osteopathic medicine distinctive and different. This philosophy and OMT should not be viewed as merely the addition of something extra to the contemporary Western medical approach (the cherry on top of the ice cream sundae). Osteopathic philosophy serves as an organizer of thought that helps the physician understand what is going on in the entire organism, allows concurrent reductionistic analysis, and then reassembles the parts into the totality of the human being (who is more than the sum of the parts).

Osteopathic diagnosis differs in that the osteopathic physician does a standard physical examination but also includes palpation and motion testing in the musculoskeletal system that is different from the standard orthopedic examination. The musculoskeletal system serves as an access point for additional diagnostic information, not only on muscle tension, but on fluid distribution and autonomic levels of activity. Well-known neurologic interactions permit a physician to conclude from musculoskeletal evidence that an underlying visceral problem may exist and should be investigated.

Four criteria are used to diagnose somatic dysfunction: tissue texture abnormalities, static or positional asymmetry, restriction of motion, and tenderness. These have been referred to by the diagnostic mnemonic *TART*. At spinal segment levels where these are noted, the knowledge of reflex relationships guides the osteopathic physician to pay more attention to both the history and physical examination of the internal organs related to that spinal cord segmental level. The musculoskeletal examination includes observation for evidence of viscerosomatic, somatovisceral, viscerovisceral, and somatosomatic reflexes. These reflexes show palpatory evidence of autonomic nervous system influence at segmental levels and are involved in abnormalities of tissue texture and muscle tone.

Treatment is also affected by this philosophy. If the nervous system and musculoskeletal system can be used for diagnosis, it is also true that an attempt may be made to reverse pathophysiology by treating the affected anatomic structures to change their physiologic performance (decreasing, for instance, inappropriate sympathetic nervous system tone and thereby enhancing homeostatic balance and adaptability). Medication or surgery may be unnecessary, depending on the severity of the problem. OMT may be used as a primary means of treatment for a problem that appears to be of nonsevere, musculoskeletal origin, as primary treatment for simple illness that requires no medication (e.g., viral upper respiratory illness), or it may be used as adjunctive therapy along with medication or surgery—again, to enhance homeostatic recovery and adaptability.

Two simple case examples are presented here. These are not complete cases, but are designed to illustrate some of the osteopathic differences in approach to diagnosis and treatment. In each example, the techniques chosen did not challenge the patients with muscular effort and were selected with homeostatic effects in mind (decrease of edema, mobilization of fluids, enhancement of respiration). In many other ambulatory cases, any of the listed treatments (e.g., HVLA thrust) could be selected based on four factors: the condition of the patient, the nature of the complaint, the goals of treatment, and the skills of the physician.

 Case Example 1

A 67-year-old black woman with a 30-pack/year history of smoking presents at the office with a productive cough that she has had for 2 weeks. She now has a fever, and the sputum is greenish. She has pain in the ribs on the left side of the thorax, and audible rhonchi when examined with the stethoscope. After a careful history and physical examination, the physician concludes that although the differential diagnosis includes a possible tumor, this is less likely than a community-acquired pneumonia. Radiographic studies indicate a left lingular pneumonitis, and there is an increased white blood cell (WBC) count with a left shift. The physician has noted on examination that pulmonary viscerosomatic reflexes are activated in the corresponding thoracic spinal region, causing limitation in range of motion and tenderness, along with tissue texture changes, at several thoracic vertebral segments. Several ribs on the left have diminished mobility, and the diaphragm has decreased excursion on the left.

The physician decides to start antibiotics immediately and treats the thoracic segments and ribs with OMT, in this case choosing counterstrain because it requires no muscular effort of the patient and there is minimal risk of injury to bones that may be osteoporotic. In patients who are coughing frequently, breathing mechanics are often disturbed. Treating the thoracic segments and ribs helps normalize the sympathetic nervous system activity and increases the efficiency and ease of breathing. The thoracic outlet, where the thoracic lymphatic duct has passage, is treated, allowing for less tissue compression to impede flow of lymphatic fluid. The diaphragm (often having impaired motion from the spasmodic motion of coughing) is treated with myofascial release, and the cervical region is treated with counterstrain to decrease any problems with the phrenic nerve (which innervates the diaphragm for respiration). A lymphatic pump concludes the treatment. Antitussives are prescribed along with the antibiotics and an expectorant. Acetaminophen may be used for fever and pain. The patient is seen again in 3 days, at which time she is greatly improved.

The rationale behind the medical treatment is obvious: kill the bacteria, decrease the viscosity of the mucus that holds them so that they can be coughed out, and give the patient a painkiller to decrease pain. This type of treatment relies on the body to recover its optimal performance once certain negatives are canceled out. The osteopathic treatment is designed to aid normal physiologic processes that augment the body's natural systems in killing the bacteria and reducing pain. The effect is to enhance the positives, not just cancel the negative effects on physiology. OMT may enable a faster recovery for the patient—or increase the odds of survival. Clearly, however, the osteopathic physician takes advantage of both possibilities, aiding the host's natural defenses while fighting the bacteria directly through use of antibiotics. The patient's comfort level is also increased by the use of the osteopathic manipulation.

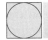 *Case Example 2*

A 19-year-old white male college student presents with an apparent sprained ankle. The injury occurred during a soccer game when he reached for the ground with his foot and made a sudden turn. There is no other relevant history. The ankle is swollen, and the patient applied ice immediately after the injury. He can walk, but he keeps most of his weight off the ankle. There is pinpoint tenderness at the posteroinferior right lateral malleolus.

The physician chooses to treat with superficial indirect myofascial release and, afterward, lymphatic techniques to decrease the edema. Treatment is specifically limited to a minimal approach, which causes the patient no pain. The patient is given a set of crutches to use for a couple of days and goes to the hospital to get an x-ray study, which is negative. He is to use ice at least three times a day and to keep his weight off the ankle, which is wrapped after the treatment with an elastic bandage. He is to keep the ankle elevated when possible, and to use acetaminophen for pain if needed. When the study shows no fracture, the physician continues the treatment 2 days later with counterstrain and lymphatic treatment, and the patient is allowed to discontinue use of the crutches.

Acetaminophen does not help the healing process directly. However, draining excess fluid and decreasing the overabundance of proinflammatory neuropeptides and other biochemicals through the use of OMT allows the hypertonic and injured tissues to return to normal more quickly. The decrease or elimination of muscle spasm allows the ankle and foot to have more normal mechanics, therefore promoting more normal lymphatic and venous drainage. Again, the osteopathic treatment is designed to enhance the body's own methods of healing, promoting a rapid return to more normal homeostatic balance by removing dysfunction.

WHY IS MANIPULATION A CRITICAL ASPECT OF OSTEOPATHIC PHILOSOPHY?

If osteopathy is a philosophy, why is the use of manipulation in the practice of medicine considered its hallmark and a necessary, integral part of osteopathic medicine? The answer lies in the original osteopathic philosophy, which relates to the interaction between structure (anatomy) and function (physiology) in the human species, and how we can effect changes in the human body. It can be found at two levels, the macroscopic and the microscopic.

At the macroscopic level, it is easy to see that if there is abnormal pressure on a joint, nerve, or blood vessel, there may be resulting changes in tissue over time. For instance, if there is more pressure on the medial aspect of the right knee, over time there will be changes in the cartilage and bone to compensate. There will also be changes in the gait as the body attempts to balance itself in the best equilibrium possible to use the least amount of energy for posture and gait. Thus local dysfunction can induce global dysfunction. Manipulation, which has local effects of adjusting the balance in the musculoskeletal system, also has global effects at a gross level.

At a microscopic level, we must analyze cellular physiology. The original one-celled organisms were bathed in a solution of seawater, which contained needed oxygen and nutrients and also took away toxic waste products and carbon dioxide as they were produced and ejected from the cell. Multicellular organisms such as the human being contain an internal ocean with the same functions. This internal fluid system is the cardiovascular system, delivering oxygen and nutrients to each individual cell and clearing carbon dioxide and waste products (as well as excessive proteins through lymphatic drainage).

If this system is impeded in any way, cells, followed by tissues, organs, and entire systems, decrease their level of function. This form of physiologic stress then makes the organism vulnerable to disease. To offer an analogy, a good fluid delivery and clearance system is like an open, clean, flowing stream or river. If the flow is blocked, we have the potential for developing a swamp. Stagnant water allows the buildup of noxious products, and the local environment is completely changed. If the blockage is cleared through manual effort, the stream reestablishes good flow and removes the toxic elements that had begun to build up. When these tissue tensions are readjusted toward the norm,

the body's own elimination systems can clear toxic waste products produced by cellular damage and allowed to build up by inappropriate tissue tensions.

Osteopathic manipulation is therefore a means not only of decreasing or eliminating pain, but also of adjusting the involved structures. This adjustment helps prevent direct noxious stimulus (through compression or excessive stretching) at a macroscopic level and toxic conditions (through lack of appropriate oxygen and nutrient delivery and inadequate waste clearance) in cells at a microscopic level. Manipulation is therefore a central issue for osteopathic medicine: although it cannot cure all illness, manipulation is used to help the body function at an optimal level, enhancing its ability to heal itself. The body is capable of amazing feats of self-recovery and may perform these feats more quickly and thoroughly if assisted.

Manipulation, like all forms of medical treatment, has limitations. It is possible that the body's functional levels have been so negatively altered that the use of manipulation alone will not enhance the body's self-adjusting systems enough (or perhaps not within an acceptable time) for it to regain good health without the additional assistance of medication or surgery. It may also be necessary to integrate direct psychosocial intervention to achieve recovery.

Medicines and surgery are used to effect changes in two circumstances: (1) when we believe that preventive measures or manipulation alone will not be able to accomplish our total goal of health (e.g., when use of insulin in a type 1 diabetic patient or narcotics in a terminally ill cancer patient are necessary), or (2) when speed is of the essence and it would be dangerous to the patient to rely solely on manipulation and wait for the body's self-healing responses (e.g., use of antibiotics in overwhelming infection).

Osteopathic physicians who do not use manipulation but who treat patients in a holistic manner are ignoring a main premise of osteopathic philosophy: eliminating structural impediments that diminish normal physiologic function in order to promote the body's self-healing capabilities.

LEVELS OF IMPLEMENTATION OF OSTEOPATHIC PHILOSOPHY

There have been conspicuous differences in the evolution of Still's ideas in the United States and other parts of the world. In the United States, there is a vast spectrum of application of osteopathic principles in the practice of medicine by DOs. Internationally, the application of osteopathic philosophy has been different from that in the United States and involves two levels of training.

In the United States, DOs have always been physicians. Current practitioners implement the osteopathic medical philosophy at various levels along a continuum of medical care. Initially, all osteopathic physicians believed in the efficacy of manipulation to affect the physiology of the body in a positive way. In fact, this has been the hallmark of the osteopathic profession, and Still's development of osteopathic structural diagnosis and treatment was the original reason for the osteopathic profession's existence.

At one end of the continuum, we find the practitioner who practices the pure, classical form of osteopathy, using either manipulation or surgery but no medications whatsoever. This type of practitioner is a historical footnote in the development of osteopathic practice in America, and this author knows of no such practitioners at this time. Some physicians accept the importance of manipulation for treatment of pain but do not see it as having any value in visceral problems. A very few who use manipulation also integrate the homeopathic approach into their practice of medicine.

A small number of osteopathic physicians have chosen to specialize in neuromusculoskeletal medicine, also giving treatment for medical cases in conjunction with treatment by surgical or internal medicine specialists. Some of these practitioners use a minimum of medications, preferring to refer patients who need more intensive medical or surgical care to physicians who likewise specialize in those forms of medical care, including family practice doctors.

Even among manipulative specialists, some apply osteopathic techniques in a reductionistic manner, for example, treating only the neck if there is neck pain. This of course negates the osteopathic concept of wholeness and implies that the physician has not understood that an area of pain may be an area of compensation for a primary problem, rather than being the source of the problem. The physician is neglecting the many muscle and connective tissue connections between the thoracic region and the neck, as well as the sympathetic chain ganglia in the upper thoracic region that help set the tone for the cervical musculature. Although such an approach often works, it is often insufficient. The patient may complain of pain in a given area, but the dysfunction in that area may be compensatory in nature. It is important to address the primary problem, not just annoying symptoms.

Most osteopathic physicians practice in primary care specialties. There is a great range in the amount of OMT that these physicians use with their patients. Others who believe in the efficacy of OMT but believe they do not have time to use it with patients may use it to treat a friend or relative and will refer patients who need manipulation to physicians who specialize in its use.

Remarkably, there are a number of DOs who have no belief in the clinical efficacy of OMT. Some never accepted the osteopathic philosophy nor intended to use OMT, but attended an osteopathic medical college because it was a pathway to an unrestricted medical license. A subset of this group believes that the laying on of hands is, however, valuable to evoke either the mind/body or placebo effects. There are also physicians who do not want to be confused with chiropractors and believe that manual therapeutics are best left to doctors of chiropractic, physical therapists, and other manual therapists.

Whether or not they use OMT, virtually all osteopathic physicians in the United States share a profound respect for the body's ability to heal and approach the patient in a holistic manner, viewing the patient as a human being in a unique psychosocial milieu.

The international evolution of osteopathy has been equally complex. After leaving the Chicago College of Osteopathic Medicine (now CCOM at Midwestern University of Health Sciences), J. Martin Littlejohn returned home to the United Kingdom and founded an osteopathic profession in which practitioners used neither surgery nor medicine and which never evolved into a profession with an unlimited medical license.[10] Although these practitioners are generally excellent at treating musculoskeletal problems with the use of manipulation, they are currently trying to address their lack of medical acumen in differential diagnosis and do not have the opportunity to prescribe medicine or to perform or assist at surgery or childbirth.

Opinions on this form of evolution vary. DOs in the United States are aware of the dangers inherent when practitioners are not well trained in differential diagnosis. Such a practitioner may fail to recognize pain as an indicator of a serious underlying treatable medical or surgical condition, and appropriate treatment may be delayed until it is too late to obtain a favorable outcome. When the only available tool is a hammer, too often every problem begins to look like a nail.

International nonmedical osteopathic practitioners, however, would be quick to point out that many American DOs who have an excellent knowledge of medical diagnosis and treatment lack sufficient manipulative skills to effectively treat a patient whose problem would clearly benefit from manipulation.

The British government has recognized the value of including nonphysician osteopathic practitioners in the national health care system. They are generally perceived as specialists in musculoskeletal pain and adjunctive treatment. They are sometimes consulted if the patient has vague complaints and continuing physician efforts do not produce an organic diagnosis. Management of medical conditions is left to the physician. Generally, the public easily identifies this profession and respects the practitioners.

The British Commonwealth spread the nonphysician practice of osteopathic philosophy and manipulation through many countries, and it has been copied in other European nations. Although these practitioners are called DOs, their degree is Diploma in Osteopathy, rather than the American degree, Doctor of Osteopathic Medicine (formerly Doctor of Osteopathy). The level of training varies. Schools in certain countries have a 4- or 5-year full-time program; others have a series of weekend courses over several years for physical therapists who wish to become osteopaths.

There is another tier of international osteopathic education, in which MD equivalents from various countries take postgraduate training in osteopathic diagnosis and manipulation. These practitioners do have an unlimited medical license, and although sometimes lacking in the full knowledge of osteopathic philosophy, in general they are similar to American DOs. Many of these physicians integrate osteopathic care into general practice, rehabilitation medicine, sports medicine, rheumatology, or neurology, or they focus on the conservative treatment of musculoskeletal conditions or preoperative and postoperative care. France is one country where such training exists. Complicating the picture, French MDs have the legal right to practice osteopathy, whereas those who hold the Diploma in Osteopathy in France have been widely tolerated and are attempting to obtain practice rights through their national legislature.

CURRENT STATUS OF THE PROFESSION

Practice Rights

Osteopathic physicians in all 50 of the United States of America have the same practice rights as MDs. At the end of the nineteenth and beginning of the twentieth century, this was not the case. Some states immediately gave full practice rights to DOs; others gave partial practice rights, which varied from the right to diagnose and treat with manual medicine without prescription of medication, to the inclusion of obstetric privileges, to full medical and surgical privileges. Most states where osteopathic licensure was possible gave full practice rights.

Although the right to practice was guaranteed by law, it was not always easy for DOs to obtain hospital privileges. Even at the time of the Kline Report to the AMA (1953), many MDs were unaware that osteopathic medical education was equivalent to their own and therefore blocked access to hospital beds for patients being treated by DOs. Younger MDs were influenced in this regard by older physicians whose opinions were formed at a time when DOs did not use available medications. There was poor understanding among MDs of the rationale behind osteopathy's early rejection of medicines: that medicines in the preantibiotic era were poor in quality and generally even toxic, and that earlier in the era of allopathic medicine, use of medications was based on tradition or conjecture rather than research.

This spurred the DOs to build their own hospitals, thus forming a network of their own for accreditation standards. At times they used a wing of another hospital, such as the osteopathic wing of the Los Angeles County Hospital, which became the women's wing after the osteopathic state medical association amalgamated with the California Medical Association following the election in 1962. By the end of the twentieth century, many hospitals closed or merged under the pressures of managed care and health maintenance organizations. The number of osteopathic hospitals declined in the face of these changing economic conditions, and also because DOs were freely granted privileges in regular hospitals, making independent osteopathic hospitals less necessary for patient care.

Requirements for Matriculation

Prospective students who wish to apply to osteopathic medical schools should have completed a bachelor's degree with a high grade point average and successful scores on the Medical College Aptitude Test. Interviewers at the osteopathic colleges look for students who are successful at academic tasks. Preference may be given to those who also have sought relevant medical experience, such as working as a volunteer at a hospital emergency department or other medical facility, holding a job in a related field such as a hospital laboratory, or participating in medical research. Such experience suggests that an applicant has observed the work of physicians and does not have extreme difficulty with the sight of blood, sick patients, or patients in pain.

The interview at an osteopathic medical school generally includes informal assessment of the student's ability to empathize with people. Because most osteopathic physicians are in general or family practice, it is a cultural value of the osteopathic profession to look for applicants who are "people persons," meaning individuals who can interact easily with others. It is believed by DOs that this characteristic enables a physician to communicate with patients in ways that elicit information more easily and encourage better compliance. This does not mean that an introvert will not be accepted; however, the interviewers place a high value on empathy.

Interviewers often also pay attention to whether a student has been interested enough to study the history and philosophy of osteopathic medicine.

Current Status of Schools

The 19 osteopathic medical schools or colleges functioning in 2001 include a core of 5 surviving original private osteopathic schools from the nineteenth or beginning twentieth century and 14 colleges of osteopathic medicine that have been founded since 1969, composing a mix of public and private schools. All AOA-accredited osteopathic medical schools are listed by the World Health Organization (WHO) in their official list of United States medical schools. Table 1-1 provides additional information about these institutions.

Postgraduate Education

Medical and surgical postgraduate education consists of internships and residencies, which are training programs for general medicine, such as internal medicine or family practice, or for specialty medicine, such as cardiothoracic surgery. Throughout the twentieth century, generalists have increased the time they spend in postgraduate programs and demanded recognition for the practice of general medicine as a specialty itself, distinguishing their practices from those who did only an internship.

The rotating internship has been a hallmark of the osteopathic medical profession, with the understanding among osteopathic physicians that the best specialist has a good foundation as a generalist. The osteopathic concept of postgraduate training has been that competence in general medicine allows more integrated assessment of the patient's needs and decreases the amount of "falling through the cracks" that is possible when the patient is seeing only a series of specialists. This concept remained in effect for osteopathic postgraduate programs through the last half of the twentieth century, a time when most MD specialists entered their specialty training directly after medical school. A number of states required candidates for licensure as an osteopathic physician to complete a rotating internship. However, the AOA has responded to needs of graduates by creating *tracking internships,* or internships that retain a level of general training while decreasing some of the previous requirements, to allow more time within the internship for specialization. The internship is then credited as the first year of postgraduate training in the appropriate specialty. The end result is that there is still an extra requirement of general medicine/surgery in the AOA tracking internships compared with the Accreditation Council for Graduate Medical Education postgraduate year 1 programs in specialties.

Throughout the twentieth century, the osteopathic profession maintained that most physicians should be family doctors practicing general medicine and attracted students who implemented this philosophy in their choice of specialties. A number of state legislatures therefore became convinced that it was in the interest of their citizens to fund an osteopathic medical college to supply more generalists and family physicians to underserved and rural areas.

One result of the mix of students favored during recruitment (e.g., students who had osteopathic physicians as role models, informal assessment of ap-

TABLE 1-1

The Nineteen Colleges of Osteopathy

College	Location	Affiliated university	Founding date	Public or private	URL
Kirksville College Of Osteopathic Medicine	Kirksville, MO	Freestanding	1892	Private	http://www.kcom.edu
Philadelphia College of Osteopathic Medicine	Philadelphia, PA	Freestanding	1899	Private	http://www.pcom.edu
College of Osteopathic Medicine	Des Moines, IA	Des Moines University	1898	Private	http://www.dsmu.edu
College of Osteopathic Medicine	Kansas City, MO	University of the Health Sciences	1916	Private	http://www.uhs.edu/
Chicago College Of Osteopathic Medicine	Chicago, IL	Midwestern University	1900	Private	http://www.midwestern.edu/
College of Osteopathic Medicine	Tulsa, OK	Oklahoma State University	1972	Public	http://osu.com.okstate.edu/osucom.html
College of Osteopathic Medicine	East Lansing, MI	Michigan State University	1969	Public	http://www.com.msu.edu
Pikeville College of Osteopathic Medicine	Pikeville, KY	Pikeville College	1997	Private	http://pcsom.pc.edu
West Virginia School of Osteopathic Medicine	Lewisburg, WV	Freestanding	1972	Public	http://www.wvsom.edu
College of Osteopathic Medicine	Athens, OH	Ohio University	1975	Public	http://www.oucom.ohiou.edu
Texas College of Osteopathic Medicine	Fort Worth, TX	University of North Texas Health Science Center, Fort Worth	1970	Public	http://www.hsc.unt.edu/education/tcom

School	Location	University	Year	Type	Website
San Francisco College of Osteopathic Medicine	Vallejo, CA	Touro University	1995	Private	http://www.tucom.edu/
Lake Erie College of Osteopathic Medicine	Lake Erie, PA	Freestanding	1992	Private	http://www.lecom.edu
Nova Southeastern University College of Osteopathic Medicine	Fort Lauderdale, FL	NOVA/SECOM University	1980	Private	http://medicine.nova.edu
New York College of Osteopathic Medicine	Old Westbury, NY	New York Institute of Technology	1977	Private	http://www.nyit.edu/nycom
College of Osteopathic Medicine	Biddeford, MN	University of New England	1978	Private	http://www.une.edu
College of Osteopathic Medicine of the Pacific	Pomona, CA	Western University of Health Sciences	1977	Private	http://www.westernu.edu
School of Osteopathic Medicine	Cherry Hill, NJ	University of New Jersey School of Osteopathic Medicine and Dentistry	1976	Public	http://som.umdnj.edu
Arizona College of Osteopathic Medicine	Phoenix, AZ	Midwestern University	1995	Private	http://www.midwestern.edu/

plicants for people skills) and the encouragement given to medical school students to choose primary care specialties has been that fewer students were recruited who showed interest in pursuing a career of medical research.

Although the osteopathic medical profession has participated marginally in medical research from its inception, the bulk of its contribution to American health care has been through patient care. With the recent rapid increase in the number of osteopathic medical colleges, increase in state funding, and increase in the number of osteopathic physicians, more attention has begun to be paid to the profession's responsibility for contributing to medical research.

This research falls into three categories. Most research at osteopathic institutions is in either basic science or standard medical care. A small amount of research is on the effects of osteopathic structural diagnosis and treatment. Historically, individuals such as Irvin Korr, Steadman Denslow, Louisa Burns, Viola Frymann, and Beryl Arbuckle represent a significant portion of the effort of the profession to validate the scientific and clinical basis of osteopathic manipulation. More recently, an Osteopathic Research Center has been established at the University of North Texas, Texas, College of Osteopathic Medicine for the purpose of conducting clinical and basic research into this question. The third category focuses on the effects of complementary medical practices, with the goal of integrating into standard medical practice what can be proven nonharmful and effective.

In fairness, much of the medical research in the United States is controlled by those who are paid by or affiliated with the pharmaceutical industry. It is not surprising that pharmaceutical companies are not inclined to fund research that might prove that the use of less medication is better or that natural practices are more likely to avoid side effects of medication. Added to this is the political nature of award grants. Another factor has been the reliance on double-blind studies. It is very difficult to do a double-blind study on the use of manual medicine because the physician knows whether he or she is using a true treatment, even if the patient is naive and has no knowledge as to whether he or she received a true or sham treatment. The increasing use of outcome studies and cost-effectiveness of treatment studies has promoted additional interest in doing research on OMT, which was the distinguishing characteristic and hallmark of the osteopathic medical profession from its beginning.

SUMMARY

Osteopathic medicine is based on a philosophy, a system of logic for medical diagnosis and care with rich roots extending back to Hippocrates and beyond. Andrew Taylor Still, MD, DO, a pioneer physician in Kansas and Missouri, developed the basic tenets of osteopathy and elaborated on them in his writings, which were adopted by the ASO (now Kirksville College of Osteopathic Medicine).

The development of scientifically validated efficacious medicines aided in the evolution of classical osteopathic philosophy to its current form, contemporary osteopathic medical philosophy. The work of Irvin Korr, PhD, a medical physiologist, further elaborated and explained osteopathic theory, including an expanded focus on preventive care and healthful practices.

Osteopathic philosophy uses a holistic approach to begin the analysis of the patient, continuing with a reductionistic approach to focus on aspects of anatomic and physiologic dysfunction. One goal of this system of logic is to remember throughout diagnosis and treatment that it is a fellow human being with whom we work, even as we use tests that zoom in on the smallest microscopic details of that person. No cell or system in the body is seen as acting in isolation, and the importance of structure and function at each level is always kept in mind. Central to this philosophy is a tremendous respect for the innate capacity of the human being to heal, and the physician attempts to work with the patient's physiologic and psychologic processes to obtain an optimal level of homeostasis and function.

OMT, the hallmark of osteopathic treatment as developed by Still, is used in patient care either alone or in conjunction with medicines and surgery, as appropriate. OMT is recognized as having beneficial effects not only in the treatment of pain, but also to decrease physiologic stress and assist the body's self-healing mechanisms.

The application of contemporary osteopathic medical philosophy varies from country to country. There are vast differences in its application not only here in the United States as opposed to foreign lands, but also among practitioners in the United States, where osteopathy originated as a distinctive American philosophy and system of medical care.

As the osteopathic profession has evolved both in and outside of the United States, it has changed significantly. The original osteopaths practiced very differently from standard or allopathic physicians at the end of the eighteenth century. Still developed the osteopathic approach because the medications of his time were not only ineffective but also toxic and were based on tradition or conjecture rather than research. His important contribution to medicine was the idea that by adjusting (normalizing) anatomic functional abnormality, a physician could enhance natural physiologic function; that by enhancing the delivery and clearance of blood, lymphatic fluid, and neurotrophic elements, a physician could promote delivery of endogenous substances; and that these endogenous substances were able to do more than the medicines of his time to normalize physiology, eliminate illness, and reestablish health. His development and teaching of OMT was designed not only to do this, but also to eliminate pain and improve biomechanical (physiologic) function in body systems other than the neuromusculoskeletal system, such as the respiratory system.

American osteopathic physicians continued to address full medical, obstetric, and surgical care of patients. Each succeeding generation of DOs adopted the use of researched medications and decreased the use of OMT for anything but neuromusculoskeletal complaints, so that at the present time, a significant number of American DOs do not use the manipulative skills they learned in osteopathic medical school. Internationally, osteopathy developed in a manner that did not incorporate surgery, obstetrics, or the use of medication. This form of osteopathy continues to rely on endogenous substances for treatment, and the presenting complaints of its patients are generally neuromusculoskeletal pain or movement problems.

The twentieth century saw the development of scientifically researched, efficacious medications (this chapter does not elaborate on the accompanying side effects or fatalities associated with these same medications). As these medications became the standard of allopathic care, they were also adopted by osteopathic physicians. Increasing numbers of osteopathic medical students were attracted to the profession, not by the difference that OMT could make in patient outcomes but by the availability of the full scope of medical and surgical possibilities and a full license to practice as they saw fit. The osteopathic profession in the United States ceased to have a distinct identification in the mind of the American public, and many patients were unaware that their doctors came from a different tradition. This evolution has followed a standard sociologic pattern wherein an offshoot of a main group initially diverges, makes a contribution by developing an idea or skill that fills a vacuum not addressed by the main group, then reconverges with the mainstream as changes in both groups make them more similar. Other factors affecting the evolution of osteopathy have included recruitment demographics, advances in science and technology, and limitations on a patient's ability to chose a medical provider (as instituted by Medicare, medical insurance plans, health maintenance organizations, physician organizations, and managed care). The development of a specialty in osteopathic neuromusculoskeletal medicine, as well as widespread dispersion of osteopathic treatment methods through many health care professions, has helped address medical needs that are unrecognized by modern training in allopathic medical colleges.

References

1. American Osteopathic Association: *Yearbook and directory of osteopathic physicians,* Chicago, 1998, The Association.
2. Gleick J: *Chaos,* New York, 1987, Viking Penguin.
3. Hildreth A: *The lengthening shadow of Dr. Andrew Taylor Still,* Paw Paw, Mich, 1942, privately published.
4. Holmes OW: *Medical essays, 1842-1882,* Boston, 1892, Houghton Mifflin.
5. Northup GW: *Osteopathic medicine: an American reformation,* ed 2, Chicago, 1966, American Osteopathic Association.
6. Schiowitz S: Facilitated positional release. In Ward RC, Jerome JA, Jones JM, editors: *Foundations of osteopathic medicine,* Philadelphia, 1997, Lippincott, Williams & Wilkins.
7. Singer C, Underwood EA: *A short history of medicine,* ed 2, New York, 1962, Oxford University Press.
8. Still AT: *Autobiography of Andrew T. Still,* Kirksville, Mo, 1897, Author.
9. Still AT: *The philosophy and mechanical principles of osteopathy,* Kirksville, Mo, 1902, Author.
10. Still AT: *Osteopathy, research, and practice,* Kirksville, Mo, 1910, Author.
11. Trowbridge C: *Andrew Taylor Still,* Kirksville, Mo, 1991, Thomas Jefferson University Press.
12. Van Buskirk RL: A manipulative technique of Andrew Taylor Still as reported to Charles Hazzard, DO, in 1905, *J Am Osteopath Assoc* 96(10):597-602, 1996
13. Webster GV, editor: Sage sayings of Still. In *Year book of the AOA,* Los Angeles, 1935, Wetzel Publishing.

Chiropractic

DANIEL REDWOOD

orn in the American Midwest a century ago, chiropractic has evolved and matured toward mainstream status while largely preserving its essential tenets. The contemporary chiropractic profession is in the unusual position of having in many ways scaled the walls of the health care establishment (with licensure, an increasingly strong scientific research base, widespread insurance coverage, and approximately 27 million patients per year in the United States), while maintaining strong roots in the "alternative" or holistic health community (with a philosophy that emphasizes healing without drugs).

Chiropractic is the third largest independent health profession in the Western world, following al-lopathic medicine and dentistry. Its practitioners are portal-of-entry providers, licensed for both diagnosis and treatment. Unlike dentistry, podiatry, and optometry, chiropractic practice is limited not by anatomic region but by procedure. The chiropractor's scope of practice excludes surgery and pharmaceutic therapy, and has as its centerpiece the manual adjustment or manipulation of the spine.

The United States is home to 65,000 of the world's approximately 90,000 chiropractors.[13] Chiropractors are licensed throughout the English-speaking world and in an increasing number of other nations. Rigorous educational standards are supervised by government-recognized accrediting agencies, including the Council on Chiropractic Education in the

United States. After fulfilling their prechiropractic college science prerequisites, chiropractic students must complete a 4-year chiropractic school program, which includes a wide range of coursework in anatomy, physiology, pathology, and diagnosis, as well as spinal adjustment, nutrition, physical therapy, and rehabilitation.

Nearly 90% of chiropractic patients present as neuromusculoskeletal cases[60]—principally back pain, neck pain, and headaches—the conditions for which spinal manual therapy (SMT) is most effective. Current chiropractic research seeks to further define the role of SMT in the management of various musculoskeletal conditions and to evaluate its effectiveness for visceral disorders such as infantile colic, otitis media, dysmenorrhea, hypertension, and asthma.

In 1998 the National Institutes of Health (NIH) founded the Consortial Center for Chiropractic Research (CCCR) under the auspices of the NIH Office of Alternative Medicine (now the National Center for Complementary and Alternative Medicine) and the National Institute of Arthritis and Musculoskeletal and Skin Diseases. Based at the Palmer Center for Chiropractic Research in Davenport, Iowa, CCCR is a joint venture by five chiropractic schools, one medical school, and a school of veterinary medicine. CCCR's mission is to support a multidisciplinary group of researchers and clinicians to perform basic, preclinical, clinical, epidemiologic, and health services research on chiropractic. It also aims to develop an environment for training future scientists and to encourage collaboration between basic and clinical scientists and between the chiropractic and conventional medical communities.

PRECURSORS IN WESTERN TRADITIONS

Spinal manipulation has been practiced for millennia in cultures throughout the world. Chiropractic's forebears have included some of the prominent figures in the history of medicine.

Hippocrates was an early practitioner of spinal manipulation.[79] According to some scholars, he used manipulation "not only to reposition vertebrae, but also thereby to cure a wide variety of dysfunctions."[40] Galen, a Greek-born Roman physician who lived in the second century AD, and whose approach to healing set the officially recognized standard in Western medicine

for 1500 years after his death, also used spinal manipulation and reported the successful resolution of a patient's hand weakness and numbness through manipulation of the seventh cervical vertebra.[42]

As Europe endured what later would be known as the Dark Ages, these healing traditions were preserved in the learning centers of the Middle East by the ascendant Arabic civilization. Later this body of knowledge returned to Europe, and the works of Hippocrates and Galen helped form the foundations of Renaissance medicine. Ambroise Paré, sometimes called the "father of surgery," used manipulation to treat French vineyard workers in the sixteenth century.[42,58]

In the centuries that followed, up to the dawn of the modern era, manipulative techniques were passed down from generation to generation within families. These "bonesetting" methods, transmitted not only from father to son but often from mother to daughter, played an important role in the history of nonmedical healing in Great Britain, and similar methods are common in the folk medicine of many nations.[5]

In the second half of the nineteenth century, the United States was a vibrant center of natural healing theory and practice. Two manipulation-based healing arts, osteopathy and chiropractic, trace their origins to that era. Both began in the American Midwest.

BEGINNINGS OF A NEW PROFESSION

Daniel David Palmer (Figure 2-1), a self-educated healer in the Mississippi River town of Davenport, Iowa, founded the chiropractic profession in 1895 with two fundamental premises: that vertebral subluxation (a spinal misalignment causing abnormal nerve transmission*) is the cause of virtually all disease, and that chiropractic adjustment (a manual manipulation of the subluxated vertebra) is its cure.[57] This "one cause–one cure" philosophy has played a central role in chiropractic history—first as a guiding principle and later as a historical remnant, providing a target at which the slings and arrows of organized medicine have repeatedly been hurled.

---

* This definition differs from the medical definition of subluxation, which, according to *Dorland's Illustrated Medical Dictionary,* is "an incomplete or partial dislocation."

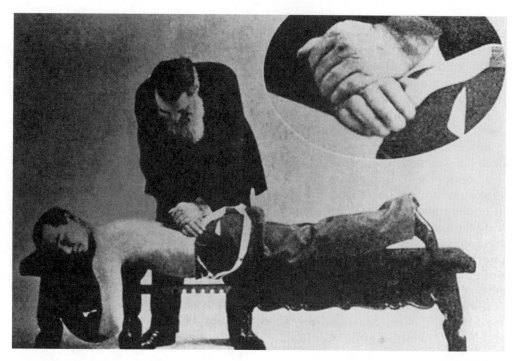

Figure 2-1 Daniel David Palmer, the founder of chiropractic, adjusting a patient, ca. 1906. (Courtesy Palmer College of Chiropractic.)

Although few if any contemporary chiropractors endorse such a simplistic and all-encompassing formulation, it nonetheless remains true that the *raison d'être* of the chiropractic profession is the detection and correction of spinal subluxations. Chiropractors may in fact do much more, but it is their ability to do this one thing well that has allowed their art to survive for a century under a constant barrage of medical opposition, some of it justified, most of it not.

One cause–one cure adherents among early chiropractors had two major political effects on the development of the profession. First, their deep faith in the truth of their message, combined with the positive results of chiropractic adjustments, created a strong and steadily growing activist constituency of chiropractic supporters. In their zeal, they generated a grassroots movement that ensured the survival of the profession through some very stormy years in the first half of the twentieth century. Civil disobedience was an integral part of the early development of the chiropractic profession, as it would later become in the American civil rights movement. Hundreds, including the founder himself, went to jail, charged with practicing medicine without a license (Figure 2-2). Incarcerated in 1906, Palmer said, "I have never considered it beneath my dignity to do anything to relieve human suffering."[57]

That chiropractic would prove controversial was evident from its inception. The first chiropractic adjustment was for a patient who sought relief from back pain; he attained results that far exceeded his expectations. Harvey Lillard, a janitor who was deaf, worked in the building where Palmer had an office. Lillard came to Palmer bent over with acute back pain. Noting an apparent spinal misalignment in Lillard's upper back, Palmer administered the first chiropractic adjustment, after which Lillard stood up straight. Lillard was free of back pain and was able to hear for the first time in many years. In this singular event are contained the two chief symptomatic benefits ascribed to the chiropractic art of healing: relief of musculoskeletal pain and disability (which is now well accepted), and restoration of proper internal organ function (which remains unresolved).

At first, there was hope that Palmer had discovered a cure for deafness, but similar results were not

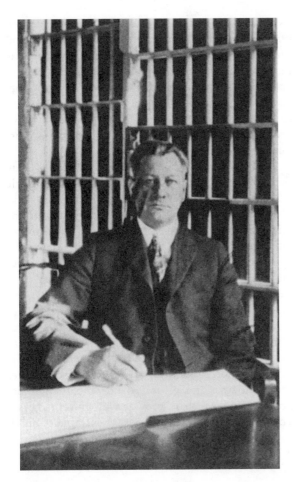

Figure 2-2 Hundreds of chiropractors served time in jail to secure the right to freely practice their healing art. Pictured here is Dr. D.S. Tracy, behind bars in Los Angeles, California. (Courtesy Palmer College of Chiropractic.)

forthcoming when other deaf people sought his assistance. There have been other reports through the years of hearing restored as a result of spinal manipulation, including one by a Canadian orthopedist,[8] but these have been rare. The story of Lillard's dramatic recovery has been used repeatedly to disparage chiropractic, with disdainful charges by critics that such an event is impossible because no spinal nerves supply the ear.

Current knowledge of neurophysiology provides a credible theoretic basis for this and other visceral organ responses to chiropractic adjustments. The underlying physiologic mechanism is the somatoautonomic reflex. Chiropractors and osteopaths assert that signals initiated by spinal manipulation are transmitted via autonomic pathways to internal organs.

In the case of Palmer's first adjustment, the relevant nerve pathway begins in the thoracic region, coursing up through the neck and into the cranium along sympathetic nerves that eventually lead to the blood vessels of the inner ear. Normal function of the hearing apparatus depends on an adequate blood supply, which in turn depends on a properly functioning sympathetic nerve supply.

Legacy of Contention: Chiropractic and Allopathic Medicine in the United States

All nascent healing arts face serious challenges. Prominent among these challenges is the need to maintain the enthusiasm generated by positive therapeutic results while clearly and consistently distinguishing among the proven, the probable, and the speculative. Some of the harshest criticism of chiropractic has been in reaction to the tendency of some chiropractors to "globalize,"[28] making broad overreaching claims on the basis of limited, although powerful, anecdotal evidence.

The American medical profession over the years established distinctly negative policies regarding the chiropractic profession that resulted in impediments to its development and have at times even threatened its very existence. Generations of allopathic medical students were taught that chiropractic was harmful, or at best worthless, and they in turn inculcated these prejudices in their patients.

That such a fiercely antichiropractic policy was pursued by the American Medical Association (AMA) is no longer in dispute. In 1990, the U.S. Supreme Court affirmed a lower court ruling in which the AMA was found guilty of antitrust violations for having engaged in a conspiracy to "contain and eliminate" the chiropractic profession.[77] The process that culminated in this landmark decision began in 1974 when a large packet of confidential AMA documents was left anonymously on the doorstep of the International Chiropractors Association's headquarters. As a result of the ensuing *Wilk v. AMA* case, the AMA reversed its longstanding ban on interprofessional cooperation between medical doctors and chiropractors, agreed to publish the full findings of the court in the *Journal of the American Medical Association,* and paid a substantial penalty, most of which was earmarked for chiropractic research on visceral disorders.

This has not completely undone the effects of organized medicine's antichiropractic activities, but it is nonetheless a milestone on the long road toward reconciliation. Although the swords of contention have not yet been beaten into plowshares of amity, the pace of progress is accelerating as men and women of goodwill in both professions strive to inaugurate a new era in which their patients are the beneficiaries of their mutual cooperation.

Seeds of Interprofessional Cooperation

Although relations between the medical and chiropractic professions outside the United States have also historically been less than cordial, they have in certain instances been sufficiently productive to permit closer collaboration between chiropractors and allopathic physicians. This has had particularly beneficial effects for research. Many of the key clinical trials that began to establish chiropractic's scientific credibility were conducted in Europe and Canada.

The tide is now turning in the United States as well. Research projects funded by the federal government have encouraged an atmosphere of growing medical–chiropractic cooperation, and multidisciplinary organizations such as the American Back Society also reflect a newfound common ground.

Agency for Health Care Policy and Research Guidelines: A Historic Breakthrough

The 1994 guidelines for acute lower back pain,[6] developed for the Agency for Health Care Policy and Research (AHCPR, now the Agency for Healthcare Research and Quality [AHRQ]) of the U.S. Department of Health and Human Services by a blue-ribbon panel primarily composed of physicians and chaired by an orthopedic surgeon (2 of the 23 members were chiropractors), included an endorsement of spinal manipulation.

The guidelines concluded that SMT "hastens recovery" from acute low back pain (LBP) and recommended it either in combination with or as a replacement for nonsteroidal, antiinflammatory drugs (NSAIDs). The panel also rejected as unsubstantiated numerous methods (including bed rest, traction, and various other physical therapy and pharmaceutic modalities) that for many years constituted the foundation of allopathic medicine's approach to acute LBP, and endorsed the use of self-care measures, including exercise, ergonomic seating, and wearing low-heeled shoes. In addition, the panel cautioned against lumbar surgery except in the most severe cases.

Perhaps most significantly, the guidelines state that spinal manipulation offers both "symptomatic relief" and "functional improvement." Because none of the other recommended nonsurgical interventions offers both of these benefits, it might be reasonably inferred that for acute LBP cases in which none of the guidelines' diagnostic red flags (e.g., fractures, tumors, infections, cauda equina syndrome) are present, SMT is now one of the treatments of choice.

The release of the AHCPR guidelines was a landmark event in chiropractic history. Federal government standards for the treatment of LBP, the nation's most prevalent musculoskeletal ailment and the most common cause of disability for persons under age 45, now assign a pivotal role to spinal manipulation, 94% of which is provided by chiropractors.[65] This is an excellent contemporary example of an alternative health care method achieving entry into the health care mainstream.

INTELLECTUAL FOUNDATIONS

The history of chiropractic, like all healing arts, is largely one in which an empiric process preceded theoretic formulation. From the earliest days, practitioners have applied new treatment methods on an intuitive, observational basis; noted that some methods were more effective than others; and then theorized about the underlying physiologic mechanisms on the basis of these findings. The resultant body of chiropractic theory, philosophy, and practice draws from principles in the common domain shared by all natural healing arts.

Common Domain Principles

Fundamental principles of natural healing, which have been part of chiropractic from the beginning and are incorporated into the curricula at chiropractic training institutions, include the following precepts:

1. Human beings possess an innate healing potential, an "inner wisdom" of the body.
2. Maximally accessing this healing system is the goal of the healing arts.
3. Addressing the cause of an illness should in most cases take precedence over suppressing its surface manifestations.
4. Pharmaceutic suppression of symptoms can in some instances compromise and diminish the body's ability to heal itself.
5. Natural, nonpharmaceutic measures (including chiropractic spinal adjustments) should generally be an approach of first resort, not last.
6. A balanced, natural diet is crucial to good health.
7. Regular exercise is essential to proper body function.

These principles, endorsed and elucidated by chiropractors for a full century, are recognizable today as the foundation of the emerging holistic health or wellness paradigm in Western medical practice (see Chapter 1).

CORE CHIROPRACTIC PRINCIPLES

In addition to precepts shared with other natural healing arts such as osteopathy, homeopathy, and naturopathy, core theoretic constructs composing the underpinning of chiropractic are as follows:

1. Structure and function exist in intimate relation with one another.
2. Structural distortions can cause functional abnormalities.
3. Vertebral subluxation is a significant form of structural distortion and dysfunction, and leads to a variety of functional abnormalities.
4. The nervous system occupies a preeminent role in the restoration and maintenance of proper bodily function.
5. Subluxation influences bodily function primarily through neurologic means.
6. Chiropractic adjustment is a specific and definitive method for the correction of vertebral subluxation.

Note the similarity of these precepts with those of osteopathic medicine.

These chiropractic principles reveal something unexpected: Although chiropractic is best known for its success in the relief of musculoskeletal pain, its basic axioms do not directly address the question of pain relief. Instead, they focus on the correction of structural and functional imbalances, which in some cases cause pain. This fundamental paradox—that a profession renowned for the relief of musculoskeletal pain does not define its basic purpose in those terms—has been a persistent and sometimes discordant theme in chiropractic history.

DIVERGENT INTERPRETATIONS: TRADITIONALISTS AND MODERNISTS

Historically, a dichotomy has existed within the profession between groups that have sometimes been called *straights* and *mixers*. Central to this controversy is the degree to which chiropractic practice should focus on symptom relief. Traditionalist intended chiropractors see their approach as being subluxation-based rather than symptom-driven, and largely confine their role to analyzing the spine for subluxations and then manually adjusting the subluxated vertebrae. Such traditionalists, a minority within the profession, reject the use of symptom-oriented ancillary therapies such as heat, electrical stimulation, and dietary supplementation. A few jurisdictions limit chiropractors to this circumscribed scope of practice.

Both groups agree that spinal adjusting is the paramount feature of chiropractic practice, and that advising patients on exercise and natural diet is appropriately within the chiropractor's scope. The chief philosophic difference between them is that whereas traditionalists seek to treat the cause and not the symptom (some even reject the term *treat* as excessively allopathic), broad-scope modernists seek to treat both the cause and the symptom. Although broad-scope chiropractors share their traditionalist colleagues' appreciation of spinal adjusting, they contend that patient care is in some instances enhanced by such adjuncts as electrical physical therapy modalities, hands-on muscle therapies, acupuncture, and nutritional regimens, including supplementation with vitamins, minerals, and herbs.

THEORETIC CONSTRUCTS AND PRACTICAL APPLICATIONS

Bone-Out-of-Place Theory

Pioneer-era chiropractors, following Palmer's lead, assumed that their adjustments worked by moving misaligned vertebrae back into line, thereby relieving pressure caused by direct bony impingement on spinal nerves. The standard explanation given to patients in the early days was the analogy of stepping on a garden hose—if you step on the hose, the water can't get through; when you lift your foot off the hose, the free flow of water is restored. Similarly, the explanation went, chiropractic adjustment removes the pressure of bone on nerve, thus allowing free flow of nerve impulses.

Based on the information available at the time, such nineteenth century concepts were plausible. Chiropractors were able to feel interruptions in the symmetry of the spinal column with their well-trained hands, and in many cases could verify this on x-ray examination. More often than not, when they adjusted the subluxated vertebra with manual pressure, patients reported significant functional improvements and healing effects.

However, there are problems with this theory, which are most simply and directly illustrated by noting that, after an adjustment resulting in dramatic relief from headaches or sciatica, an x-ray study rarely shows any discernible change in spinal alignment. (Such comparative x-ray studies are now considered inappropriate because of the unnecessary radiation exposure.) Positive health changes have not been convincingly correlated with vertebral alignment.

Motion Theory and Segmental Dysfunction: The New Paradigm

Alternative hypotheses are needed to replace the bone-out-of-place concept. Chief among these is the dominant chiropractic paradigm of our era, the theory of intervertebral motion and segmental dysfunction (SDF). (Note again the similarity between chiropractic and osteopathic terminology.) Although advocated by a small minority of chiropractors for many decades, this model first achieved profession-wide attention among chiropractors in the 1980s, and now enjoys broad acceptance in chiropractic college curricula throughout the world. This theory has the advantage of allowing a coherent explanation of chiropractic and the subluxation complex to be communicated in terms familiar to medical practitioners and researchers.

Motion theory contends that loss of proper spinal joint mobility, rather than positional misalignment, is the key factor in the subluxation complex. It posits that subluxation always involves more than a single vertebra, and that subluxation mechanics involve SDF, an interruption in the normal dynamic relationship between two articulating joint surfaces.[63] Anatomically, the vertebral motor unit or motion segment consists of an anterior segment, with two vertebral bodies separated by an intervertebral disc, and a posterior segment, consisting of two adjacent articular facets, along with muscles, ligaments, blood vessels, and nerves, interfacing with one another in an intricate choreography. Restriction of joint motion, a common feature of the manipulable lesion or subluxation, is termed a *fixation*. Fixation subluxations are the clinical entity most amenable to SMT.

Former Palmer College of Chiropractic president and vice president for Professional Affairs of the American Chiropractic Association J.F. McAndrews, DC, an early advocate of motion theory and practice, offers the following visual model of spinal motion principles:

View it as a mobile hanging from the ceiling, with many strings on which ornaments are suspended. As the mobile hangs there, it is in a state of dynamic equilibrium. Then, if you cut one of the strings, the whole mobile starts moving, because its balance has been upset. Eventually, it slows down and reaches a new state of dynamic equilibrium. But things have changed. It doesn't look the same. All those ornaments have shifted, in relation to the central axis and also in relation to each other.

The body's musculoskeletal system works in much the same way (Figure 2-3). If its normal balance is disrupted, it must compensate. Structural patterns will be altered to a greater or lesser degree, depending on the nature and intensity of the forces that threw off the old pattern of balance. ❧

Leach[40] describes the following triad of signs classically accepted as evidence for the existence of SDF: (1) point tenderness or altered pain threshold to pressure in the adjacent paraspinal musculature or over the spinous process; (2) abnormal contraction or tension within the adjacent paraspinal musculature, and (3) loss of normal motion in one or more planes. These criteria represent three of the four elements that define the osteopathic diagnosis of somatic dysfunction. Chiropractic education includes extensive training in the development of the psychomotor skills necessary to diagnose the subluxation complex and SDF and to perform the manipulative maneuvers best suited to its correction.

More problematic than fixations are those subluxations involving joint hypermobility, characterized by ligamentous laxity often caused by trauma. Hypermobility is clinically diagnosed by eliciting a repeated click when a joint is moved through its normal range of motion. Hypermobile joints should not be forcibly manipulated (because this can further increase the degree of hypermobility), but nearby articulations that have become fixated to compensate for the hypermobile joint should be manipulated, and muscles in the area should be strengthened and toned to minimize the workload of the overstressed hypermobile joint.

The motion segment is the initial focus of chiropractic therapeutic intervention, and is the site where the most direct and immediate effects of SMT are likely to be noted. However, more far-reaching effects are possible through neural facilitation.

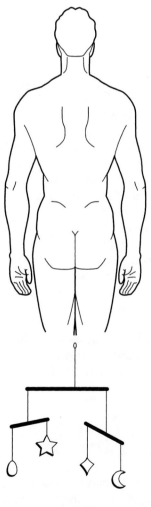

Before

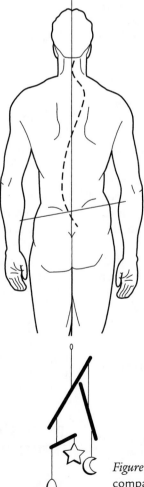

After

Figure 2-3 Visual model of spinal motion principles comparing mobile hanging from ceiling to body's musculoskeletal system before and after imbalance is introduced.

Facilitation

Segmental facilitation has been defined as a lowered threshold for neuronal firing in a spinal cord segment, caused by sensory (afferent) bombardment of the dorsal horn of the cord associated with structural spinal lesions.[39] Once a segment has become facilitated, consequent effects can take the form of local somatic pain or visceral organ dysfunction. Segmental facilitation is the dominant hypothesis proposed as the neurophysiologic basis by which the vertebral subluxation complex or SDF influences autonomic function. The autonomic nervous system contains two distinct and antagonistic divisions, the sympathetic and parasympathetic. These two divisions normally function in dynamically balanced equilibrium, although they have opposite effects on the organs and tissues they innervate.

Some models for the specific mechanisms of facilitation postulate that inflammation is a key factor,[21,27,51] whereas others have proposed neurologic models through which such facilitation can occur even in the absence of inflammation.[38,59] Inflammation, when present, alters the local milieu of the nerve, causing chemical, thermal, and mechanical changes; inflammation surrounding a nerve is likely to compromise its function. Researchers theorize that such aberrant nerve activity can disrupt the homeostatic mechanisms essential to normal visceral organ function.

A facilitated segment may result in either parasympathetic dominance or excessive sympathetic output. As Leach[40] concludes, "It appears that SDF is capable of initiating segmental facilitation and that certainly this is the most logical explanation for the use of [chiropractic] adjustment . . . for other than pain syndromes; certainly the segmental facilitation hypothesis is gaining greater acceptance and is based upon a large body of acceptable scientific research."

RATIONALE FOR THE CHIROPRACTIC ADJUSTMENT: INDICATIONS AND CONTRAINDICATIONS

The central focus of chiropractic practice is the analytic process for determining when and for whom SMT is appropriate and, secondarily, the type of adjustment most appropriate in a given situation.

Proposed algorithms for this process[40] detail procedures whereby the chiropractor, after arriving at an overall diagnostic impression (not limited to the spine) and methodically ruling out pathologies that contraindicate SMT, proceeds to evaluate SDF to arrive at a specific chiropractic diagnosis (Figure 2-4). This diagnostic process takes into account subluxations that are present, along with other clinical entities (e.g., degeneration, disc involvement, carpal tunnel syndrome) that in certain cases require treatment additional to SMT or affect the style of SMT that is appropriate.

For example, the presence of advanced degenerative joint disease does not render SMT inappropriate, but certainly rules out all forms of SMT that introduce substantial amounts of force into the arthritic joint. According to the Guidelines for Chiropractic Quality Assurance and Practice Parameters,[29] the high-velocity, low-amplitude thrust (HVLA) adjustment, the most common form of chiropractic SMT, is "absolutely contraindicated" in anatomic areas where the following occur:

1. Malignancies
2. Bone and joint infections
3. Acute myelopathy or acute cauda equina syndrome
4. Acute fractures and dislocations, or healed fractures and dislocations with signs of ligamentous rupture or instability
5. Acute rheumatoid, rheumatoidlike, or nonspecific arthropathies, including ankylosing spondylitis characterized by episodes of acute inflammation, demineralization, and ligamentous laxity with anatomic subluxation or dislocation
6. Active juvenile avascular necrosis
7. Unstable os odontoideum
8. Moderate to severe osteoporosis

These guidelines also rate, in descending order of severity, conditions listed in the following categories:

- Relative to absolute contraindication
- Relative contraindication
- Not a contraindication

Chiropractic diagnosis is geared toward evaluating where each case falls on this spectrum, and then proceeding with appropriate medical referral, chiropractic treatment, or concurrent care.

TYPES OF MANUAL THERAPY USED BY CHIROPRACTORS

HVLA, also known as *osseous adjustment* or *mobilization with impulse,* is performed by manually moving a joint to the end-point of its normal range of motion

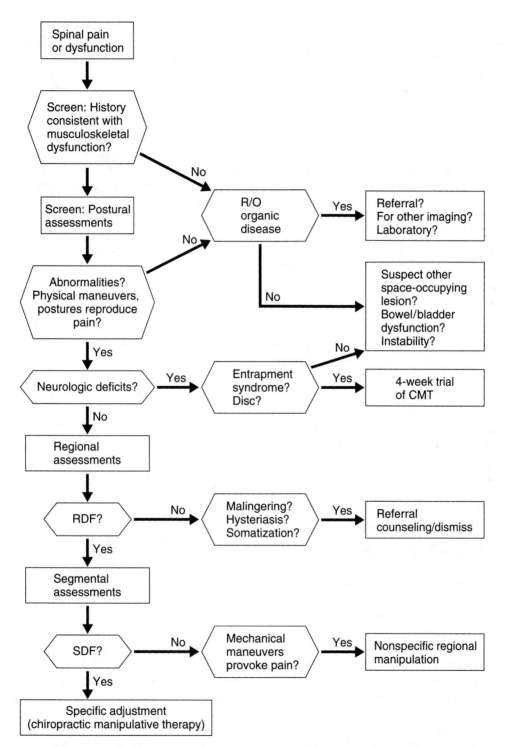

Figure 2-4 Proposed algorithm for the assessment of regional and segmental dysfunction. *R/O,* Rule out; *CMT,* chiropractic manipulative therapy; *RDF,* regional dysfunction; *SDF,* segmental dysfunction. (Adapted from Leach RA: An algorithm for chiropractic management of spinal dysfunction. In *The Chiropractic Theories: Principles and Clinical Applications,* ed 3, Baltimore, 1994, Williams & Wilkins.)

(ROM), isolating it by local pressure on bony prominences, and then imparting a swift, specific, low-amplitude thrust, which is often accompanied by a sound (presumably indicating joint cavitation) as the joint moves into the "paraphysiologic space" between normal ROM and the limits of its anatomic integrity. Properly applied, the adjustment generally is a painless procedure.

A variety of other adjusting methods enjoy wide application in the profession, including the following methods:

- High-velocity thrust with recoil
- Low-velocity thrust
- Flexion-distraction (originally an osteopathic technique for lumbar disc syndrome)
- Adjustment with mechanically assisted drop-piece tables
- Adjustment with compression wave instruments
- Various light-touch techniques

Some of these procedures are low-force methods, developed to help chiropractors manage cases in which standard HVLA adjustment is either contraindicated or otherwise undesirable. Nonadjustive manual measures also used by chiropractors, generally to supplement rather than replace SMT, include trigger-point therapy, joint mobilization, and massage.

CLINICAL SETTINGS AND METHODOLOGIES

Independence Born of Necessity

Because of chiropractic's long-time role as a dissenting wing of European-American healing arts, its practitioners have functioned almost entirely within the context of freestanding private practice. Similarly, chiropractic educational facilities have been private institutions, functioning almost entirely without public funding.

This outsider status is gradually changing. Chiropractors now serve on the staffs of a small but growing number of hospitals, and state (provincial) universities in Quebec, Australia, and Denmark now include chiropractic departments. Chiropractors serve in official capacities at the Olympic Games, and play an increasingly prominent role in the treatment of sports and workplace injuries. In 1993, J.R. Cassidy became the first chiropractor to be named research director of a university hospital orthopedics department, at the University of Saskatchewan in Canada, and in 1994 John Triano became the first member of the profession to join the staff of the Texas Back Institute, in the dual role of staff chiropractor and clinical research scientist.

Such developments bode well for the future, but remain more the exception than the rule. Evolving outside the mainstream has been a constant struggle, although this struggle has strengthened many who have committed themselves to the cause. By far the most serious negative effect of chiropractic's peripheral status has been that most patients who could benefit from chiropractic treatment have not received it because referrals from allopathic physicians to chiropractors remain far more rare than referrals to other medical practitioners or physical therapists.

The most salient positive effect of operating outside the establishment for so many years has been that the creativity of individual chiropractors has been encouraged rather than curtailed. Among the greatest challenges currently facing the profession is developing uniform practice standards (the 1993 Guidelines for Chiropractic Quality Assurance and Practice Parameters,[29] the "Mercy Document," is an initial effort) while maintaining the innovative atmosphere that has characterized the profession since its beginnings.

Diagnostic Logic

In the clinical setting, the chiropractic model demonstrates similarities and differences when compared with the standard medical approach. First and foremost, chiropractors seek to evaluate individual symptoms in a broad context of health and body balance, not as isolated aberrations to be suppressed. This holistic viewpoint shares much in common with both ancient and newly emerging models elsewhere in the healing arts.

Chiropractors recognize the need for thorough evaluation of symptoms, and are trained to take histories and perform physical examinations in a manner that would not seem out of place at the typical medical office. However, the chiropractic paradigm does not hold the elimination of symptoms to be the sole or ultimate goal of treatment. Health is not just the absence of disease symptoms. The true goal is sustainable balance, which is recognized by chiropractors and other holistically oriented health practitioners.

Chiropractors are trained in state-of-the-art diagnostic techniques, and chiropractic examination procedures overlap significantly with those used by orthodox (medical) physicians, but chiropractors evaluate the information gleaned from these methods from a perspective that places greater emphasis on the intricate structural and functional interplay between different parts of the body (Figure 2-5).

Chiropractic and Medical Approaches to Pain

The contrasting medical and chiropractic approaches to pain provide a case in point. Allopathic physicians tend to engage in symptom suppression far more than chiropractors, and also more commonly assume that the site of a pain is the site of its cause. Thus knee pain is generally assumed to be a knee problem, shoulder pain is assumed to be a shoulder problem, and so forth. This pain-centered diagnostic logic of-

ten leads to increasingly sophisticated and invasive diagnostic and therapeutic procedures. If physical examination of the knee fails to clearly define the problem, an x-ray study of the knee is taken. If the x-ray study fails to offer adequate clarification, a magnetic resonance imaging (MRI) study of the knee is performed. In some cases, a surgical procedure follows.

Like their allopathic colleagues, chiropractors use diagnostic tools such as x-ray studies and MRIs. The point here is not to criticize these useful technologies but to present an alternative diagnostic model. Chiropractors are all too familiar with cases in which this high-tech diagnostic scenario is played out, after which the knee problem is found to be a compensation for a mechanical disorder in the lower back, a common condition that too often remains outside the medical diagnostic loop.

A lower back that is mechanically dysfunctional and in need of spinal manipulation often can place unusual stress on one or both knees. In cases of this sort, allopathic physicians can, and in many instances do, spend months or years medicating the knee symptoms or performing surgery without ever addressing the source of the problem.

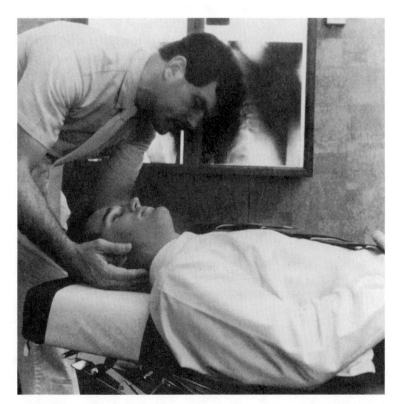

Figure 2-5 Contemporary chiropractors use state-of-the-art diagnostic and therapeutic methods.

Regional and Whole-Body Context: Neurology and Biomechanics

The chiropractic approach to musculoskeletal pain involves evaluating the site of pain in a regional and in a whole-body context. Shoulder, elbow, and wrist problems can of course be caused by injuries or pathologies in the shoulder, elbow, and wrist—but pain in and around each of these joints can also have as its source SDF in the cervical spine. In like manner, symptoms in the hip, knee, and ankle can also originate at the site of the pain—but in many cases the source lies in the lumbar spine. Other neurologically mediated symptoms such as paresthesia also can have a similar cause. The need to consider this chain of causation is built into the core of chiropractic training.

Chiropractors from Palmer forward have intentionally refrained from assuming that the site of a symptom is the site of its cause. They assume instead that *the source of the pain should be sought along the path of the nerves leading to and from the site of the symptoms.* Thus pain in the knee might come from the knee itself, but tracing the nerve pathways between the knee and the spine reveals possible areas of causation in and around the hip, in the deep muscles of the buttocks or pelvis, in the sacroiliac joints, or in the lumbar spine.

Furthermore, if joint dysfunction does exist, for example at the fourth and fifth lumbar levels, it might have its primary source at L4-5, or it might represent a compensation for another subluxation elsewhere in the spine, perhaps in the lower or middle thoracics, or in a mechanical dysfunction of the muscles and joints of the feet. Such an integrative, whole-body approach to structure and function is of great value.

Once contraindications to SMT have been ruled out, chiropractic diagnostic logic for patients whose presentation involves visceral organ symptoms includes evaluation of the spine with particular attention to those spinal levels providing autonomic nerve supply to the involved area, along with consideration of possible nutritional, environmental, and psychologic factors.

Criteria for Referral to Allopathic Physicians

Chiropractic practice standards[29] mandate timely referral to an allopathic physician for diagnosis and/or treatment for conditions beyond the chiropractor's domain, or when a reasonable trial of chiropractic care (current standards in most cases limit this to about 1 month) fails to bring satisfactory results.

In addition, chiropractors often seek second opinions in less dramatic cases if chiropractic treatment, although helpful, fails to bring full resolution. Referrals from chiropractors to neurologists, neurosurgeons, orthopedic surgeons, internists, and other medical specialists are common. Referrals to complementary practitioners such as acupuncturists, massage therapists, homeopaths, and naturopaths also occur, when appropriate, in areas where such practitioners are available.

Ethics of Referral

The medical profession has long had a clearly defined set of ethics for *intra*professional referral—a report is sent to the referring physician, and the patient remains the patient of the referring physician. During the era when the medical establishment prohibited collegial relations with chiropractors, physicians receiving referrals from chiropractors often failed to extend such professional courtesies in return. In a declining number of instances, this is still the case.

The most insidious effect of this remnant of the old antichiropractic bias is that it exerts a subliminal, if not overt, pressure on chiropractors not to refer. Ethical chiropractors of course resist the pressure. Such a vestige of the old order has no place in the modern health care arena, and must be rooted out with all deliberate speed. At a time when many chiropractic patients still elect not to inform their allopathic physicians that they are seeing a chiropractor,[23,24] the need for breaking down all such barriers should be readily apparent.

RESEARCH

For years, chiropractors were attacked for offering only anecdotal evidence in support of their methods. By the early 1990s, only those ignorant of the scientific literature could still make such claims. Spinal manipulation has now been shown by reputable researchers to be an effective treatment for LBP. More than 40 randomized trials have compared SMT to other forms of treatment for LBP.[1,65] All of these trials have shown SMT to be at least equal to and in some cases superior to the other procedures, and none of the studies have shown it to be less effective than the comparison approaches or a control group. Additional studies have demonstrated the effectiveness of chiropractic care for an increasing number of conditions including neck pain, headaches, and infantile colic.

Research Priorities: Musculoskeletal and Visceral Disorders

A 1979 New Zealand government commission of inquiry on chiropractic[18] drew an instructive distinction between musculoskeletal and visceral disorders. The initially skeptical commissioners concluded that chiropractic was safe and effective for musculoskeletal problems, which, in their definition, included back pain and associated leg symptoms, neck pain and associated arm symptoms, and migraine headaches.

Regarding visceral disorders, the commission stated that although credible instances of therapeutic benefit from chiropractic treatment were undeniable, response to chiropractic for such visceral organ problems was far less predictable than for musculoskeletal disorders, and further research was necessary before any definitive conclusions could be reached.

In the intervening years, a chiropractic research agenda has coalesced around the need to thoroughly document the effectiveness of SMT for both musculoskeletal and visceral disorders. Understandably, because approximately half of chiropractic patients present with lower back pain as their primary complaint, the initial research goal was to document chiropractic's effectiveness for that condition. The 1994 AHCPR guidelines indicate that this goal has now been largely achieved.

Early Chiropractic Research

B.J. Palmer, son of the founder of chiropractic and for many years a major force in the profession, was among the premier early chiropractic researchers.[56] He was one of the first in any health profession to use diagnostic x-ray studies. He also devised the neurocalometer (a thermographic instrument that detects paraspinal heat variances) and developed a specialized method for adjusting the upper cervical spine.

Other researchers and developers noted for their seminal contributions to the field include Henri Gillet, who formulated and refined motion theory[53]; Joseph Janse and Fred Illi, whose anatomic dissections and cineroentgenographic studies of spinal and pelvic mechanics provided crucial documentation for that theory[2]; Clarence Gonstead, for his system of x-ray analysis; Major Bertrand De Jarnette, for advances in postural analysis; and George Goodheart, for his elaboration of manual muscle testing (see Chapter 6).

The University of Colorado Project

Beginning in the 1970s, first with grants from the International Chiropractors Association and later with added financial support from the American Chiropractic Association and the federal government, Chung Ha Suh and colleagues at the Biomechanics Department of the University of Colorado undertook a series of studies that provided an extensive body of chiropractic-related basic science research.

It is worth noting that Suh, the first American college professor willing to defy the AMA boycott to pursue chiropractic research, was a native of Korea, where he was not subjected to the same lifelong antichiropractic bias as his American colleagues. In launching this research, he had to withstand intense pressure from powerful political forces within the American medical and academic establishments that condemned chiropractic for lack of scientific underpinning, while doing everything in their considerable power to prevent chiropractors from ever obtaining the funding and university connections necessary for the development of such a research base.[77]

Suh's team pursued research in two major areas. In one, a computer model of the cervical spine was developed that allowed a deeper understanding of spinal joint mechanics and their relationship to the chiropractic adjustment.[70] The other involved a number of studies on nerve compression and various aspects of neuronal function. One study demonstrated that minuscule amounts of pressure on a nerve root (10 mm Hg), resulted in up to a 50% decrease in electrical transmission down the course of the nerve supplied by that root.[33,44-46,64,72]

Research on Manual Adjustment for Low Back Pain

A substantial body of research has addressed the efficacy of SMT in the treatment of LBP. Consensus panels evaluating the data have consistently placed it on the short list of recommended procedures for acute, uncomplicated LBP.[6,62,66] These reports are based on controlled clinical trials, which at the turn of the twenty-first century number approximately 40.

The most influential trial to date was conducted by British orthopedic surgeon T.W. Meade with over 700 patients.[48,50] Meade compared chiropractic manipulation with standard hospital outpatient treatment for LBP, which consisted of physical therapy and wearing a corset. He concluded that "for patients with low-back pain in whom manipulation is not contraindicated, chiropractic almost certainly confers worthwhile, long-term benefit in comparison to hospital outpatient management." Describing the applicability of these findings for primary care physicians (PCPs), he stated, "Our trial showed that chiropractic is a very effective treatment, more effective than conventional hospital out-patient treatment for low-back pain, particularly in patients who had back pain in the past and who [developed] severe problems. So, in other words, it is most effective in precisely the group of patients that you would like to be able to treat. One of the unexpected findings was that the treatment difference—the benefit of chiropractic over hospital treatment—actually persists for the whole of that three-year period [of the study]. The treatment that the chiropractors give does something that results in a very long-term benefit."[48]

Meade's study was the first large randomized clinical trial to demonstrate substantial short-term and long-term benefits from chiropractic care. Because it dealt with both acute and chronic LBP patients, Meade's data support the use of SMT for both populations.

Perhaps the most widely publicized study reaching more negative conclusions about the use of SMT for LBP is the 1998 trial conducted by Cherkin and colleagues comparing chiropractic manipulation, Mackenzie extension exercises, and an instructional booklet.[14] The chiropractic group had less severe symptoms than the booklet group at 4 weeks, and there was a trend toward less severe symptoms in the physical therapy group. There was also greater dysfunction in the booklet group at one year follow-up. These differences were judged by the investigators to be minimal. There were no significant differences between the physical therapy and chiropractic groups and no significant differences among any of the groups in the numbers of days of reduced activity, missed work, or recurrences of back pain. Patients receiving care from the chiropractors and physical therapists reported far greater levels of satisfaction than those receiving the booklets. Costs were significantly higher for the chiropractic and physical therapy groups than for the booklet group.

Methodologic controversies in this study include the fact that the chiropractors were not permitted to recommend extension exercises (as would be the case in typical chiropractic practice) and were limited to one form of high-velocity manipulation without regard to clinical diagnostic differences among the patients. In addition, the physical therapists received intensive training from the founder of the Mackenzie technique during the week immediately preceding the trial. No comparable training was offered to the chiropractors.

Acute Versus Chronic Low Back Pain

Consensus panels and meta-analyses have not fully resolved the question of whether the literature supports recommending spinal manipulation for both chronic and acute LBP patients. In the main, there is strong agreement that SMT is appropriate for many acute LBP cases,[6] but the jury is still out regarding chronic LBP.* The perceived current insufficiency of data favoring SMT for chronic LBP has led some analysts to rate it as inappropriate for chronic LBP.

When Shekelle and colleagues rated the "appropriateness" of decisions to initiate manipulative therapy in a 1998 *Annals of Internal Medicine* article,[68] they deemed manipulation inappropriate for all cases of chronic lower back pain. Although this lowered the percentage of cases in which chiropractic was considered appropriate, both Shekelle's group and an accompanying editorial by Micozzi[52] aptly noted that the study offered solid justification for PCPs to refer many more of their LBP patients to chiropractors.

---

* A minority view can be found in the work of van Tulder, Koes, and Bouter,[75] who conclude that the evidence supports SMT for chronic but not acute cases.

Evidence for Manual Methods in Chronic Cases

Seeing that manipulation is considered "inappropriate" for chronic LBP, physicians and other health practitioners might logically conclude that until further convincing evidence emerges, they should not refer chronic LBP cases to chiropractors. However, physicians often refer chronic LBP patients to physical therapists based on perceptions of its effectiveness and appropriateness that vastly exceed its research documentation.[16] Because a PCP's decision about whether and to whom to refer LBP cases hinges on which treatments are expected to yield the most satisfactory outcomes, a summary of studies on spinal manipulation for chronic LBP may aid the decision-making process.

Aside from Meade's work, cited earlier,[49,50] perhaps the most impressive of these is a prospective study[34] performed at the University of Saskatchewan hospital orthopedics department by Kirkaldy-Willis, a world-renowned orthopedic surgeon, and Cassidy, the chiropractor who later became the department's research director. The approximately 300 subjects in this study were "totally disabled" by LBP, with pain present for an average of 7 years. All had gone through extensive, unsuccessful medical treatment before participating as research subjects. After 2 to 3 weeks of daily chiropractic adjustments, more than 80% of the patients without spinal stenosis had good to excellent results, reporting substantially decreased pain and increased mobility. After chiropractic treatment, more than 70% were improved to the point of having no work restrictions. Follow-up a year later demonstrated that the changes were long lasting. Even those with a narrowed spinal canal, a particularly difficult subset, showed a notable response. More than half improved, and about one in five were pain free and on the job 7 months after treatment.

In a randomized trial of 209 patients, Triano and colleagues[73] compared SMT with education programs for chronic LBP, which they defined as pain lasting 7 weeks or longer, or more than 6 episodes in 12 months. These investigators found greater improvement in pain and activity tolerance in the SMT group, and noted that "immediate benefit from pain relief continued to accrue after manipulation, even for the last encounter at the end of the 2-week treatment interval." They concluded that "there appears to be clinical value to treatment according to a defined plan using manipulation even in low back pain exceeding 7 weeks duration."

Koes and colleagues[36] compared manipulation with physiotherapy (PT) and treatment by a general practitioner (GP) in a randomized trial of 256 chronic cases that included back and neck pain. PT included exercises, massage, heat, electrotherapy, ultrasound, and short-wave diathermy. GP care included medication (analgesics, NSAIDs) and advice about posture, rest, and activity. In this study, the data indicated that both manipulation and PT were far more effective than GP treatment, with SMT marginally surpassing PT. This advantage was sustained at 12-month follow-up.

Another randomized trial by Bronfort and colleagues[11] compared the effects of SMT and NSAID treatments, each combined with supervised trunk exercise for 174 chronic LBP patients. Both regimens were found to produce similar and clinically important improvement over time that was considered superior to the expected natural history of longstanding chronic LBP. The SMT and trunk-strengthening exercise group showed a sustained reduction in medication use at 1-year follow-up. Also, continuation of exercise during the follow-up year was associated with better outcomes for both groups.

Preventing Acute Cases from Becoming Chronic

Because the prognosis for acute LBP is better than for chronic cases, high priority must be accorded to preventing acute conditions from becoming chronic. Unfortunately, a key factor leads physicians to minimize this concern: the conventional wisdom that 90% of LBP resolves on its own within a short time. Recent findings published in the *British Medical Journal* call for urgent reassessment of the assumption that most LBP patients seen by PCPs attain resolution of their complaints. Contrary to prevailing assumptions, researchers Croft and colleagues found that *at 3- and 12-month follow-ups, only 21% and 25%, respectively, had completely recovered in terms of pain and disability.*[20] However, only 8% continued to consult their physician for longer than 3 months. In other words, the oft-quoted 90% figure actually applied to the number of patients who stopped seeing their doctors, not the number who recovered from their back pain. Patients' dissatisfaction with PCP care found by Croft and colleagues was also reminiscent of earlier work by Cherkin.[15,17] Lead researcher Croft had this to say:

We should stop characterizing low-back pain in terms of a multiplicity of acute problems, most of which get better, and a small number of chronic long-term problems. Low-back pain should be viewed as a chronic problem with an untidy pattern of grumbling symptoms and periods of relative freedom from pain and disability interspersed with acute episodes, exacerbations and recurrences. This takes account of two consistent observations about low-back pain: firstly, a previous episode of low-back pain is the strongest risk factor for a new episode, and, secondly, by the age of 30 years almost half the population will have experienced a substantial episode of low-back pain. These figures simply do not fit with claims that 90 percent of episodes of low-back pain end in complete recovery.

The subjects in Croft's study were not referred for manual manipulation, and most became chronic. Based on the AHCPR guidelines, which emphasize the functionally restorative qualities of SMT, it seems reasonable to expect that early chiropractic adjustments could have prevented this progression in many cases. Recall that follow-up in both the Meade (1-year and 3-year)[49,50] and the Kirkaldy-Willis and Cassidy (1-year)[34] studies showed that the beneficial effect of manipulation was sustained for extended periods. The decision not to refer patients to chiropractors may mean that many LBP patients will develop longstanding problems that could have been avoided.

Low Back Cases with Leg Pain

Differential diagnosis is crucial for cases in which LBP radiates into the leg. Specifically, motor, sensory, and reflex testing should be used to screen for signs of radicular (nerve root) and cauda equina syndromes. However, a recent British study of primary care practitioners[41] found that most of these physicians do not examine routinely for muscle weakness or sensation, and 27% do not routinely check reflexes. Such factors play a central role in determining which patients should be referred directly for surgical consultation and which should be referred for manual manipulation.

The AHCPR guidelines state that manipulation is appropriate for acute LBP cases that include non-radicular pain radiating into the lower extremity.[6] However, in patients in whom radicular signs such as muscle weakness or decreased reflex response are present, there is now preliminary evidence[4,19] that chiropractic can yield beneficial results. In a series of 424 consecutive cases, J.M. Cox[19] reports that 83% of 331 lumbar disc syndrome patients completing care (13% of whom had previous low back surgeries) reported good to excellent results. (Excellent was defined as >90% relief of pain and return to work with no further care required. Good was defined as 75% relief of pain and return to work, with periodic manipulation or analgesia required.) There was a median of 11 treatments and 27 days to attain maximal improvement.

D.J. BenEliyahu[4] followed 27 patients receiving chiropractic care for cervical and lumbar disc herniations, most being lumbar cases. Pretreatment and posttreatment MRIs were performed. Good clinical outcome was reported for 80% of the patients, and 63% of the posttreatment MRIs showed herniations either reduced in size or completely resorbed.

In a study of 14 patients with lumbar disc herniation, Cassidy and colleagues[12] reported that all but one patient obtained significant clinical improvement and relief of pain after a 2- to 3-week regimen of daily side posture manipulation of the lumbar spine directed toward improving spinal mobility. All patients underwent computed tomography (CT) scanning before and 3 months after treatment. In most cases, the appearance of the disc herniation on CT scan remained unchanged after successful treatment, although in five cases there was a small decrease in the size of the herniation, and in one case a large decrease.

Headaches: Chiropractic Compared with Conventional Medicine

Probably the most noteworthy chiropractic research to emerge from the United States by the year 2000 is the ongoing work on headaches conducted at Northwestern College of Chiropractic in Minnesota,[7,54] in which chiropractic has been shown more effective than the tricyclic antidepressant amitriptyline for long-term relief of headache pain.

During the treatment phase of the first trial,[7] pain relief among those treated with medication was comparable with the SMT group. However, the chiropractic patients maintained their levels of improvement after treatment was discontinued, whereas those taking medication returned to pretreatment status in an average of 4 weeks following its discontinuation. This strongly implies that although medication suppressed the symptoms, chiropractic addressed the problem at a more causal level.

A subsequent trial by this group of investigators,[54] using a similar protocol for patients with migraine headaches, demonstrated that migraines were similarly responsive to chiropractic, and that adding amitriptyline to chiropractic treatment conferred no additional benefit.

In a more recent migraine study, Tuchin and colleagues[74] conducted a 6-month, randomized, controlled trial with 127 subjects, in which one group received SMT and the other group received detuned interferential therapy. Of the SMT group, 22% reported a more than 90% reduction of migraines as a consequence of 2 months of treatment, and another 49% reported significant improvement in the morbidity of each episode. An additional finding was that 59% reported a full remission of neck pain as a result of 2 months of SMT.

Further Musculoskeletal Data

Additional noteworthy findings relating to musculoskeletal conditions include the following:

- An Australian study[22] showed that LBP patients treated by chiropractors lost four times fewer work days than those who were treated by medical doctors.
- A cost-comparison study in the *Journal of Occupational Medicine*[32] demonstrated that the compensation costs for lost work time were ten times higher for those receiving standard, nonsurgical medical care than for those treated by chiropractors.
- A study of Florida workers' compensation cases[80] indicated that patients receiving chiropractic care were temporarily disabled for half the length of time, were hospitalized at less than half the rate, and accrued bills less than half as high as patients receiving medical care for similar conditions.
- A RAND Corporation study on the appropriateness of SMT for LBP[65,67] declared spinal manipulation an appropriate treatment for some patients; the RAND protocol involved a multidisciplinary panel, headed by an allopathic physician, that conducted an extensive review of the scientific literature and a consensus process among the participants to determine areas of agreement.
- An independent study commissioned by the Ontario provincial government (the Manga report[47]) found chiropractic in general to be safer and more effective than medical care for LBP. The report stated, "On the evidence, particularly the most scientifically valid clinical studies, spinal manipulation applied by chiropractors is shown to be more effective than alternate treatments for low-back pain." Addressing the pressing economic issues that precipitated the government's request for the report, Manga and colleagues concluded, "There seems to be a comprehensive body of evidence, which can fairly be described as overwhelming, for the cost-effectiveness of chiropractic over medical management of patients with low-back pain." They recommended "a shift in policy to encourage and prefer chiropractic services for most patients with LBP," and called for placing chiropractors on the staffs of all hospitals.

Visceral Disorders Research

Infantile Colic: Two Studies

Although the bulk of recent and current chiropractic research still focuses on musculoskeletal disorders, by the early 1990s leading chiropractic clinicians and academics had concluded that for the profession to survive and thrive with more than a limited musculoskeletal scope of practice, research on visceral disorders must be expedited.

In late 1999 the first breakthrough study on chiropractic treatment of visceral disorders was published in the *Journal of Manipulative and Physiological Therapeutics*. This randomized controlled trial by chiropractic and medical investigators at Odense University in Denmark demonstrated chiropractic spinal manipulation effective for treating infantile colic.[76]

Fifty participants were subjected to a 2-week trial of either dimethicone or spinal manipulation by a chiropractor. (Dimethicone, which decreases foam in the gastrointestinal tract, is prescribed for colic, although several controlled studies have shown it no better than a placebo.[31,43]) The main outcome measure was the percentage of change in the number of hours of infantile colic behavior per day as registered in the parental diary, an instrument whose reliability has been validated in previous studies.

The 25 infants randomized to the chiropractic group were given a routine case history and a physical examination that included motion palpation of the spinal vertebrae and pelvis. "Those articulations found to be restricted in movement were manipulated/mobilized with specific light pressure with the fingertips for a period of up to 2 weeks (3 to 5 treatment sessions) until normal mobility was found in the involved segments." The areas treated were primarily in the upper and midthoracic regions, the source of sympathetic nerve input to the digestive tract.

The mean daily hours of colic in the chiropractic group were reduced by 66% on day 12, which is virtually identical to the 67% reduction in a previous prospective trial.[35] In contrast, the dimethicone group showed a 38% reduction.

The Danish study on infantile colic was the first randomized controlled trial to demonstrate effectiveness of chiropractic manipulation for a disorder generally considered nonmusculoskeletal. Addressing this issue, the authors conclude that their data lead to two possible interpretations: "Either spinal manipulation is effective in the treatment of the visceral disorder infantile colic or infantile colic is, in fact a musculoskeletal disorder."

In a later randomized trial,[55] Norwegian investigators compared infants receiving spinal manipulation against a group of infants who were held for 10 minutes per session by a nurse. Both groups experienced substantial decreases in crying, the primary outcome measure. Of the SMT group, 70% improved, compared with 60% of those held by nurses. Because the researchers defined the group held by nurses as a placebo group, and there was no statistically significant difference between the two groups, they concluded that "chiropractic spinal manipulation is no more effective than placebo in the treatment of infantile colic."[55]

Other Visceral Disorders Research

- A pilot study by Fallon, a New York pediatric chiropractor, evaluating chiropractic treatment for children with otitis media demonstrated improved outcomes compared with the natural course of the illness. Using parental reports and tympanography with a cohort of more than 400 patients, these data suggest a positive role for spinal and cranial manipulation in the management of this challenging condition.[25,26]

- Two small, controlled clinical trials evaluating the effects of chiropractic manipulation on primary dysmenorrhea showed encouraging results. Both pain relief and changes in certain prostaglandin levels have been noted. However, a larger randomized, controlled trial failed to demonstrate significant benefits from SMT.[30,37,71]

- A randomized, controlled clinical study demonstrated that diastolic and systolic blood pressure decreased significantly in response to chiropractic adjustments of the thoracic spine (T1-T5), whereas placebo and control groups showed no such change.[81] This showed short-term effects of SMT on blood pressure, and indicated a need for research on longer term effects. No larger trials have been published.

- A study at the National College of Chiropractic showed a marked increase in the activity levels of certain immune-system cells (polymorphonuclear leukocytes and monocytes) after thoracic spine manipulation.[10] The increases were significantly higher than in control groups that were given either sham manipulation or soft-tissue manipulation. To date, no large trials on possible effects of SMT on the immune system have been published.

Methodologic Challenges in Chiropractic Research

The most challenging methodologic issues in chiropractic research are as follows:

- What constitutes a genuine control or placebo intervention?
- How can we properly interpret data collected in trials that compare active and control treatments?

These questions apply not only to chiropractic but to a broad range of procedures, particularly nonpharmaceutic modalities such as massage, acupuncture, physical therapy, and therapeutic touch. Depending on how the placebo is defined, the same set of research data can be interpreted as supporting or refuting the value of the therapeutic method under study.[61]

Two recent widely publicized studies illustrate the potential difficulties of defining the placebo or control too broadly. In their research on children with mild to moderate asthma, Balon and colleagues[3] randomly assigned patients to either active manipulation or simulated manipulation groups. Both groups experienced substantial improvement in symptoms and quality of life, reduction in the use of β-agonist medication, and statistically insignificant increases in peak expiratory flow. But because these two groups did not differ significantly from each other with regard to these improvements, the researchers concluded that "chiropractic spinal manipulation provided no benefit."

If the simulated manipulation had no beneficial effect, this is a reasonable conclusion. However, a closer reading of the article's text reveals the following information:

For simulated treatment, the subject lay prone while soft-tissue massage and gentle palpation were applied to the spine, paraspinal muscles and shoulders. A distraction maneuver was performed by turning the patient's head from one side to the other while alternately palpating the ankles and feet. The subject was positioned on one side, a nondirectional push, or impulse, was applied to the gluteal region, and the procedure was repeated with the patient positioned on the other side; then the subject was placed in the prone position, and a similar procedure was applied bilaterally to the scapulae. The subject was then placed supine, with the head rotated slightly to each side, and an impulse applied to the external occipital protuberance. Low-amplitude, low-velocity impulses were applied in all these nontherapeutic contacts, with adequate joint slack so that no joint opening or cavitation occurred. Hence, the comparison of treatments was between active spinal manipulation as routinely applied by chiropractors and hands-on procedures without adjustments or manipulation.[3]

The validity of this study entirely hinges on the assumption that these procedures are therapeutically inert. The following questions may be helpful in evaluating this claim:

1. Would osteopathic physicians or massage therapists view these hands-on procedures as nontherapeutic?
2. Would acupuncturists or practitioners of shiatsu concur that direct manual pressure on multiple areas rich in acupuncture points is so inconsequential as to allow its use as a placebo?
3. Perhaps most significantly, would the average chiropractor agree that these pressures, impulses, and stretches are an appropriate

placebo, particularly in light of the fact that they overlap with certain low-force chiropractic methods?

The authors of the study dismiss these concerns as follows: "We are unaware of published evidence that suggests that positioning, palpation, gentle soft-tissue therapy, or impulses to the musculature adjacent to the spine influence the course of asthma." However, a reasonable alternative interpretation of this study's results is that various forms of hands-on therapy, including joint manipulation and various forms of movement and soft tissue massage, appear to have a mildly beneficial effect for asthmatic patients.[61]

A second study that raises similar questions is Bove and Nilsson's work on manipulation for episodic tension-type headache (ETTH), published in *The Journal of the American Medical Association.*[9] Patients were randomly assigned to two groups. One group received soft tissue therapy (deep friction massage on the neck) plus spinal manipulation, and the other group (the "active control" group) received soft tissue therapy plus application of a low-power laser to the neck. All treatments were applied by one chiropractor. Both groups had significantly fewer headaches and decreased their use of analgesic medications. As in the asthma study, differences between the two groups did not reach statistical significance. Thus the authors concluded that "as an isolated intervention, spinal manipulation does not seem to have a positive effect on tension-type headache."

Unlike the asthma study cited above, Bove and Nilsson's carefully worded conclusion *is* justified by their data. However, it would have been more informative to affirm an equally accurate conclusion—that hands-on therapy, whether massage or manipulation plus massage, demonstrated significant benefits. Shortly after his paper's publication, Geoffrey Bove noted in a message to an Internet discussion group, "Our study asked one question [whether manipulation as an isolated intervention is effective for ETTH] and delivered one answer, a hallmark of good science. We stressed that chiropractors do more than manipulation, and that chiropractic treatment has been shown to be somewhat beneficial for ETTH and *very* beneficial for cervicogenic headache. The message was that people should go to chiropractors with their headaches, for diagnosis and management."

The mass media's reporting on Bove and Nilsson's headache study illustrates why defining the placebo or control correctly is more than an academic curiosity. Media reports on this study put forth a message quite different than Bove's nuanced analysis, with headlines concluding that chiropractic does not help headaches. Reports on the asthma study were similar. Moreover, future Medline searches will include the authors' tersely stated negative conclusions, with no mention of any controversy surrounding their interpretation.

The best way to avoid such confusion in the future is to emphasize increased usage of other valid methodologies, particularly direct comparisons of complementary and alternative medicine (CAM) procedures and standard medical care. Comparative studies have shown spinal manipulation equal or superior to conventional medical procedures, with fewer side effects.[7,48,50,54,78] If well constructed, such studies may yield data that allow health practitioners and the general public to place CAM procedures in proper context. Comparing chiropractic and other nonpharmaceutic procedures against highly questionable placebos confuses the issue.

CHIROPRACTIC IN THE HEALTH CARE SYSTEM OF THE FUTURE

The greatest issue facing chiropractic in its first century was survival—whether it would remain a separate and distinct healing art, succumb to the substantial forces arrayed against it, or be subsumed into the great maw of allopathic medicine. The question of survival has been resolved. Chiropractic has survived.

The key question for the next century, or at least the next generation, is this: How can chiropractic best be integrated into the mainstream health care delivery system, so that chiropractic services are readily available to all who can benefit from their application? A corollary question is this: How can such integration be achieved without diluting chiropractic principles and practice to the point that chiropractic becomes a shadow of its former self?

It appears that an overwhelming majority of chiropractors do not wish to pursue the path toward becoming full-scope allopathic physicians. Moreover, they will not willingly opt for any system in which chiropractic services are available only on medical referral. Chiropractors will gladly function as contributing members of the health care team, but will not voluntarily surrender either their political independence or the holistic, wisdom-of-the-body philosophy that has always been the core of their practice. How then can the desired integration be achieved for the benefit of many millions of current and future patients?

To answer this question in a manner satisfactory to chiropractors, allopathic physicians, and the general public, a mutually agreed on framework of common goals is essential. Fortunately, a common purpose does exist—all parties seek to create the most effective, efficient health care system possible for the greatest number of people. A framework for implementation also exists, at least in theory, based on the "level playing field" concept. This concept is a synthesis of two principles, democracy and hierarchy, coexisting in dynamic harmony.

The democracy of clinical science is one in which equal opportunity is enjoyed by all, and all hypotheses are innocent until proven guilty. Blind prejudice on the part of allopathic doctors, chiropractors, or anyone else has no place in this environment. All methods, whether presently considered conventional or alternative, must prove themselves therapeutically effective and cost effective, and must also demonstrate minimal iatrogenic (physician-induced) effects. Approaches presently enjoying the imprimatur of the mainstream medical establishment should in no way be exempt from this scrutiny.

Hierarchy also has a place on the level playing field, as long as it is based on demonstrable skills and proven methods. In those areas in which conventional Western medicine has clearly established its superior quality (e.g., trauma care, certain surgeries, and the treatment of life-threatening infections), this expertise should be honored and deferred to. However, this is a two-way street. If a complementary method such as chiropractic is proven superior (LBP is the first sphere in which this has occurred), chiropractors must be accorded a similar role. Hierarchy in this sense does not imply a control and domination model. This is a horizontal application of hierarchic construct rather than a vertical one, a relationship among equals in which precedence is based on quality, which in turn is determined through adherence to mutually agreed on standards.

To facilitate the integration of chiropractic into the mainstream, there is an immediate and pressing need to broaden lines of communication between the chiropractic and medical professions, on a one-to-one basis and in small and large groups, with the goal of offering to all patients the gift of their doctors' cooperation. Each side must learn to recognize its own strengths and weaknesses, as well as the strengths and weaknesses of the other. No one has all the answers, and humility befits our common role as seekers after truth.

At present, although chiropractors have clear guidelines for when to refer to medical doctors, neither the medical profession as a whole nor its various specialty groups have developed formal guidelines indicating when to refer patients for chiropractic care. Given the legacy of contention surrounding chiropractic, this is not surprising. But in the post-AHCPR guidelines era, such criteria are essential for informed decision making. The time for creating these guidelines is now. At a bare minimum, these guidelines should recommend referral to chiropractors for LBP patients who do not meet the AHCPR's tightly circumscribed criteria for surgical referral.

The future need not mirror the worst aspects of the past. It is incumbent upon all health care providers, and wholly consonant with our role as healers, that we heal not only sickness but also old rifts among ourselves. We now have an unprecedented opportunity to do so.

References

1. Anderson R, Meeker WC, Wirick BE et al: A meta-analysis of clinical trials of spinal manipulation, *J Manipulative Physiol Ther* 15(3):181-194, 1992.
2. Baker WJ: A clinical reformation in chiropractic: the research of Dr. Fred Illi, *Chiropr Hist* 5:59-62, 1992.
3. Balon J, Aker PD, Crowther ER et al: A comparison of active and simulated chiropractic manipulation as adjunctive treatment for childhood asthma, *N Engl J Med* 339(15):1013-1020, 1998.
4. BenEliyahu DJ: Magnetic resonance imaging and clinical follow-up: study of 27 patients receiving chiropractic care for cervical and lumbar disc herniations, *J Manipulative Physiol Ther* 19(9):597-606, 1996.
5. Bennett GM: *The art of the bonesetter,* Isleworth, England, 1981, Tamor Pierston.
6. Bigos S, Bowyer O, Braen G: *Acute lower back pain in adults, clinical practice guideline, quick reference guide number 14,* Rockville, Md, 1994, US Department of Health and Human Services, Public Health Service, Agency for Health Care Policy and Research, AHCPR Pub. No. 95-0643.
7. Boline PD, Kassak K, Bronfort G et al: Spinal manipulation vs. amitriptyline for the treatment of chronic tension-type headaches: a randomized clinical trial, *J Manipulative Physiol Ther* 18(3):148-154, 1995.
8. Bourdillion JF: *Spinal manipulation,* ed 3, East Norwalk, Conn, 1982, Appleton-Century-Crofts.
9. Bove G, Nilsson N: Spinal manipulation in the treatment of episodic tension-type headache: a randomized controlled trial, *JAMA* 280(18):1576-1579, 1998.
10. Brennan PC, Kokjohn K, Kaltinger CJ et al: Enhanced phagocytic cell respiratory burst induced by spinal manipulation: potential role of substance P, *J Manipulative Physiol Ther* 14(7):399-408, 1991.
11. Bronfort G, Goldsmith CH, Nelson CF: Trunk exercise combined with spinal manipulative or NSAID therapy for chronic low back pain: a randomized, observer-blinded clinical trial, *J Manipulative Physiol Ther* 19(9):570-582, 1996.
12. Cassidy JD, Thiel HW, Kirkaldy-Willis WH: Side posture manipulation for lumbar intervertebral disk herniation, *J Manipulative Physiol Ther* 16(2):96-103, 1993.
13. Chapman-Smith DA: *The chiropractic profession,* West Des Moines, Iowa, 2000, NCMIC Group.
14. Cherkin DC, Deyo RA, Battie M et al: A comparison of physical therapy, chiropractic manipulation, and provision of an educational booklet for the treatment of patients with low back pain, *N Engl J Med* 339(15):1021-1029, 1998.
15. Cherkin DC, Deyo RA, Berg AO: Evaluation of a physician education intervention to improve primary care for low back pain I: impact on physicians, *Spine* 16(10):1168-1172, 1991.
16. Cherkin DC, Deyo RA, Wheeler K et al: Physician views about treating low back pain: the results of a national survey, *Spine* 20(1):1-9, 1995.
17. Cherkin DC, MacCornack FA: Patient evaluations of low back pain care from family physicians and chiropractors, *West J Med* 150(3):351-355, 1989.
18. Chiropractic in New Zealand: *Report of the Commission of Inquiry,* Wellington, New Zealand, 1979, PD Haseelberg, Government Printer.
19. Cox JM, Feller JA: Chiropractic treatment of low back pain: a multicenter descriptive analysis of presentation and outcome in 424 consecutive cases, *J Neuromuscu-loskel Syst* 2:178-190, 1994.
20. Croft PR, Macfarlane GJ, Papageorgiou AC et al: Outcome of low back pain in general practice: a prospective study, *BMJ* 316(7141):1356-1359, 1998.
21. Dvorak J: Neurological and biomechanical aspects of pain. In Buerger AA, Greenman PE, editors: *Approaches to the validation of spinal manipulation,* Springfield, Ill, 1985, Charles C. Thomas.
22. Ebrall PS: Mechanical low back pain: a comparison of medical and chiropractic management within the Victorian WorkCare scheme, *Chiropr J Australia* 22(2):47-53, 1992.

23. Eisenberg DM, Davis RB, Ettner SL et al: Trends in alternative medicine use in the United States, 1990-1997: results of a follow-up national survey, *JAMA* 280: 1569-1575, 1998.

24. Eisenberg DM, Kessler RC, Foster C et al: Unconventional medicine in the United States: prevalence, costs, and patterns of use, *N Engl J Med* 328(4):246-252, 1993.

25. Fallon J: The role of the chiropractic adjustment in the care and treatment of 332 children with otitis media, *J Clin Chiropr Ped* 2(2):167-183, 1997.

26. Fallon J, Edelman MJ: Chiropractic care of 401 children with otitis media: a pilot study, *Altern Ther Health Med* 4(2):93, 1998.

27. Gatterman MI, Goe DR: Muscle and myofascial pain syndromes. In Gatterman MI, editor: *Chiropractic management of spine related disorders,* Baltimore, 1990, Williams & Wilkins.

28. Gellert G: Global explanations and the credibility problem of alternative medicine, *Adv Mind Body Med* 10(4):60-67, 1994.

29. Haldeman S, Chapman-Smith D, Peterson DM, editors: *Guidelines for chiropractic quality assurance and practice parameters: proceedings of the Mercy Center Consensus Conference,* Gaithersburg, Md, 1993, Aspen.

30. Hondras MA, Long CR, Brennan PC: Spinal manipulative therapy versus a low force mimic maneuver for women with primary dysmenorrhea: a randomized, observer-blinded, clinical trial, *Pain* 81(1-2):105-114, 1999.

31. Illingworth RS: Infantile colic revisited, *Arch Dis Child* 60:981-985, 1985.

32. Jarvis KB, Phillips RB, Morris EK: Cost per case comparison of back injury claims of chiropractic versus medical management for conditions with identical diagnostic codes, *J Occup Med* 33(8):847-852, 1991.

33. Kelly PT, Luttges MW: Electrophoretic separation of nervous system proteins on exponential gradient polyacrylamide gels, *J Neurochem* 24:1077-1079, 1975.

34. Kirkaldy-Willis W, Cassidy J: Spinal manipulation in the treatment of low back pain, *Can Fam Physician* 31:535-540, 1985.

35. Klougart N, Nilsson N, Jacobsen J: Infantile colic treated by chiropractors: a prospective study of 316 cases, *J Manipulative Physiol Ther* 12(4):281-288, 1989.

36. Koes BW, Bouter LM, van Mameren H et al: A blinded randomized clinical trial of manual therapy and physiotherapy for chronic back and neck complaints: physical outcome measures, *J Manipulative Physiol Ther* 15(1):16-23, 1992.

37. Kokjohn K, Schmid DM, Triano JJ et al: The effect of spinal manipulation on pain and prostaglandin levels in women with primary dysmenorrhea, *J Manipulative Physiol Ther* 15(5):279-285, 1992.

38. Korr IM: Proprioceptors and the behavior of lesioned segments. In Stark EH, editor: *Osteopathic medicine,* Ac-

ton, Mass, 1975, Publication Sciences Group.

39. Korr IM: The spinal cord as organizer of disease processes: some preliminary perspectives, *J Am Osteopath Assoc* 76:89-99, 1976.

40. Leach RA: *The chiropractic theories: principles and clinical applications,* ed 3, Baltimore, 1994, Williams & Wilkins.

41. Little P, Smith L, Cantrell T et al: General practitioners' management of acute back pain: a survey of reported practice compared with clinical guidelines, *BMJ* 312:485-488, 1996.

42. Lomax E: Manipulative therapy: a historical perspective from ancient times to the modern era. In Goldstein M, editor: *The research status of spinal manipulation,* Washington, DC, 1975, Government Printing Office.

43. Lucassen PL, Assendelft WJ, Gubbels JW et al: Effectiveness of treatments for infantile colic: a systematic review, *BMJ* 316:1563-1569, 1998.

44. Luttges MW, Kelly PT, Gerren RA: Degenerative changes in mouse sciatic nerves: electrophoretic and electrophysiological characterizations, *Exp Neurol* 50:706-733, 1976.

45. MacGregor RJ, Oliver RM: A general-purpose electronic model for arbitrary configurations of neurons, *J Theor Biol* 38:527-538, 1973.

46. MacGregor RJ, Sharpless SK, Luttges MW: A pressure vessel model for nerve compression, *J Neurol Sci* 24: 299-304, 1975.

47. Manga P, Angus D, Papadopoulos C et al: *A study to examine the effectiveness and cost-effectiveness of chiropractic management of low-back pain,* Ottawa, 1993, Ministry of Health, Government of Ontario.

48. Meade TW: Interview on Canadian Broadcast Corporation. In *Chiropractic: a review of current research,* Arlington, Va, 1992, Foundation for Chiropractic Education and Research.

49. Meade TW, Dyer S, Browne W et al: Low back pain of mechanical origin: randomised comparison of chiropractic and hospital outpatient treatment, *BMJ* 300(6737):1431-1437, 1990.

50. Meade TW, Dyer S, Browne W et al: Randomised comparison of chiropractic and hospital outpatient management for low back pain: results from extended follow up, *BMJ* 311(7001):349-351, 1995.

51. Mense S: Considerations concerning the neurobiological basis of muscle pain, *Can J Physiol Pharmacol* 69:610-616, 1991.

52. Micozzi MS: Complementary care: When is it appropriate? Who will provide it? *Ann Intern Med* 129:65-66, 1998.

53. Montgomery DP, Nelson JM: Evolution of chiropractic theories of practice and spinal adjustment, 1900-1950, *Chiropr Hist* 5:71-76, 1985.

54. Nelson CF, Bronfort G, Evans R et al: The efficacy of spinal manipulation, amitriptyline and the combination of both therapies for the prophylaxis of migraine

headache, *J Manipulative Physiol Ther* 21(8):511-519, 1998.

55. Olaffsdottir E, Forshei S, Fluge G et al: Randomised controlled trial of infantile colic treated with chiropractic spinal manipulation, *Arch Dis Child* 84:138-141, 2001.

56. Palmer BJ: *Chiropractic clinical controlled research,* Davenport, Iowa, 1951, Palmer School of Chiropractic.

57. Palmer DD: *Text-book of the science, art, and philosophy of chiropractic,* Portland, Ore, 1910, Portland Printing House.

58. Paré A: *The collected works of Ambroise Paré,* New York, 1968, Milford House.

59. Patterson MM, Steinmetz JE: Long-lasting alterations of spinal reflexes: a potential basis for somatic dysfunction, *Manual Med* 2:38-42, 1986.

60. Plamondon RL: Summary of 1994 ACA annual statistical study, *J Am Chiropr Assoc* 32(1):57-63, 1995.

61. Redwood D: Same data, different interpretation, *J Altern Complement Med* 5(1):89-91, 1999.

62. Royal College of General Practitioners: *Clinical guidelines for management of acute low back pain,* London, 1997, Royal College of General Practitioners.

63. Schafer RC, Faye LJ: *Motion palpation and chiropractic technique,* Huntington Beach, Calif, 1989, Motion Palpation Institute.

64. Sharpless S: Susceptibility of spinal roots to compression block. In Goldstein M, editor: *The research status of spinal manipulation,* Washington, DC, 1975, Government Printing Office.

65. Shekelle PG, Adams AH: *The appropriateness of spinal manipulation for low back pain: project overview and literature review,* Santa Monica, Calif, 1991, RAND, Report No. R-4025/1-CCR-FCER.

66. Shekelle PG, Adams AH et al: *The appropriateness of spinal manipulation for low-back pain: project overview and literature review,* Santa Monica, Calif, 1991, RAND, Report No. R-4025/1-CCR/FCER.

67. Shekelle PG, Adams AH, Chassin MR et al: Spinal manipulation for low-back pain, *Ann Intern Med* 117(7):590-598, 1992.

68. Shekelle PG, Coulter I, Hurwitz EL: Congruence between decisions to initiate chiropractic spinal manipulation for low back pain and appropriateness criteria in North America, *Ann Intern Med* 129(1):9-17, 1998.

69. Simske SJ, Schmeister TA: An experimental model for combined neural, muscular, and skeletal degeneration, *J Neuromusculoskel Syst* 2:116-123, 1994.

70. Suh CH: The fundamentals of computer aided x-ray analysis of the spine, *J Biomech* 7:161-169, 1974.

71. Thomasen PR, Fisher BL, Carpenter PA et al: Effectiveness of spinal manipulative therapy in treatment of primary dysmenorrhea: a pilot study, *J Manipulative Physiol Ther* 2:140-145, 1979.

72. Triano JJ, Luttges MW: Nerve irritation: a possible model of sciatic neuritis, *Spine* 7:129-136, 1982.

73. Triano JJ, McGregor M, Hondras MA et al: Manipulative therapy versus education programs in chronic low back pain, *Spine* 20:948-955, 1995.

74. Tuchin PJ, Pollard H, Bonello R: A randomized controlled trial of spinal manipulative therapy for migraine, *J Manipulative Physiol Ther* 23(2): 91-95, 2000.

75. van Tulder MW, Koes BW, Bouter LM: Conservative treatment of acute and chronic nonspecific low back pain: a systematic review of randomized controlled trials of the most common interventions, *Spine* 22: 2128-2156, 1997.

76. Wiberg JM, Nordsteen J, Nilsson N: The short-term effect of spinal manipulation in the treatment of infantile colic: a randomized controlled clinical trial with a blinded observer, *J Manipulative Physiol Ther* 22(8): 517-522, 1999.

77. *Wilk v. AMA:* 895 F2D 352 Cert den, 112.2 ED 2D 524, 1990.

78. Winters JC, Sobel JS, Groenier KH et al: Comparison of physiotherapy, manipulation, and corticosteroid injection for treating shoulder complaints in general practice: randomised, single blind study, *BMJ* 314(7090): 1320-1325, 1997.

79. Withington ET: *Hippocrates,* vol 3, Cambridge, Mass, 1959, Harvard University Press.

80. Wolk S: *Chiropractic medical care: a cost analysis of disability and treatment for back-related worker's compensation cases,* Arlington, Va, 1987, Foundation for Chiropractic Education and Research.

81. Yates RG, Lamping DL, Abram NL et al: Effects of chiropractic treatment on blood pressure and anxiety: a randomized, controlled trial, *J Manipulative Physiol Ther* 11(6):484-488, 1988.

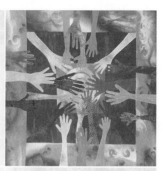

3

Massage Therapy
TouchAbilities™

IRIS BURMAN
SANDY FRIEDLAND

MASSAGE THERAPY

From the beginning of human history, massage as therapy was used for self-care and the support of others. It might have involved rubbing a tired muscle, squeezing a cut, holding an aching belly, or nurturing a wounded spirit. This has not changed over time. What is different today is the sophistication and organization of techniques that reflect humankind's ongoing process of discovery and understanding of the human body.

Each culture developed its own particular version of massage based on its unique psychologic, social, and spiritual constructs. Techniques evolved that were consistent with the philosophy of the culture.

These skills were passed down from one generation to the next, first orally and then in written form. Touch was used as part of an approach to healing along with diet, nutrition, exercise, meditation, plant medicines, and prayer.

Each generation shifted and changed the techniques. Interpretations, translations, and further sophistication, along with life experiences and society's needs, established an environment of mutual influence.

Intermingling and exchanging ideas between cultures was limited to trade routes and the occasional adventurer. Relative isolation kept healing practices within a culture essentially pure as they were transmitted through the generations. This changed in the nineteenth and twentieth centuries when developments in communication, transportation, and other technologies provided instant and distant connection, making the world a much smaller place.

BODYVIEWS

Modalities are created as practitioners are inspired to focus their work on a particular population, situation, or condition. Practitioners establish a philosophic basis for this focus and an intended outcome for the work, and identify and develop the techniques that best serve this outcome. Acquiring knowledge and employing a process of discovery (trial and error) brings sophistication and organization to the developing system.

There are hundreds of bodywork modalities, most of which are variations on similar themes. Each modality is organized around a general approach through which to "see" the body; in other words, *Body Views*. The categorization of these philosophic and theoretic "views" is inspired by the ideas presented in Mirka Knaster's book, *Discovering the Body's Wisdom*. Knaster identifies the Structural, Functional, Movement, Energetic, and Convergent Views[5] (Box 3-1).

Structural View

The *Structural View* is based on the paradigm of the body's relationship between its flesh and bone components and the pull of gravity. Structuralists look at the way a body is held in gravitational space. Their "art of seeing" is to observe and assess the signs of fascial support. These signs are the body's manifestation of its response to physical, mental, and emotional stimuli.

BOX 3-1

Body Views

> *A general approach through which to "see" a body:*
> - Structural View
> - Functional View
> - Movement View
> - Energetic View
> - Convergent View

Fascia is a flat membrane of connective tissue with a ubiquitous presence around and between all other tissues. It is a plastic, highly adaptive material that has tensile qualities. It connects, separates, defines, and binds everything from head to toe and allows the body to retain its shape. Because fascia is everywhere and touches everything, whatever happens to any one part of the body has an effect on every other part. The goal of a structural bodyworker is to optimize and maintain efficient verticality by freeing any restrictive holding patterns within a fascial plane. Structure influences form and function.

Functional View

The *Functional View* is based on the paradigm that our personal style of movement is learned and that these movement patterns are held within our neuromuscular system. With intention we can create efficient and economic movement that more optimally serves us. It is important to become aware of inherent patterns, and select body parts and movement strategies that support sensorimotor reeducation. Functionalists look at posture, strength, range, and quality of movement to provide guidance and opportunity for action, using the least amount of effort and energy. Function affects structure.

Movement View

The *Movement View* is based on the same paradigm as the functional view, but it takes a different form of expression. It focuses on individual or interactive movement within an organized system such as dance, yoga, or the martial arts. Used therapeutically, the modalities within this view, as in the functional view, take the practitioner on a journey of kinesthetic awareness and self-sensing to discover new possibilities and more effective movement patterns.

Energetic View

The *Energetic View* is based on the paradigm that we have a deep and abiding relationship with energetic forces inherent in the universe. In this view the basis of our existence is our connection to this energy. The goal of a therapeutic application of modalities within this view is to establish and maintain an uninterrupted flow of this universal life-force energy to support balance. Each modality presents a theory regarding the manner in which energy moves through the body. These systems identify energetic pathways, flows, channels, zones, points, and pulses and introduce techniques to influence them.

Convergent View

The *Convergent View* is based on the paradigm that experiences and emotions are held in the body and that energy is expressed in physical form. In other words, the body is shaped by experiences. These are body-oriented therapies, not psychotherapies. They emphasize the somatic component of posture and movement and address the mental and emotional manifestations in living tissue. By bringing awareness to specific areas through dialogue, physical contact, and positioning, "physical manifestations of emotional issues or emotional expressions of physical issues" can be consciously resolved.[5] The systems in this view focus on the personal revelation and understanding that lead to transformation and new options for expression and behavior.

MODALITIES

Most modalities emerged out of an individual quest to solve a personal problem. Challenged to find an answer for a situation or issue, people like Per Henrik Ling, Moshe Feldenkrais, Ida Rolf, and Milton Trager were compelled to explore options for persistent health concerns. Their search led them to look beyond existing practices that did not provide solutions. They asked new questions. By challenging the edges of the known, they discovered new ways of "looking" that provided effective intervention techniques. Excited by their own discoveries, they started sharing their experiences with others. Their personal stories grew into a context for relating to the body. Modalities were born and schools developed to train others in the practice of these touch skills.

Western bodywork practices, originating in Europe in the nineteenth century, are founded in skills developed by Per Henrik Ling that are the groundwork for Swedish massage. Ling's work was popularized by Johan Mezger in the mid-1800s and brought to the United States by the Taylor brothers in the middle to late 1800s. Swedish massage features the techniques of effleurage, pétrissage, friction, vibration, tapotement, and joint mobilization. Most schools align their core curriculum with this Swedish thinking and classification of techniques. However, very few schools limit their training to these six applications. They go beyond them and present techniques other than those founded in Ling's work. Blending and cross-fertilizing techniques created derivatives of classic Swedish massage that are most commonly taught and currently practiced in this country.

No one technique is the sure-fire answer for all people under all conditions. Some people get lasting relief from chiropractic or acupuncture, while others do not. Some people get the results they need from only one body therapy, while others mix several approaches because they build on or complement each other. . . . There are infinite varieties, and you will work out your own sequence. Success has less to do with what's "right" and more to do with what's right for you and at what time.[5]

MIRKA KNASTER

Twenty-first century massage is a compilation of "the best of" whatever happened before the year 2000. The evolutionary journey and developmental process of understanding the body has moved beyond concrete physical reality and once again includes the invisible world of energetic flows and dimensions. Sophisticated technology continually reveals information that expands awareness of what it means to be alive. Practitioners are constantly learning new ways to play in many realms to improve and maintain *homeostasis*—well-being and good health.

In the new paradigm, flesh is more than flesh. Anatomy is more than structure. Physiology is more than function. Current practice recognizes that the interaction of all the elements is more dynamic and vast than our historical and even present-day understanding. Twenty-first century massage is cutting edge. Practitioners are pushing the envelope on definitions and traditional notions of touch and concepts of what is being touched.

What developed during the last 180 years in private practice, spas, resorts, health clubs, and medical centers throughout Europe and the United States appears today alongside of and integrated with bodywork approaches from the East and healing touch traditions of indigenous populations from around the world. This global fusion has created the need to identify the broader ground that forms the philosophic and technical basis for the multitude and variety of touch modalities available today.

TouchAbilities™, a foundational approach to bodywork, is the conceptual framework of this presentation of massage. TouchAbilities™ identifies and organizes the fundamental methods of interacting with or acting on and between bodies. The basic touch skills comprise 26 specific techniques in 8 categories. These techniques incorporate physical manipulation of soft tissue and dynamic interaction with the body's mental and energetic fields.

The elements of TouchAbilities™ are introduced here in a specific order—an intentional progression for learning purposes only. However, in practice the challenge for the practitioner is to creatively blend the techniques. TouchAbilities™ is nonlinear. It is an ever-changing, ongoing integration of combinations and recombinations. There is no numeric sequence, no "right" order, no fixed system. TouchAbilities™ techniques are the building blocks of the touch modalities, which are referred to as *BodyWays*.

Each of the eight categories, known as *components,* represent a set of techniques with common characteristics and shared purpose in relation to the body. The components are described as follows:

- Breathing
- Mental
- Energetic
- Compression
- Expansion
- Kinetic
- Oscillation
- Gliding

Each component contains a number of subcomponents, each of which is listed in Box 3-2.

Applying TouchAbilities™ is an experiential process, an "in the moment" dialogue between bodies to support optimal function. It is a conscious conversation (verbal and nonverbal) used to recognize and connect with the current state of an individual. Its objective is to identify areas in which actions, waves, or flows are obstructed or distorted, and to apply techniques that reestablish a more functional dynamic.

To be in a position to truly assist others with bodywork, it is essential that a practitioner first use TouchAbilities™ for *self* discovery. Through continual exposure to the power and potential of these techniques, the therapist can most competently and effectively guide others.

BOX 3-2

Components and Subcomponents of TouchAbilities™

1. Breathing Component
   - Observing
   - Directing
   - Synchronizing
2. Mental Component
   - Visualizing
   - Inquiring
   - Intending
   - Focusing
   - Transmitting
3. Energetic Component
   - Sensing
   - Intuiting
   - Balancing
4. Compression Component
   - Pressing and Pushing
   - Squeezing and Pinching
   - Twisting and Wringing
5. Expansion Component
   - Pulling
   - Lifting
   - Rolling
6. Kinetic Component
   - Holding and Supporting
   - Mobilizing
   - Letting go and Dropping
   - Stabilizing
7. Oscillation Component
   - Vibrating
   - Shaking
   - Striking
8. Gliding Component
   - Stroking
   - Rubbing

Touch is our first language. . . . Touch is our one reciprocal sense. We cannot touch another without being touched ourselves.[2]

CLYDE FORD

A body is a multidimensional field that extends into the space beyond the physical. It is an organized dynamic of *material substance* integrating with *energy fields* and incorporating physical, mental, emotional, and spiritual essence.

TouchAbilities™ is also multidimensional. What lives through and beyond technique is possibility—intention—the experiential value of relationship.

We are a multidimensional creation with coexisting 'bodies'. … Our physical body is composed of matter; our subtle body is energy, thought and emotion; and our causal body is a spiritual source of energy. Health is the integration of all aspects of our being.[5]

MIRKA KNASTER

Energy manifests on the physical plane as internal and external waves. It includes the inner waves of respiration, circulation, digestion, elimination, and thought, and the outer waveform influences of light, sound, water, weather, earth changes, and cosmic shifts.

In bodywork, the bodies of the practitioner and client interface in the *field of engagement*. This space of connection offers a window into current internal and external states, allowing for intentional therapeutic exchange. Essentially, a therapist uses TouchAbilities™ to explore patterns in material and energetic fields, interacting with waves and reverberations to establish balance and enhance vitality and wholeness.

We not only can experience nature in terms of particle (form and structure) and the wave (movement and vibration), but can also experience the interface where they meet—standing in a strong wind, leaning into a tree, or at any interface where movement meets form.[11]

FREDRICK SMITH

BREATHING COMPONENT

Breath is life, the link between our corporal body and our spirit essence. It animates our physical being. It provides the fuel for every vital function. It is the *carrier wave* for life force, movement, and flow. It is an involuntary mechanism that allows for some voluntary control. Each and every moment, with or without our awareness, the body meets the physical demands of all its systems. We can consciously override these autonomic patterns to influence the speed, power, depth, rhythm, location, and duration of breath and the muscular activity involved in breathing.

Respiration drives an essential exchange of nutrient and waste gases through the lungs. Inhalation into the lungs brings nutrient gases to the blood and heart. The heart propels these gases to every cell in the body. Inversely, metabolic waste is carried through the blood to the heart and lungs and is expelled through exhalation.

We take thousands of breaths each day. The mechanics of breathing involve the diaphragm, muscles of the ribs and neck, and various other muscles, tissues, and organs. The movement of these structures during breathing creates waves that affect every system of the body. This effect translates to pulsation, excitation, movement, vitality, motility, and connection. The three primary techniques that can be applied when using breath as a therapeutic tool are observing, directing, and synchronizing.

Observing

Observing is taking notice of the pattern of inhalation and exhalation—the breath wave. It means to study, explore, scan, and scrutinize the way breath moves through the body. Ideally, the passage of air is animated and expressed in a free and easy respiratory cycle. Optimal breathing requires a body that is flexible, elastic, responsive, and vital. By following the breath through the nose and mouth, neck and throat, chest, back, and belly, down to the pelvis, both the practitioner and the client can note its path—which areas expand first, which ones follow, and which ones are restricted. The locations where inconsistencies are noted can indicate areas of "holding" on any level: physical, emotional, mental, and spiritual. Observing depth, breadth, rhythm, effort, restrictions, and irregularities enables the therapist to identify the focus and purpose for therapeutic intervention. Breathing patterns often change as other shifts occur in the body. Observing the breath throughout a session helps verify a person's response to various techniques and other stimuli.

Breathing is the one function of the body which is directly responsive to both our voluntary and autonomic nervous systems, and it is a key bridge between the conscious and unconscious. The breath is a primary source of our energy and vibration. … The response of the breath pattern is a direct signal of the energy shifts in the body.[11]

DR. FRITZ SMITH

Directing

Directing is used to consciously and intentionally influence the flow of inhalation and exhalation. This process can be initiated by the client or guided by the therapist. Engaging, inviting, encouraging, leading, regulating, managing, and controlling the breath wave produces numerous and varied effects on the tangible and intangible aspects of the body. On a core level, it supports oxygenation and vitalizes life-force energy. Directed breathing can be instrumental in releasing held tensions and stresses and correcting respiratory pattern distortions. It supports self-awareness, shifts consciousness and brain wave activity, and connects a person to sacred realms and the energy of the universe. It is a dynamic way to use the compressive and expansive forces of the breathing mechanism within the body itself to access and affect internal structures.

Synchronizing

Synchronizing is a technique whereby the therapist coordinates his or her breath with that of the client. Matching inhalations and exhalations, the practitioner entrains to, follows, and uses the client's breath wave or creates and exaggerates his or her own breath wave to influence the client. By matching breath patterns, the therapist can come into harmony and resonance with the client. This connection allows the therapist to "step into the client's being" to gain insight into his or her state. This establishes a relationship on the most primal level and sets the baseline from which the therapist responds. Synchronized breathing can carry an intention, or information, anywhere on or in the body. It can support the client to become aware of his or her own breath. It can soften the intensity or heighten and amplify the effects of a particular treatment application. It can also be used with directed breathing to support a shift in breath pattern. Box 3-3 lists BodyWays that feature breathing Component techniques.

Entrainment . . . involves the ability of the more powerful rhythmic vibrations of one object to change the less powerful vibrations of another object and cause them to synchronize their rhythms with the first object.[3]

JONATHAN GOLDMAN

BOX 3-3

BodyWays Using Breathing Component Techniques

Breathing Component techniques can be incorporated into any therapeutic relationship and combined with any modality. However, there are BodyWays that feature these techniques as an integral part of their system. The following are examples of such BodyWays: Holotropic Breathwork, Structural Integration, Neuromuscular Therapy (NMT), Pranayama Yoga, Rebirthing, Natural Childbirth, Past-life Regression, Feldenkrais, Tai Chi, Waterdance, Chi Kung, Meditation, Body Logic, Toning, Multidimensional Movement Arts (MDMA), and Body Rolling.

The correct use of the breath is central to both the quality of life itself and all healing work. The very word "pneuma," or breath, has the same Greek root as "psyche"—the words are basically synonymous. "Spiritus," from the Latin, is used to denote breath and soul both. The Huni Kui believed that the most powerful force coming from any live being was its breath and that words emanating from the breath were a creative force.[9]

HUGH MILNE

MENTAL COMPONENT

Mental techniques can greatly enhance and magnify the affect of all physical manipulations. These techniques arise from the mind, which is distinct from the brain. The *brain* is a physical structure located in the body, whereas *mind* is intangible and beyond the limits of the physical construct. The world is experienced through images that appear on our mental screen. Thought "waves" and mental images carry ideas, information, and intentions. Humans can communicate and interact with all living forms using these waves and images to manipulate and affect reality. Thoughts, ideas, prayers, and dreams, for example, are nonlocal and can be used to cause effects over distance and time.

Inquiring, Intending, Visualizing, Focusing, and *Transmitting* are the mental tools for assessment, enhancement, modification, and change. Applied alone or in combination with touch, they can have a profound effect on the way a person experiences himself or herself in the universe.

A good practitioner is helping the client to learn how to "control the controls" of our essentially conservative yet radically open-ended sensorimotor creativity. . . . New images suggest new kinds of movement and new possible strategies . . . [that] challenge the parameters of previous beliefs . . . [and] can alter not only the specific instances in which a specific resistance is encountered, but a whole world view that creates resistance per se. . . . It is clear that bodywork must reach the mind in order to effect genuine and lasting changes of this kind.[4]

DEAN JUHAN

Visualizing

Visualizing is creating a picture in the mind. A person can conceive an idea, develop a vision, imagine a goal, or conjure up a mental image. This technique can assist in manifesting a dream or bringing a concept into concrete reality, such as when an artist sees the finished sculpture in the raw piece of marble or an entrepreneur sees a store filled with stock before renting the space.

Envisioning possibilities allows a person to more easily recognize opportunities as they appear. Visualizing allows the therapist, client, or both to use a mentally held image for self-discovery, healing, relaxation, problem solving, pain management, and behavioral and functional modification. It promotes shifts in the body, such as when a person slows his or her breathing by imagining himself or herself in a relaxed situation. It can cause change on a cellular level, such as when a cancer patient holds an image of a vacuum consuming the tumor. It can assist in healing a condition, such as when a person with a heart ailment holds an image of a healthy heart muscle. During a massage treatment, Visualizing can be effective when focused on releasing a trigger point, lengthening a muscle, or opening an energy pathway.

Our language for describing physical sensation lends itself to somatic imaging. We are accustomed to using metaphors to describe our physical condition. A "stabbing" pain, a "wrenched" neck, a "churned up" stomach, a "burning" sensation, a "shooting" pain, a "pins and needles" sensation, a "tight" muscle are examples of the images embedded within commonly used phrases.[2]

C. FORD

Inquiring

Inquiring encompasses the quest for truth, knowledge, and information. It is the verbal and nonverbal act of asking. The words examine, interrogate, probe, scrutinize, analyze, check, test, study, investigate, search, seek, and check out exemplify the concept of inquiring. To "bring a question to the table" in a bodywork session is to be open to "what is so" in the moment. It includes a therapist interviewing a client to gather information and set an *Intention* for the session. (How do you feel? What would you like to accomplish in today's session? Is there an area you want to focus on?) It helps identify qualities and boundaries of physical and energetic fields. (What is the pliability of this tissue? How does this move and stretch? What is attached to the part or parts being moved? How far can this joint be mobilized? Did you feel the energy expand through this part?) A therapist or client can "hold a question" as an underlying impetus for observing, assessing, and responding to what is taking place. The therapist may ask the following questions: What area or parts are not moving that should? What can be freer, lighter, easier? As this lets go, where else can I take it? This is not releasing; what else can I try? The client may hold the following questions: Where am I holding? How can I let go? What does this mean to me?

This powerful interactive tool can be used throughout a session to establish and maintain a line of communication for discovery and feedback. How is the pressure of my contact? Are you aware of this restriction? Tell me how you feel now? Did you notice that release?

All bodywork is essentially a conversation between two intelligent systems. That conversation—especially when it is nonverbal—takes place in the language of relationship. . . . We do not "fix" people, no matter how good we get; we inform their bodies, and they organize themselves into "better."[8]

TOM MEYERS

Intending

Intending gives impetus to create and provides purpose for our actions. It is an essential and integral part of a conscious bodywork session. Intending establishes a purpose or plan; it directs effort toward a determined goal. It is used to develop strategies and design, aim toward, set one's sights on, have in mind, or predetermine a desired outcome. This goal can be vocalized, written, or held as a thought in the mind. *Intentions* define the nature of the client-practitioner relationship. They can be for the moment, session, or course of treatment. They can be localized to a specific point of focus or can be more generalized, involving an area or an entire field. They can be singular or multiple and can change moment to moment. Flexibility is a key to effective outcomes. It is essential in responding to the new influences that are always stimulating change and shifting the current state of things. Setting a goal provides an ideal by which to measure client progress. During a session, the therapist can observe the current state of the client and compare this with the intended outcome. For example, if an intention is to expand the range of motion (ROM) of a joint, the therapist occasionally checks the mobility of that joint to see whether the work is effective and when the goal is reached. Using intention in this way helps the therapist recognize when and how to modify the application or course of action or when a session is complete. The benefits are intensified when an intention is co-created by both therapist and client and established and directed toward the highest good for all concerned. This technique empowers the work and facilitates the process toward balance, homeostasis, and health on physical, emotional, mental, and spiritual levels.

Focusing

Focusing concentrates awareness on a selected point of attention. It delineates and specifies a site to which we can deliver ideas, information, and intentions. It is the act of taking aim at a target. Focusing is used to localize physical manipulations, dissipate tension or pain, or integrate a part to the whole. It is a directive of where to place attention onto any sensation, idea, or location, such as a trigger point, prior experience, or body process. This is helpful when Transmitting an image of health or an affirmation for change. The act of Focusing allows a person to center on, emphasize, distinguish, highlight, and bring consciousness and awareness to sensations experienced in a particular area. Then mental images can be directed to that specific location. For example, when treating a tight muscle, the therapist can focus touch on that location and direct a client's attention to the exact point of discomfort. The client is then guided to breathe into that

BOX 3-4

BodyWays Using Mental Component Techniques

> Mental Component techniques can be incorporated into any therapeutic relationship and combined with any modality. However, the following BodyWays feature these techniques as an integral part of their system: Progressive Relaxation, Visualization, MDMA, Reiki, Imagery, Trager, Craniosacral, Feldenkrais, Lomi Lomi, Meditation, Somatosynthesis, Focusing, Hypnosis, and Affirmations.

area, focus on it during the in-breath, and dissipate the sensation during the out-breath. Progressive Relaxation is another example of Focusing whereby a client is guided through his or her body and led to sequentially contract and release specific muscles.

Transmitting

Transmitting is about communicating and connecting—sending out a signal in the form of a thought, image, feeling, idea, intention, color, or sound. As intangible waves, these signals broadcast, transfer, convey, and otherwise make connections. Transmitting is the active principle that links the signal to its destination. It is a delivery mechanism and actualizing vehicle for mental and other techniques. It is the bridge between the intention and the focus. Transmissions can influence the body biomechanically, mentally, and energetically. Delivering signals, a therapist can highlight or modify the current state of or introduce something new to a system. These signals, which bounce back with information regarding the client's status, are perceived through *Sensing*. Using this feedback, modifications can then be made by adding, subtracting, amplifying, distorting, or introducing something new to the body by Transmitting colors, waves, or vibrations. Box 3-4 lists BodyWays that feature Mental Component techniques.

As surely as we "call" with our skilled touch, the client "calls" back and is responding at every moment in a completely unique way. . . . It is out of the mysterious dialogue of this mostly nonverbal call-and-response that understanding arises. Therefore, the actual practice of therapy has much more to do with the graceful back and forth swing of call-and-response than it does with the unidirectional approach of diagnosis and treatment.

When we touch, we are moving within the person's structural body and energy field. Our movements, as we understand the client better and better, become more appropriate responses. When we understand each other, we say we feel in synch.[6]

DAVID LAUTERSTEIN

ENERGETIC COMPONENT

Energy is the carrier wave of life force. It rides the breath wave into and throughout the body. Energy animates the body and is commonly known as *Chi, Ki, Prana, Mana, Orgone,* or *Kundalini.* In his writings, scientist James Oschman, PhD, identifies six energetic systems: electromagnetic, elastic, acoustic, thermal, gravitational, and photonic. Practitioners influence these systems by integrating and balancing the body in the direction of homeostasis by applying the techniques of *Sensing, Intuiting,* and *Balancing.*

On the basis of what is now known about the roles of electrical, magnetic, elastic, acoustic, thermal, gravitational and photonic energies in living systems, it appears that there are many energetic systems in the living body and many ways of influencing them. What we refer to as the "living state" and as "health" are all of these systems, both known and unknown, functioning collectively, cooperatively and synergistically. The debate about whether there is such a thing as "Healing Energy" or life force is being replaced with the study of the interactions between the biological energy fields, structures and functions.[10]

JAMES OSCHMAN, PHD

Energy is expressed in matter through the vitality and motility of structure. Discordant energy patterns appear in the body as stress and distortion. Because energetic fields are influenced by interaction with the many distinctive wave patterns inherent in the world, energy techniques are effective in manipulating these distortions and supporting the body to establish balance. A body in balance can be supported to a higher level of wellness by using these techniques to expand, support, and fine-tune existing patterns.

Sensing

Sensing is perceiving or receiving impressions from internal and external stimuli. We experience this through our own internal and external sense mechanisms. Internally, these are our receptors for touch, pressure, pain, temperature, and stretch. We sense the external world through the mechanisms of sight, hearing, smell, taste, and touch. It is through proprioception that we sense the rhythms and states of the electromagnetic, elastic, acoustic, thermal, gravitational and photonic energetic systems. *Proprioception* is "the awareness of posture, movement and changes in equilibrium and the knowledge of position, weight and resistance of objects in relation to one's own body."[12] Through sensing, a practitioner can feel, detect, discern, and experience; that is, become conscious of the current state of the body. In the electromagnetic system the practitioner can sense rhythms in the form of pulses (respiratory, circulatory, cranial) and waves (brain, breath). In the elastic system states of density, tension, distortion, fibrocity, plasticity, resistance, mobility, and congestion, and the rhythm of motility can be sensed. In the acoustic system practitioners can sense vibrations as expressed through the rhythms of amplification, frequency (range, timing), and pattern (formation). In the thermal system practitioners can sense the state of temperature. In the gravitational system practitioners can sense the state of weight, motion, tension, and position (alignment). Finally, in the photonic system practitioners can sense color and light.

Intuiting

Intuiting means to innately "know" through core knowledge or insight; to sense that which is not apparent or visible. It enables what is known on the level of the unconscious to be incorporated with and become a part of consciousness. Intuition, also known as *revelation, moment of illumination,* or *premonition,* allows for intangible, nonlinear connections and understandings. This kind of direct perception links to truths that extend beyond the structure and predictability of the known. Intuition is often identified as a gut feeling, impression, instinct, hunch, "sixth sense," epiphany, or flash of insight. This source of inner wisdom leads to clarification and new perspectives. As practitioners, we use intuition to know which techniques to apply, when to shift techniques or place of focus, and when to customize speed, alter rhythm, change depth, modify pressure, or adjust angle.

BOX 3-5

BodyWays Using Energetic Component Techniques

Energetic Component techniques can be incorporated into any therapeutic relationship and combined with any modality. However, there are BodyWays that feature these techniques as an integral part of their system. Some examples of these BodyWays are Acupuncture, Acupressure, Shiatsu, Anma, Ayurveda, Espira (formerly Light Touch), Kinergetics, Lomi Lomi, MDMA, Polarity, Reiki, Reflexology, Therapeutic Touch, Watsu, and Zero Balancing.

Balancing

Balancing is both a technique and a state. As a technique, it is the act of supporting, aligning, and harmonizing energetic flow. As a state, it is an energetic experience of support, alignment, and harmony. Balancing means to synchronize, stabilize, integrate, connect, coordinate, adjust, equilibrate, normalize, correlate, or complement. *Homeostasis* refers to the balance of the internal environment of the body (microcosm) and the body's dynamic relationship with the external environment (macrocosm). Using balance as an intention, a therapist can assist movement toward homeostasis on all levels: physical, emotional, mental, and spiritual. The ultimate goal is for optimal function, a smooth interface, and a supportive relationship for all body parts and processes. Some modalities use concepts such as chakras, meridians, zones, doshas, elements, or paired segments in the body as focal points or pathways for balance. Box 3-5 lists BodyWays that feature Energetic Component techniques.

Our bodies are continually in a state of change and movement, but we are rarely aware of the thousands of small, subliminal alterations that are regularly occurring. When the physical body and the energy body are in harmony, there is an experience of "balance." When we stimulate an energy flow and change its movement within the body, there will be internal shifts as the person adjusts to those changes and establishes new equilibrium. This period of internal rearrangement to an energetic shift is what I call the "working state," and means that the body/mind/spirit is responding, reorganizing, and reintegrating during or following a shift of balance or vibration.[11]

F.F. SMITH

Compression Component

Compression creates the carrier wave of centripetal force. Compression techniques move energy toward the core of the body. The resulting dynamic of interfacing forces and pressures produces waves that can be used to stabilize, obstruct, reverse, and exaggerate existing wave patterns in and beyond the field of engagement. By imposing a force on the body, the practitioner influences its inherent flows and moves energy into many directions within and beyond the contact site. These techniques deal with intentions of distortion, interference, resistance, and support. They can be used to explore and assess the state of the body. Compression creates change by challenging defined edges, occluding flows, and remodeling shapes and boundaries. Collectively these techniques can be used to initiate or assist and to obstruct or block flows. They can initiate, assist, or resist movement of bones, organs, tissues, energies, and fluids. They can be used to flatten, stretch, reshape, or separate fascia, muscles, tendons, ligaments, and other tissues. Compressive techniques can also stimulate or override nerve impulses to dissipate trigger points, release contracted muscles, and influence neurologic patterns. All Compression Component techniques share a similar set of intentions. The differences in their application produce variations in outcome. Each technique, as presented, is a progressive sophistication of the technique preceding it. They all affect the cavities, tubes, tissues, bones, flows, and pulses of the body in some manner. They are identified in this particular way to highlight their subtle differences.

Pressing and Pushing

Pressing and *Pushing* are grouped because of their similarities. They are presented as two variations because of their differences. Both techniques involve placing force against an object. The distinction is found in the delivery of the application. Pressing applies pressure to, puts force on, or bears down onto or into a body. It can compress, compact, condense, approximate, or anchor the target area. Pushing, on the other hand, moves something aside, away, or ahead using steady pressure or contact. It sets in motion, advances, nudges, prods, intrudes, propels, thrusts, or shoves the target area. Pushing is actually Pressing with movement. A practitioner might compress a fluid vessel by Pressing, thus occluding it, blocking its flow. Pushing the same structure can move the flow forward (ahead of the source of force, in the direction of the vector), encouraging a draining effect. Both techniques can be used as assessment tools to examine tissues for resilience, hardness, fibrosis, mobility, tension, resistance, receptivity, and strength. They provide a proprioceptive awareness of depth and layers of tissue and energy. A practitioner can either Push or Press to initiate, assist, or resist movement of bones, organs, tissue, energy, fluids, or gases. Depending on the application, these techniques can stretch, reshape, and separate fascia with a resultant effect on muscles, ligaments, organs, and other structures. Pressing and Pushing can override nerve impulses and dissipate energy at tissue lesions, otherwise known as *tender points, trigger points* (see Neuromuscular Therapy), or *tsubos* (see Chapter 4).

Squeezing and Pinching

Squeezing and *Pinching* are derivations of Pressing and Pushing using opposing forces. They are closely related techniques with subtle variations in application. In this case the differences are a matter of refinement. Squeezing is the compression of an object between two forces that close or tightly press together. This is accomplished using the fingers, palms, entire hands, fists, or elbows. This action compacts, occludes, or constricts the target area. Pinching, more specifically, is a hard squeeze between the ends of fingers and thumb, as in crushing or nipping. As with all compressive techniques, Squeezing and Pinching affect fluid and gas movement, override nerve impulses, release tissue lesions, assess tissue qualities, and affect tissue patterns. Because of a more pointed, specific contact, these techniques are well suited to stimulate the nervous system.

Twisting and Wringing

Twisting and *Wringing* add a turning movement to the Compression Component. Each technique features its own unique style. Twisting creates a revolving, winding, rotation wave in the body. This wave can produce shearing forces that stretch, separate, and distort layers of tissue (e.g., muscle, organ, fascia). It can also involve turning, coiling, pivoting, and spinning joints, segments, or entire body parts. It can be

---

BOX 3-6

BodyWays Using Compression Component Techniques

> Compression Component techniques can be incorporated into any therapeutic relationship and combined with any modality. However, there are BodyWays that feature these techniques as an integral part of their system. Some examples of these BodyWays are Trigger Point Release, Swedish Massage, MDMA, Acupressure, Shiatsu, Amma, Craniosacral Therapy, Sports Massage, Thai Massage, Applied Kinesiology, Structural Integration, NMT, Reflexology, Positional Release, Muscle Energy Technique, Feldenkrais, Hoshino, and Lymphatic Drainage, among others.

used specifically to release unconscious patterns and armoring as well as to challenge and release adhesions. Wringing, on the other hand, combines Twisting and Squeezing. Specifically, it compresses from two opposing sides while Twisting. This combination distorts, contorts, presses out, or milks an area of focus. In addition to the general intentions of compression, Twisting and Wringing offer challenges and options to usual daily movement patterns. Common patterns are primarily along the sagittal plane (flexion and extension). Twisting and Wringing add the dimension of rotation in the horizontal plane, which creates a shearing action. They even go beyond that to combine the horizontal plane with the coronal plane to produce spiraling. Box 3-6 lists BodyWays that feature Compression Component techniques.

Expansion Component

Expansion moves in the opposite direction from Compression and is the carrier wave of centrifugal force. Expansion techniques draw matter and energy away from the core of the body. Expansion and Compression are complementary and integral to one another. Tissues "expand" around the area of Compression, and it is typical to grasp tissue with Compression to accomplish Expansion. Although Compression and Expansion techniques are at the opposite ends of a continuum, their intentions and outcomes are similar. These components are an example of how totally different ways of handling the body elicit similar results and responses. They can initiate or assist flows and initiate, assist, or resist movement of body parts. They can also stretch, reshape, or separate fascia, muscles, tendons, ligaments, and other tissues. Furthermore, they can stimulate or override nerve impulses, dissipate trigger points, release contracted muscles, and influence neurologic and behavioral patterns. However, some distinctions do exist. Expansion techniques open up the spaces within and between structures. This creates greater mobility, relieves impingement, and makes room for unobstructed free flow of fluids, gases, energy, and information. The immediate effect of Expansion is to open and separate structure. Its secondary effect is a rebound or trampoline response of tissue bouncing back toward the body. The immediate effect of Compression, on the other hand, is the reduction of space between structures. Its secondary effect is the resultant rebound and expansion or opening of these compressed areas.

Pulling

Pulling creates space by separating, drawing apart, opening up, and lengthening structures and energies. This is accomplished by exerting a tugging force to change the state of the body. Structurally, this technique addresses the condition and connection of tissue layers. It can be used to stretch, separate, and elongate muscle fibers and enhance the elasticity of soft tissues. Pulling can separate layers of tissue (e.g., skin from muscle, muscle from muscle, muscle from bone, bone from bone). It can also be used to assess the status of soft tissue and its rebound response and to expand the layers of the energetic field.

Lifting

Lifting elevates or raises something from a lower to a higher place. Lifting to reposition a body part can create comfort for the client. It can provide a therapist easier access to a client's body. Elevation can also be used to modify circulatory flow.

Rolling

This is another intricate and multidimensional technique. Mechanically, *Rolling* is a combination of Lift-

ing and Squeezing while Pushing or Pulling. It is applied to the skin, tissues, and segments of the body to expand movement and space between layers of tissue and increase flexibility at joints. Rolling means to undulate, turn over, and move in a circular or wavelike pattern. This technique is used to mobilize tissue (separate, disorient, and reeducate) and to soften and mold, thereby expanding resting options for fascia. Skin and Tissue Rolling create heat and encourage circulation and oxygenation of mobilized tissues. Box 3-7 lists BodyWays that feature Expansion Component techniques.

KINETIC COMPONENT

Kinetics is "a branch of dynamics that deals with the effects of forces upon the motions of material bodies."[12] As applied here, kinetics is an umbrella term for a collection of techniques that focus on the movement relationship between segments of the body. *Intention* determines outcome because these techniques are used to access information, address conditions, and assess treatment progress and effect. In the subtle realm, this component reveals body receptivity to touch and support. Moving on a continuum from stillness to the edge of a client's ROM, whether active, passive, resistive, or assistive, the practitioner can assess the state of a joint and its surrounding tissues. The following questions are helpful in making such an assessment. Is there acceptance of the practitioner's presence and holding? Is there fluid mobility of the parts consistent with their action potential? Does the articulation feel dry or gritty and in need of hydration? Are there holding patterns, habitual or otherwise, originating in the physical, mental, or emotional fields? Is the ROM less

BOX 3-7

BodyWays Using Expansion Component Techniques

Expansion Component techniques can be incorporated into any therapeutic relationship and combined with any modality. However, there are Body-Ways that feature these techniques as an integral part of their system, including Swedish Massage, MDMA, Trager, Sports Massage, Body Logic, Myofascial Release, Active Isolated Stretching, Thai Massage, Phoenix Rising, and Yoga.

than optimal? Are there bony or soft tissue limitations to the movement?

The therapist may observe a healthy structure and choose to play with its capacity or move on to another area of focus. With less than optimal conditions the therapist may choose to apply the same kinetic techniques used for assessment to provide a therapeutic influence or test responsiveness to the work. Ease and flexibility of movement are the ultimate goals, and can be reached through the techniques known as *Holding, Supporting, Mobilizing, Letting go, Dropping*, and *Stabilizing*.

Holding and Supporting

Holding is the act of grasping, cradling, or holding on to, whereas *Supporting* actually bears the weight of or suspends a body segment. Holding is gripping, handling, clasping, embracing, and sustaining, whereas Supporting involves propping, bolstering, carrying, or holding up. These two related techniques are used to sense the state of the person and his or her structure, to connect, to nurture, and to assess the client's response to touch. Holding and Supporting can create stillness and establish trust. They can also take over the job of muscles in maintaining a body position or posture. This is a vehicle for both therapist and client to experience proprioceptive awareness. The practitioner can lift and take the weight of a part, and identify client patterns of allowing and surrendering. These techniques can promote heat transfer and, through stimulation, sedation, or reprogramming, influence the nervous system. They can be used to contact specific points in the body, making connections between them and beyond, to integrate with universal energy. Both Holding and Supporting soothe the spirit and encourage release of mental, emotional, and physical tensions.

Mobilizing

Mobilizing plays with the movement potential of the body. This ranges from the subtlest, quietest signs of ease or bind between the bony structures to the largest movement currently available at a joint or joints. Mobilizing is a way to assess and treat articulations and the surrounding tissues. This encompasses all manner of movement in any direction, through all planes and elevations, for example, raising, lowering, rotating, rolling, manipulating, dislodging, and moving side-to-side. This active technique can be used as a tool to sense and identify resistance or restriction in movement patterns. It can also be used to reveal limitations and remind the body of its movement potential. Resisting movement at a joint can be used to assess and build strength and develop surrounding tissues. Separating bones at articulations lengthens the muscles, tendons, and ligaments that surround or attach to those bones. Opening, closing, and otherwise manipulating articulations creates a pumping action that stimulates the natural hydration of the joint capsule. This promotes venous, lymphatic, and synovial circulation. To best use mobilization, the therapist must have a good working knowledge of the structure and function of the skeletal/articular and muscular systems. He or she must also have developed the kinesthetic or palpatory sense to recognize, identify, and respond to his or her perceptions. A competent practitioner knows the optimal ROM appropriate for each articular relationship, the types of tissues that interface in the joint space, and the ligamentous structures that bind the skeletal segments together. The basic mobilization techniques are categorized as active, passive, resistive, and assistive. In *active mobilization* clients move on their own. In *passive mobilization* the therapist moves the client—the client makes no effort. In *resistive mobilization* the therapist offers resistance to the efforts of the client. *Assistive mobilization* involves movement by the client with the help of the therapist.

Letting Go and Dropping

Appropriate reactions, the crucial result of clear sensations, accurate perception and the functional organization of accumulated experience, hinge upon three prerequisites within each organism:
(1) Free anatomical ranges of motion, unrestricted by habituated limitations or unnecessary defensive inhibitions;
(2) The ability to preserve and repeat movements and sequences that have proved in the past to be effective under recognizable conditions; and
(3) The additional—and quite separate—ability to react with open-ended, creative flexibility to all sorts of novelties, both enhancing and destructive.[4]

DEAN JUHAN

BOX 3-8

BodyWays Using Kinetic Component Techniques

Kinetic Component techniques can be incorporated into any therapeutic relationship and combined with any modality. However, there are Body-Ways that feature these techniques as an integral part of their system. Some examples of these BodyWays are Supportive Touch, Swedish Massage, MDMA, Thai Massage, Positional Release, Sports Massage, Proprioceptive Neuromuscular Facilitation (PNF), Tai Chi, Chi Kung, Yoga, Feldenkrais, Alexander Technique, Trager, Craniosacral Therapy, Active Isolated Stretching, Pilates, and Connective Tissue Unwinding, among others.

Letting go is releasing a hold or loosening a grip, that is, disengaging, yielding, or unhanding a body segment. By letting go, a practitioner breaks physical and energetic contact, allowing for repositioning and movement to a different location on the body. The act of relinquishing and unclasping might signal the completion of an application. It also permits the flow, expansion, and rebound that are secondary effects of a compression application. *Dropping* allows or causes a structure to fall. It implies that a structure is elevated and the therapist withdraws support, causing it to drop. This is valuable for discovering and challenging holding patterns and for inducing "surrender." Dropping can free articulations and affect proprioception through space-time disorientation.

Stabilizing

Stabilizing grounds energy and limits motion. It steadies an articulation. It is used to secure, fix, or anchor a joint, creating a fulcrum for motion or leverage. For instance, immobilizing or limiting the movement of one segment or muscle optimizes movement in other areas. Any point or segment of the body can be held motionless to control or direct mobility in related tissue. Stabilizing is core to the use of isometric resistance and specific proprioceptive neuromuscular facilitation (PNF) techniques that release tension or increase muscle length. Stabilizing can also be used in resistive and resistive assistive mobilizations to con-

dition, rehabilitate, and strengthen. Box 3-8 lists BodyWays that feature Kinetic Component techniques.

OSCILLATION COMPONENT

Everything vibrates and is connected and related to everything else. All matter exists as an expression of, and is distinguished by, its unique oscillation pattern, its vibratory "signature." A healthy body is in vibrational harmony. Each aspect of the body, material as well as energetic, has its own optimal frequency. *Oscillation* techniques link us with the vibratory waves that animate the body and all its systems. Some wave patterns produce stress and various disharmonious conditions. Other wave patterns support homeostasis, the return to balance and harmony. Frequencies, from an internal or external source, can shift the vibrations of an organism—they can exaggerate, minimize, or otherwise alter them. These new rhythms affect digestion, respiration, circulation, thoughts, and emotions. It is possible to introduce waves or use existing waves to break up rigidity—to loosen, open, soften, and align. Oscillations initiate reverberation, ripple, and rebound responses. As if "surfing," both the client and practitioner "ride the waves" of tissues and energetic fields. These waves run through the body, from head to toe, in all directions: horizontally, vertically, and circumferentially. A therapist extends sensors and feelers to slip into these waves, noticing their paths and patterns. Sensations of rhythm, flow, and swing typify this exploration of motion. What is moving? What is not moving? It is all about momentum, flow, and consistency of rhythm. What feels dull and solid? What feels soft and receptive? Ideally and optimally, waves move freely through structure. *Vibrating, Shaking,* and *Striking* are the techniques of this component. They are different in form and delivery, but they each have a similar influence on the body—they generate waves. What distinguishes one from another is that each creates a different kind of wave. The energy trajectories of Vibrating and Shaking run along a path parallel to the body surface, whereas the energy trajectory of Striking runs perpendicular to the body surface.

Striking is a staccato technique characterized by intermittent and broken contact. In contrast, Vibrating and Shaking maintain continuous contact. Vibrating is the more subtle form of the two. It is a refined and focused movement with laserlike affect that penetrates deep into the tissues. Shaking, on the other hand, is a larger movement with a broader, more superficial effect.

Vibrating

Vibrating is the application of fine, tremulous, rhythmic motions to the body. This oscillating technique can be modified by the various qualities of touch, such as speed, rhythm, duration, and intensity. Vibrations pulsate, throb, and tremble their way through the body. As true balancing influences, they may stimulate or sedate. This technique appeals to the body's ability to self-regulate, using any and all waves and pulses to establish and maintain homeostasis.

When an organ or another part of the body is in a state of health, it will be creating a natural resonant frequency that is harmonious with the rest of the body. However, when disease sets in, a different . . . pattern is established in that part of the body which is not vibrating in harmony. Therefore, it is possible, through use of externally created [oscillations] . . . projected in the diseased area, to reintroduce the correct harmonic pattern into that part of the body which is afflicted and effect a curative reaction. Through the principle of resonance . . . [oscillation] can be used to change disharmonious frequencies of the body back to their normal, healthful vibration.[3]

JONATHAN GOLDMAN

Shaking

Shaking is a gross expression of Vibrating. Jiggle, rock, sway, flutter, jostle, bounce, and waggle are subtle variations of Shaking. Shaking means moving something side to side or to and fro or swinging it back and forth with varying speed and intensity. Once again, the overall intention is to engage and harmonize the body. With Shaking, the practitioner can loosen, soften, open, and release holding patterns, congestion, emotions, and more. This technique introduces rhythms that can reveal and reorganize inherent patterns. It can disorient and reorient the proprioceptive awareness of tissues and body parts. It can move energy along channels and tubes.

BOX 3-9

BodyWays Using Oscillation Component Techniques

Oscillation Component techniques add another dimension to the conversation regarding "attunement" of the body. They can be incorporated into any therapeutic relationship and combined with any modality. However, there are BodyWays that feature these techniques as an integral part of their system. Some examples are Trager, Swedish Massage, Craniosacral Therapy, Sound Therapy, MDMA, Water Therapy, Do-In and the use of "tuning forks," and light pulsations and electrical frequency machines (e.g., vibrators, Vega, transcutaneous electrical nerve stimulation [TENS]).

Striking

Striking creates wave patterns via repetitive broken contact. Brisk blows, ranging from gentle to strong, send waves radiating from the point of connection. Striking is like drumming, which creates rhythms and waves that run like signals throughout the body, communicating, entraining, balancing, and aligning. Striking is applied with a loose hand that adds control and rhythm to the delivery. The nuances of the Striking technique are graphically expressed by such actions as hitting, percussing, slapping, thumping, rapping, pounding, beating, tapping, hacking, and flicking. Striking is used to, among other things, stimulate the nervous system, decongest the lungs, loosen attachments, and create specific rhythms.

Collective Intentions of Vibrating, Shaking, and Striking

Vibrating, Shaking, and Striking, by their effect, have shared intentions. Individually and collectively they create radiating waves to support a wide variety of goals. These waves become signals and patterns of information for every system and every aspect of the body.

Each technique moves energy. This softens tissues and loosens attachments. Each initiates rhythms and waves. This activates, sedates, or reprograms the nervous system, which then communicates back to the body to release physical and emotional holding patterns. As they undulate through the body, waves affect physiology and anatomy. The therapist can shake organs, vibrate muscle spindles, activate proprioceptors, and beat out rhythms for support or change. Vibrating, Shaking, or Striking can stimulate or sedate organs, reveal existing patterns, create movement, and open joints. Box 3-9 lists BodyWays that feature Oscillation Component techniques.

GLIDING COMPONENT

Gliding techniques are an interesting mix. As the name implies, they slide. The fingers, hands, arms, elbows, and feet are used to sense and follow the contours of skin, muscle, tendon, ligament, and bone. The quality of liquidity in this technique allows a practitioner to ride the waves of the body and experience and transmit a sense of flowing movement. Gliding can be used to sculpt, mold, and trace. It can also be used to direct, guide, and explore. Whatever the intention, it is truly about the engagement of bodies in a fluid dance. Gliding is expressed along convergent continuums of opposites, for example, superficial and deep, soft and hard, short and long, fast and slow, rhythmic and erratic, and vertical and horizontal. Gliding along the skin surface, a practitioner can spread a lubricant, gather information about the general quality of tissue, and identify palpable irregularities. Gliding is a tool for locating and distinguishing one type of tissue from another and detecting temperature, texture, tension, density, resistance, and shape. It can also be used to affect attitudes and emotions or to stimulate or sedate the nervous system. To affect below skin level, a practitioner engages the fascia of descending strata of tissues and glides the more superficial layers over the deeper layers. Gradually increasing pressure progressively deepens contact. These techniques can separate adhesions between and within body layers and release tension patterns to support freedom of movement. Gliding at these levels addresses the subcutaneous fascia, intramuscular or intermuscular fascia, blood and lymph vessels, tendons, and ligaments, all the way down to the periosteum of bone. In addition to soft tissue influences, gliding powerfully affects the subtle dimensions of the body. It is a specific type of exploration that gives insight into the strength of (and allows bodyworkers to influence vital elements of) chi, thermal variation, wave pattern, and biomagnetic attraction–repulsion.

Stroking

Stroking delivers the energy of fluidity. The act of Stroking is a continuous slide across a surface without pause. It looks like skating, sculpting, smoothing, soothing, skimming, whisking, or swirling. It can be applied superficially or more deeply into the subcutaneous layers of functional and structural tissue. Deeper stroking elongates fibers and moves fluids and gases. It stimulates, sedates, defines, separates, stretches, releases, explores, connects, propels, and nurtures. Stroking can be used to shape, caress, and define body parts and contours. It is a flowing, continuous technique, which travels at varying depths and speeds along the edges of bone. It slides into crevices and fleshy spaces following the directions of muscle fibers. Stroking is a powerful tool for assessing texture, temperature, elasticity, skin quality, and receptivity to touch. It is a primary vehicle to express nurture and support palliative care. Stroking over bare skin can be enhanced with the use of lubricants. Strokes can be applied off the surface of the physical body to influence the energetic field.

Rubbing

Rubbing weaves itself through many healing traditions as the "fire-maker." It carries the energy of fire. To rub is to move back and forth across a structure with pressure. This produces different effects depending on depth, angle, direction, speed, rhythm, and location. Rubbing is a friction-producing move that ranges from spread, polish, and shine to buff, scour, or burnish. Whether gentle or forceful, rubbing generates warmth and heat. Superficial rubbing can be expressed as a chafing or scuffing action, much as in scratching an itch. It could be a scraping or scrubbing movement to exfoliate the skin or stimulate activity in the sebaceous or sudoriferous glands. On deeper levels, rubbing warms and softens fascial layers and muscle fibers to allow for elongation, separation, and greater flexibility. The friction produced by rubbing can soften, reduce, or release an adhesion, trigger point, or tsubo. It can also affect shifts in tension patterns. Box 3-10 lists BodyWays that feature Gliding Component techniques.

BOX 3-10

BodyWays Using Gliding Component Techniques

> Gliding Component techniques can be incorporated into any therapeutic relationship and combined with any modality. However, there are Body-Ways that feature these techniques as an integral part of their system. Some examples of these Body-Ways are Swedish Massage, Lymphatic Massage, Lomi Lomi, Cyriax, Chua Ka, Myofascial Release, MDMA, Rolfing, NMT, Sports Massage, and Body Rolling.

[Our] perspective values self-responsibility, authentic self-exploration, self-expression and the healing relationship . . . this means the individual person plays an active, responsible role in his or her healing and preventive healthcare. . . . Practitioners . . . will be a valuable resource to individuals who are actively engaged in composing their lives, defining their personal visions of health, and learning from and responding to life's adversities.[1]

ELLIOT DACHER

There is a natural progression in manual therapy from the gross to the subtle, from the fascial matrix to the energy matrix, from working on someone to working with someone, from overcoming resistance to establishing trust. As one learns to listen . . . a whole new world of subtle rhythms and forces is revealed.[7]

TOM MCDONOUGH

TRAINING AND CERTIFICATION

Although basic education in massage therapy in the United States is available in every state, the length, depth, quality, and focus vary greatly. For the most part, professional training requires from 500 to 1000 hours and includes studies in anatomy, physiology, pathology, basic massage techniques, and hygienic practice. In addition, some schools provide classes in hydrotherapy, business development, personal growth, and introductions to specific modalities. Many schools have some form of clinic where

BOX 3-11

TouchAbilities™ User Guidelines

> Remember to use this information nonlinearly.
> Everything is connected.
> Everything connects.
> Be sure to mix and match.
> Create, deconstruct, and recreate your own relationship to the concepts presented in this chapter.

students work with the general public to practice their developing skills. The foundational skills as taught in most schools today are based in Swedish style techniques because that form of massage is the most widely recognized by both recipients and employers. During the last 25 to 30 years, the United States has experienced an infusion of many styles of bodywork from other parts of the world, particularly from the East and Europe. Many innovative practitioners have created new approaches or variations on old approaches that have become known modalities. Today, there are many entry-level schools that present a modality other than Swedish as their base curriculum, such as Shiatsu, Pfrimmer, NMT, and Polarity. In these schools the bodywork philosophy is geared to a particular modality, and specific techniques are stressed more than, or to the exclusion of, others in support of the school's focus. Minimum education requirements vary from state to state. In the United States they range from the 250 hours required in Texas to the 1000 hours required in Nebraska and New York. The most common state requirement is 500 hours.

Licensure

As of this printing, 29 states and the District of Columbia currently offer some type of credential to professionals in massage and bodywork—usually licensure, certification, or registration. Most of the 29 regulating states require a written examination. Six states require a practical examination in addition to a written examination. Tennessee, Maine, and West Virginia require only schooling or apprenticeship. Of the states that require a test, 23 require or accept the National Certification Exam from the Na-

Glossary

Body A multidimensional field extending beyond the physical plane. This *field* incorporates the physical, mental, emotional, and spiritual essence, integrating anatomy, physiology, and energy; a living form that is defined and animated by its amorphous, ever-changing energetic nature and the vibrating, pulsating, dynamic mechanisms of its physicality.

BodyViews General approaches through which to "see" a body:
- Energetic View
- Functional View
- Movement View
- Structural View
- Convergent View

BodyWays The selection and organization of techniques, based on a particular viewpoint or organizing principle, applied to a body to effect an outcome. BodyWays include a variety of philosophic approaches, theoretic frameworks, and specific combinations of techniques. These systems are known as *modalities* within the bodywork profession.

Bodywork As a *profession*, Bodywork is characterized by the collection of systems (modalities) designed to interact with the body in support of balance and good health; as an *action*, it is the skillful, intentional application of the techniques of any of the modalities within the profession.

Carrier wave A wave or current whose modulations are used to carry signals through and between bodies.

Contraindication A symptom or particular circumstance that leads a therapist to cautiously apply or refrain from applying a therapeutic procedure. Metaphorically, a contraindication translates to a "yellow light" for caution and a "red light" for avoidance.

Domain A distinctly defined sphere of knowledge or activity; one's peculiar and exclusive function or field of active cultivation and responsibility.

Field A realm of forces in dynamic interplay; a coherent realm with identifiable qualities and specific characteristics.

Field of engagement An interpersonal field established between beings; a place of interfacing edges; the point of connection between individuals where the composite elements of their bodies interact.

Holarchy An order of increasing holons—of increasing wholeness and integrative capacity. A principle popularized in the cosmology of holistic philosopher Ken Wilber, meaning, "Everything is simultaneously a part of something larger than itself (a higher whole), and a whole in its own right is made up of its own smaller parts. Everything is a holon, in the sense that it is a whole in one context and a part in another."

Homeostasis The balance within the internal environment of the body (microcosm); and the dynamic relationship between the body and the universal environment (macrocosm).

Indication A symptom, signal, or particular circumstance that supports the necessity for a therapeutic procedure; metaphorically, indications are "green lights" to apply techniques in response to what a client presents.

Kinetics A branch of dynamics that deals with the effects of forces upon the motions of material bodies[12]; an umbrella term for a collection of techniques that focus on the movement relationship between segments of the body.

Mobility The capacity for and facility of movement.

Modality A BodyWays system comprising a selection and organization of touch techniques, based on a particular viewpoint or organizing principle and used to effect an intended outcome.

Motility The vital wave of life that animates tissue; the power to move spontaneously.

Multidimensional Relating to or marked by several dimensions. A dimension is a unit comprising qualities, aspects, and variables.

Proprioception The awareness of posture, movement, and changes in equilibrium and the knowledge of position, weight, and resistance of objects in relation to one's own body.[12]

Proprioceptive Neuromuscular Facilitation (PNF) Specific techniques that activate the body's own "receptors" to shift muscle tone, promote relaxation, and support lengthening.

Qualities of touch The tangible and intangible influences that create the distinctions, intentions, and character of a particular technique, for example, speed, duration, location, direction, rhythm, angle, depth, pressure, drag, intention, and scope of focus.

Glossary—cont'd

Rhythm Harmonious or orderly movement, fluctuation, or variation, with recurrences of action or situation at fairly regular intervals; a regularly recurrent quantitative change in a variable, biologic process.

State The status, mode, or condition of being; a condition or stage in the physical constitution of something.

Technique A method, procedure, process, way, or manner used to accomplish a desired aim.

TouchAbilities™ The fundamental methods of interacting with and acting on and between bodies. These methods are foundational or seminal to the development of Modalities.

Wave A rolling or undulating movement, or one of a series of such movements, passing along the surface of or through matter or air. ◞

tional Certification Board for Therapeutic Massage and Bodywork. Others states design and administer their own tests. Although some states are in the process of developing or passing legislation to regulate the practice of massage and bodywork, New Jersey has passed laws that are not yet in effect. Twenty states remain unregulated.

References

1. Dacher E: Healing values: what matters in health care, *Noetic Sci Rev* 42:10, 1997.
2. Ford C: *Where healing waters meet: touching the mind and emotion through the body,* New York, 1992, Talman.
3. Goldman J: *Healing sounds: the power of harmonics,* London, 1996, HarperCollins.
4. Juhan D: Somatic explorations, *Massage Mag* 54:62, 1995.
5. Knaster M: *Discovering the body's wisdom,* New York, 1996, Bantam Books.
6. Lauterstein D: The mind in bodywork, *Massage Ther J* 37(3):108, 1998.
7. McDonough T: *Massage Mag* 73:93, 1998.
8. Meyers T: A language revolution, *Massage Mag* 85:20, 2000.
9. Milne H: *Heart of listening: a visionary approach to craniosacral work: anatomy, technique, transcendence,* Berkeley, Calif, 1998, North Atlantic Books.
10. Oschman J: *Energy medicine: the scientific basis of bioenergy therapies,* Kent, England, 2000, Churchill Livingstone.
11. Smith, FF: *Inner bridges: a guide to energy movement and body structure,* Atlanta, 1986, Humanics Publishing Group.
12. *Webster's Third new international dictionary,* Springfield, Mass, 1986, Merriam-Webster, Inc.

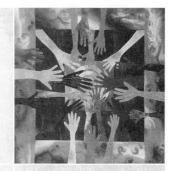

Modern Neuromuscular Techniques*

L E O N   C H A I T O W

J U D I T H   D E L A N Y

THE ROOTS OF MODERN NEUROMUSCULAR TECHNIQUES

During the last half-century, neuromuscular therapy (NMT) techniques have emerged almost simultaneously in Europe and North America. The two versions have unifying similarities in theoretic foundations and subtle differences in their hands-on applications. On both continents, NMT has bridged multiple professions and has been integrated into a variety of settings, including massage therapy, chiropractic, os-

teopathy, sports medicine, occupational therapy, physical therapy, nursing, health spas, professional sports, and conventional medicine. NMT is a therapeutic intervention to treat injury and repetitive trauma, and for postsurgical rehabilitation. It is also a preventive procedure for assessing and removing the potential sources of myofascial dysfunction.

European-style NMT first appeared between the mid-1930s and early 1940s through the work of Stanley Lief and Boris Chaitow, cousins trained in chiropractic and naturopathy. While practicing in Lief's world-famous health resort Champneys at Tring in Hertfordshire, England, they developed and refined a means of assessing and treating soft-tissue dysfunction, which they called *neuromuscular technique*. The European neuromuscular techniques have since evolved

---

*Modified from Chaitow L, DeLany J: *Clinical application of neuromuscular techniques,* vol 1, Chapter 9, Edinburgh, 2000, Churchill Livingstone.

through many osteopaths and naturopaths, including Peter Lief, Brian Youngs, Terry Moule, Leon Chaitow, and others. European NMT is now taught widely in Britain in sports massage and osteopathic settings, and is an elective module on the Bachelor of Science (BSc[Hons]) degree courses in Complementary Health Sciences, University of Westminster, London.

Just a few years after neuromuscular techniques developed in Europe, a step-by-step system began to emerge in America through the writings of Raymond Nimmo, DC, and James Vannerson, DC. In their newsletter, *Receptor Tonus Techniques,* Nimmo and Vannerson wrote of their experiences with what they termed *noxious nodules.* They called their modality *Receptor Tonus Technique,* although it is often referred to as the *Nimmo method.* Their struggle to support their theoretic platform was eased by the research and writings of Janet Travell, MD, who was later joined by David Simons, MD. Travell and Simons' work with myofascial trigger points (TrPs), rich in documentation, research, and references, provided a new field of study, and trigger points became a central focus of European and American neuromuscular techniques.

While Nimmo continued to research, write, and train practitioners to treat the noxious points, which had come to be known as *TrPs,* his students began teaching their own treatment protocols. NMT St. John Method and its offspring, NMT American Version™, became two prominent systems that still retain a strong focus on Nimmo's original techniques. Nimmo's method also survived and is used in many chiropractic offices today. Although the European and American methods of NMT have similar philosophies of health care and pain reduction, application of their hands-on techniques are somewhat different.

A comprehensive text has recently been published,[15] which offers step-by-step protocols of the application of both versions of NMT and their associated modalities, such as muscle energy techniques, positional release, and myofascial release. Although this text serves to bring the two major methods of NMT closer together, it also supports the distinctiveness of each.

WHAT IS NEUROMUSCULAR THERAPY?

In North America, the acronym NMT signifies *neuromuscular therapy* rather than the European *neuromuscular technique.* The North American style differs slightly from the slow-paced, thumb-drag method of the European style because it uses a medium-paced thumb- or finger-glide and a slightly different emphasis in the manner of applying ischemic compression to treat TrPs. To encourage lifestyle changes and the elimination of predisposing and precipitating factors that may contribute to the client's condition, both versions emphasize a home self-care program and the client's participation in the recovery process. They also have similar philosophies regarding hydrotherapies, movement, self-help therapies, awareness of postural habits, nutritional choices, work and recreational practices, and stress factors. In this chapter, the similarities between the two methods are presented as part of the philosophic discussion, and the contrast of hands-on application is presented with the discussion of techniques.

NMT attempts to assess and address a number of factors that are commonly involved in causing or intensifying pain,[14] influencing the perception of pain and its spread throughout the body, and maintaining dysfunctional conditions. These and other factors can be broadly clustered under the headings of biomechanical, biochemical, and psychosocial. Most major influences on health are found within these three categories, certain components of which are of particular concern in NMT. Factors that affect locally dysfunctional states, such as hypertonia, ischemia, inflammation, TrPs, and neural compression or entrapment are more obvious to manual practitioners. Those that affect the whole body, such as stress (physical or psychologic), posture (including patterns of use), nutritional imbalances and deficiencies, toxicity (exogenous and endogenous), and endocrine imbalances are easily overlooked unless the practitioner is trained to assess and deal with them.

The practitioner and client together may address as many influences on musculoskeletal pain as can be identified, as long as they avoid placing excessive demands on the individual's adaptive capacity. In other words, for the most comprehensive recovery to be achieved, it is necessary to remove or modify as many causal and perpetuating influences as possible.[38] However, because local and general adaptation is almost inevitably a result of each therapeutic intervention, a delicate balance in the application of techniques and principles must be maintained to produce beneficial change without overwhelming the body's adaptive mechanisms. Otherwise, results may be unsatisfactory,[16] confusing, or frustrating for both client and practitioner.

Biomechanical factors include myofascial TrPs, which are hyperirritable nodules found in taut bands of myofascial tissue. TrPs form in muscle bellies (central TrPs [CTrPs]) or in tendinous or periosteal attachments (attachment TrPs [ATrPs]). TrPs may also occur in skin, fascia, ligaments, periosteum, joint surfaces, and occasionally in visceral organs,[38] although none of these are considered *myofascial* TrPs. TrPs are painful when compressed and give rise to referred pain (and other sensations), motor disturbances, and autonomic responses in other body tissues.[38] The location of TrPs are fairly predictable, as are their target zones of referral patterns.

An integrated TrP hypothesis has been presented by Simons and colleagues[38] in an attempt to explain the mechanisms by which TrPs form. Their hypothesis postulates that CTrPs are associated with motor endplate dysfunction in myofascial tissues, resulting in excessive acetylcholine release, and that CTrPs are predictably located at the center of a muscle fiber. ATrPs are thought to result from an inflammatory process created by tension in the taut band created by CTrPs.

The NMT practitioner uses a variety of assessment techniques to identify taut bands and TrP sites and then applies compression techniques (also called *TrP pressure release*) to CTrPs. ATrPs often improve without specific treatment once the CTrPs are deactivated. Unless ATrPs show signs of inflammation, the taut fibers housing CTrPs are then lengthened by range of motion stretching of the fibers. When attachment conditions contraindicate full fiber stretching, specific myofascial release of the fiber's belly and applications of ice to the tendons may be used.

Pressure may be imposed on neural structures by vertebral, osseous or intervertebral disc elements (compression or impingement) or by muscle, tendon, ligament, fascia, and skin (entrapment). Although the underlying cause of entrapment and compression may come from overuse, abuse, misuse, or trauma, these mechanical interfaces, which interfere with normal neural transmission, may produce similar symptoms.[8] The skilled practitioner considers the entire neural pathway and assesses (or refers for assessment) when any impingement condition is suspected. Manual methods often may be used to modify or correct them and should be considered before surgical intervention.

Postural and use factors have a substantial influence on the neuromusculoskeletal components. Although many practitioners examine static posture for "correct" alignment, experts, including Feldenkrais[18] and Hanna,[21] point out that a degree of asymmetry is normal. However, clients with a small degree of imbalance should display normal functional accommodation, range of motion, and use, taking into consideration the factors of age, genetics, and body type.

Many clinicians, including Janda[24] and Lewit,[29] have noted which regions of the body most commonly adapt in compensating patterns of dysfunction. When practitioners attempt to change local restrictions in myofascial tissues, it is imperative that they consider the body as a whole and look beyond the specific area for postural compensations.

In addition, an individualized home care program is often designed to help promote a client's awareness of poor habits of use and posture and to improve those habits through appropriate stretching, retraining, and frequent breaks from long term strain. Sitting, standing, and sleeping positions are considered, as are repetitive use of involved tissues and patterns of breathing (e.g., hyperventilation tendencies, paradoxical breathing).

Biochemical factors are factors that influence local and body-wide chemistry. They include localized ischemia, dehydration, nutrition, endocrine function (or dysfunction), chemical exposure, medication, inflammatory processes, and carbon dioxide levels (pH). Manual practitioners may note that, because of limitations imposed by their scope of practice (license) or prior training, some of these factors necessitate a referral network for assessment and treatment.

Ischemia, commonly caused by muscle spasm or contracture, reduces blood flow, thus reducing delivery of oxygen and nutrients, resulting in an accumulation of metabolic waste products. As these neurologic irritants accumulate in tissue, they increase neurologic excitability,[9] which can become self-perpetuating.

The decrease of blood flow associated with ischemia results in a local energy crisis in the myofascial tissue because adenosine triphosphate (ATP) supplies drop while the tissue's energy needs rise. An integrated hypothesis presented by Simons and colleagues[38] attributes the formation of TrPs to this ATP deprivation because the actin and myosin elements are "locked" in a shortened position when the energy supply is depleted.[6]

Nutritional factors include ingestion, digestion, absorption, and assimilation of nutrients necessary for cellular metabolism, repair, and normal reproduction of cells and tissues. Proper nutrition, which is especially important for chronic pain clients, also requires avoidance of toxic agents such as harmful chemicals, caffeine, and smoke, among others, which stimulate or irritate the nervous system or create general body toxicity. Vitamin and mineral levels, hydration, breathing habits, and obvious or hidden allergies or food intolerance, which may increase nociception and lymphatic congestion,[36] should each be assessed and appropriate corrections encouraged. Nutritional imbalances may perpetuate ischemia, TrPs, postural distortions, and neuroexcitation,[15,38] and therefore may be a critical factor in pain management. Endocrine function (most particularly thyroid function in the case of myofascial pain) and local and general inflammatory processes should be assessed. In addition, the balance between oxygen and carbon dioxide, which is intimately connected to breathing patterns and has psychosocial overlays, is of critical importance.[19,30,31]

Psychosocial factors, emotional well being, and stress management influence the musculoskeletal system.[15,28] Alleviating the stress burden is ideal; however, the role of the practitioner often involves teaching and encouraging the client to handle his or her psychologic load more efficiently, or referring the client elsewhere when scope of practice and insufficient training indicate. The degree to which a client can be helped with emotional stress relates directly to how efficiently he or she is able to adapt and how much of the load can actually be removed, which depends in part on whether it is self-generated (endogenous) or externally derived (exogenous).

Because biomechanical, biochemical, and psychosocial factors are synergistic, they do not produce a single, isolated change, but multiple changes. The following list provides some examples:

- Hyperventilation creates feelings of anxiety and apprehension, modifies blood acidity, influences neural reporting (initially hyperventilation and then hypoventilation), and directly affects muscles and joints of the thoracic and cervical regions.[20]
- Hypoglycemia, acidosis, and other factors that alter chemistry affect mood directly, and altered mood (e.g., depression, anxiety) changes blood chemistry and alters muscle tone, thus (by implication) affecting TrP evolution.[7]
- Altered structure modifies function (e.g., posture alters breathing) and therefore affects chemistry (e.g., O_2-CO_2 balance; circulatory efficiency and delivery of nutrients), which affects mood.[20]

NMT assesses the person's condition for each of the above factors and offers therapeutic intervention (when appropriate) or referral to appropriate health care professionals. Because the body must adapt to any changes, intervention management is applied at appropriate levels so as not to overwhelm the body's adaptive mechanisms.

PRACTICING NEUROMUSCULAR THERAPY

Therapeutically, NMT encourages the restoration of normal function by modifying dysfunctional tissue. One focus of treatment is to deactivate focal points of reflexogenic activity, such as myofascial TrPs. NMT also strives to normalize imbalances in hypertonic or fibrotic tissues, either as an end in itself or as a precursor to joint mobilization.

When the European and American methods of NMT are compared, similarities and differences between the two methods become apparent. Although the differences lie mainly in palpation methods (discussed in the following), the similarities are foundational and philosophically encompassing. Both methods seek to normalize tissues, uncover the precipitating and perpetuating factors, and teach skills to the client to prevent recurrence. The incorporation of other modalities such as hydrotherapy and stretching are also common to both versions. In general, the following goals are common to both the European and the American styles of NMT[15]:

- Offer reflex benefits
- Deactivate myofascial TrPs
- Prepare for other therapeutic methods, such as stretching, exercise, or manipulation
- Relax and normalize tense fibrotic muscular tissue
- Enhance lymphatic drainage and general circulation
- Provide diagnostic information to the practitioner
- Teach the client to recognize behaviors and patterns of use that stress the tissues
- When possible, offer the client alternative functional patterns and choices to reduce perpetuating factors

Indications and Contraindications for Use of Neuromuscular Therapy

NMT techniques are valuable for the management of most chronic pain syndromes and for posttrauma recovery and rehabilitation. NMT can also be applied to an apparently healthy body to help prevent injury by removing structural stresses before they become painful, long-lasting dysfunctions.

NMT is contraindicated in the initial stages of acute injury. Care must be given to protect the tissues during the first 72 hours following an injury. During the acute phase, the body often produces swelling, which applies a natural "splint" to the injured area,[9] thus reducing hemorrhaging in torn tissues and preventing movement that might further traumatize the fibers. During this initial 72 hours following injury, rest, ice, compression, and elevation (RICE) are appropriate treatments. NMT techniques, which increase blood flow and allow increased mobility, should not be used on recently injured tissues while they initiate the first phase of repair. However, NMT may be applied to parts of the body that may compensate for the injured area. The client may also benefit from referral for qualified medical, osteopathic, or chiropractic care. Other techniques, such as lymphatic drainage and certain movement therapies that are appropriate for acute injuries, may be indicated.

Once the acute inflammatory stage is past and reorganization of the tissues has started, the subacute phase begins (Figure 4-1). Pain that remains at least 3 months after the injury or tissue insult is considered to be chronic[39]; subacute pain occurs between the acute and chronic stages. NMT may be carefully applied to injured tissues in the subacute phase once the initial 72 hours have passed. Supporting structures and muscles involved in compensating patterns should be assessed periodically and therapy started or continued as needed.

Whether the tissues are in the acute, subacute, or chronic stage of recovery, consultation with the attending physician is suggested if range of motion intervention is questionable (e.g., for a moderate or severe whiplash). Such consultation may help avoid further compromise to the damaged structures (e.g., cervical discs, ligaments, vertebrae). If symptoms of disc injury are present, diagnosis of current status of disc health is suggested regardless of the length of time since the injury, because deterioration may have progressed since the last assessment.

Once the traumatized tissues are no longer inflamed or particularly painful, the initial elements of treatment, which aim to reduce spasm and ischemia, encourage drainage, and cautiously elongate, tone, and strengthen tissues, can usually be safely introduced. Although these treatment elements may be introduced at the first treatment session, pain should

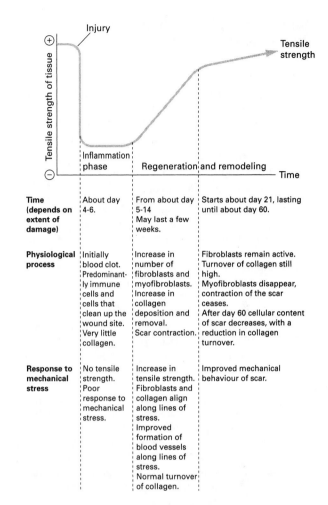

Figure 4-1 Normal phases of the process of tissue repair. (Courtesy Chaitow L, DeLany J: *Clinical application of neuromuscular techniques,* vol 1, The upper body, Edinburgh, 2000, Churchill Livingstone.)

	Injury / Inflammation phase	Regeneration and remodeling	
Time (depends on extent of damage)	About day 4-6.	From about day 5-14 May last a few weeks.	Starts about day 21, lasting until about day 60.
Physiological process	Initially blood clot. Predominantly immune cells and cells that clean up the wound site. Very little collagen.	Increase in number of fibroblasts and myofibroblasts. Increase in collagen deposition and removal. Scar contraction.	Fibroblasts remain active. Turnover of collagen still high. Myofibroblasts disappear, contraction of the scar ceases. After day 60 cellular content of scar decreases, with a reduction in collagen turnover.
Response to mechanical stress	No tensile strength. Poor response to mechanical stress.	Increase in tensile strength. Fibroblasts and collagen align along lines of stress. Improved formation of blood vessels along lines of stress. Normal turnover of collagen.	Improved mechanical behaviour of scar.

always be respected as a signal that the treatment is inappropriate in relation to the current physiologic status of the area. The discomfort scale suggested later in this chapter is the primary indicator regarding appropriate application of techniques.

When active or passive movements initiate pain, especially when that pain is elicited with little provocation, tissues associated with the movement should be treated with particular care and caution. Gentle, passive movement can usually safely accompany softtissue manipulation, and mild active movements may then be initiated with care. However, more comprehensive exercises, especially those involving resistance, should not be used until the active and passive movements cause no pain.

Sequencing of Neuromuscular Therapy Protocols

It is important to keep in mind that the stages of healing are not solely defined by the length of time since the injury but also by the degree of current pain and inflammation within the injured tissues. Box 4-1 describes the rehabilitation sequence that may begin once acute inflammation subsides.[17]

Chaitow and DeLany made the following suggestions, derived from NMT protocols[15]:

- Appropriate soft tissue techniques should be applied with the aim of decreasing spasm and ischemia, enhancing drainage of the soft tissues and deactivating trigger points.
- Appropriate active, passive and self-applied stretching methods should be introduced to restore normal flexibility.
- Appropriately selected forms of exercise should be encouraged to restore normal tone and strength.
- Conditioning exercises and weight training approaches should be introduced, when appropriate, to restore overall endurance and cardiovascular efficiency.
- Normal proprioceptive function and coordination should be assisted by use of standard rehabilitation approaches.
- Methods for achieving improved posture and body use should be taught and/or encouraged as well as exercises for restoring normal breathing patterns. Posture, body usage and breathing may be addressed at any stage.

Although the last two steps may be started at any time, in most cases the first four should be sequenced

in the order listed. Clinical experience suggests that symptoms may be prolonged and recovery compromised if an element is skipped or the order changed, except as noted. For instance, if exercise or weight training is initiated before the practitioner deactivates TrPs and eliminates contractures, the referral patterns may be intensified or new pain patterns initiated. In cases of recent trauma, deep tissue work and stretching applied too early may further damage and inflame the recovering tissues.

NMT protocols are taught as a step-by-step procedure that encourages assessment, examination, and treatment of each muscle that may be associated with a particular pain pattern, restricted movement, or chronic syndrome. These associated tissues include synergists, antagonists, and TrPs related to painful target zones. Although the protocols provide a general framework, they also offer flexibility for alternative or additional treatment approaches, the use of which depends on the practitioner's training and skill. In most situations, a number of manual techniques may effectively ease pain, improve range of motion, or release excessive tone; however, some techniques may be more effective with certain conditions. Use of synergistic modalities may significantly improve the result. On the other hand, excessive therapeutic intervention might induce a negative effect and create inflammation or reflexive spasm. Finding the right combination to "unlock" the patterns of dysfunction in each situation is sometimes the greatest challenge for the practitioner.

The following general guidelines are suggested when addressing most myofascial tissue problems[15]:

- The most superficial tissue is usually treated before the deeper layers.
- The proximal portions of an extremity are treated (softened) before the distal portions are addressed so that proximal restrictions of lymph flow are removed before distal lymph movement is increased.
- For two-jointed muscles, both joints are assessed; in multi-jointed muscles, all involved joints are assessed. For example, if triceps brachii is examined, both glenohumeral and elbow joints are assessed; if extensor digitorum longus, then the wrist and all phalangeal joints being served by that muscle are checked.
- Most myofascial trigger points either lie in the endplate zone (mid fiber) of a muscle or at the attachment sites.[38]
- Other trigger points may occur in the skin, fascia, periosteum, and joint surfaces.

BOX 4-1

Summary of Rehabilitation Sequence

- Decrease spasm and ischemia, enhance drainage, and deactivate trigger points
- Restore flexibility (lengthen)
- Restore tone (strengthen)
- Improve overall endurance and cardiovascular efficiency
- Restore proprioceptive function and coordination
- Improve postural positioning, body usage (active and stationary), and breathing

Courtesy Chaitow L, DeLany J: *Clinical application of neuromuscular techniques,* Edinburgh, 2000, Churchill Livingstone.

- Knowledge of the anatomy of each muscle, including its innervation, fiber arrangement, nearby neurovascular structures, and overlying and underlying muscles will greatly assist the practitioner in quickly locating the appropriate muscles and their trigger points.

When the client has multiple areas of pain, the following empiric rule-of-thumb is suggested:

- Treat the most proximal, most medial, and most painful TrPs first.
- Avoid overtreating either the whole structure or the individual tissues.
- Treatment of more than five active points during any one session might place an adaptive load on the client, which can prove stressful. If the client is frail or demonstrates symptoms of fatigue and general susceptibility, common sense suggests that fewer than five active TrPs should be treated at any one session.

USING NEUROMUSCULAR THERAPY PALPATION TECHNIQUES

The term *neuromuscular techniques* refers to the application of lubricated or nonlubricated gliding strokes, friction, and specialized applied pressure. Occasionally, special tools (e.g., pressure bars) or other body parts (e.g., elbows, palms, forearms, knuckles) may be used; however, most of the techniques are performed with the thumbs, fingers, or both (as in a pincer-type grasp).

NMT can be applied with the client in a variety of positions (e.g., seated, supine, prone) and can be general (postural) or local (for specific pain patterns or joint dysfunctions). Usually the sequence in which body areas are addressed is not regarded as critical as long as the proximal portion is treated before the distal and superficial layers before deeper tissues. However, the order of application may have some repercussions in postural reintegration, much as it does in Rolfing™ and Hellerwork™.

The NMT methods described here as the European version are in essence those of Stanley Lief, DC, and Boris Chaitow, DC. Regarding palpation, Dr. Chaitow writes the following:

To apply NMT successfully it is necessary to develop the art of palpation and sensitivity of fingers by constantly feeling the appropriate areas and assessing any abnor-

mality in tissue structure for tensions, contractions, adhesions, spasms. It is important to acquire with practice an appreciation of the "feel" of normal tissue so that one is better able to recognize abnormal tissue. Once some level of diagnostic sensitivity with fingers has been achieved, subsequent application of the technique will be much easier to develop. The whole secret is to be able to recognize the "abnormalities" in the feel of tissue structures. Having become accustomed to understanding the texture and character of "normal" tissue, the pressure applied by the thumb in general, especially in the spinal structures, should always be firm, but never hurtful or bruising. To this end the pressure should be applied with a "variable" pressure, i.e. with an appreciation of the texture and character of the tissue structures and according to the feel that sensitive fingers should have developed. The level of the pressure applied should not be consistent because the character and texture of tissue is always variable. The pressure should, therefore, be so applied that the thumb is moved along its path of direction in a way which corresponds to the feel of the tissues. This variable factor in finger pressure constitutes probably the most important quality a practitioner of NMT can learn, enabling him to maintain more effective control of pressure, develop a greater sense of diagnostic feel, and be far less likely to bruise the tissue.[11]

Using a Discomfort Scale

Although NMT examination and treatment effectively reduces chronic pain, it may cause discomfort to the client. Because one objective is to locate and then to introduce an appropriate degree of pressure into tender localized areas of dysfunctional soft tissue, feedback from the client during the session is crucial to the use of proper pressure. The amount of pressure used varies considerably depending on the health and reported discomfort level of the tissue. The degree of pressure also varies depending on whether a diagnostic or therapeutic objective is employed.

Palpatory feedback during applied pressure techniques relays important information to the practitioner regarding the condition of the tissues, location of taut bands, and the degree of tissue involvement. Applied compression (Box 4-2), especially that which is maintained for several seconds, has the following effects:

- Reduces inappropriate degrees of hypertonicity, apparently by releasing the contracted sarcomeres in the TrP nodule[38]

BOX 4-2

Effects of Applied Compression

Digital pressure applied to tissues produces the following simultaneous effects:

1. A degree of ischemia as a result of interference with circulatory efficiency, which reverses when pressure is released[38]
2. Neurologic inhibition (an osteopathic term) is achieved by means of the sustained barrage of efferent information resulting from the constant pressure[40]
3. Mechanical stretching of tissues occurs as the elastic barrier is reached and the process of "creep" commences[10]
4. A possible piezoelectric influence occurs, modifying relatively gel tissues toward a more solute state[2,5] because colloids change state when shearing forces are applied
5. Mechanoreceptors are stimulated, interfering with pain messages (gate theory) to the brain[33]
6. Local endorphin release is triggered along with enkephalin release in the brain and central nervous system[4]
7. Direct pressure produces a rapid release of the taut band associated with trigger points[38]
8. Acupuncture and acupressure concepts associate digital pressure with alteration of energy flow along hypothesized meridians[12]

Courtesy Chaitow L, DeLany J: *Clinical application of neuromuscular techniques,* Edinburgh, 2000, Churchill Livingstone.

- Induces a mechanical stress on the colloidal matrix, which may alter its state from that of a gel to a sol[26]
- Overrides neural reflex mechanisms, thereby reducing spasm through gating mechanisms[33,38]
- Blanches the tissues, which is followed by a flushing of blood that brings oxygen and nutrients[14]
- Releases endorphins and enkephalins[33]

The practitioner monitors any temporary discomfort produced by the applied compression, and makes adjustments as needed to avoid excessive treatment. A useful discomfort scale can be established to help encourage the application of proper pressure and to allow the client a degree of control over the process (Box 4-3). Melzack and Wall[33] suggest a scale in which 0 means "no pain" and 10 means "unbearable pain." An outline of their pain scale follows:

1. In using pressure techniques, avoid pressures that induce a report of a pain level of between 8 and 10.
2. The person should be instructed to report when the level of his or her perceived discomfort varies from what he or she judge to be a score of between 5 and 7.
3. Below 5 usually represents inadequate pressure to facilitate an adequate therapeutic response from the tissues, while prolonged pressure that elicits a report of pain above a score of 7 may provoke a defensive response from the tissues, such as reflexive shortening or exacerbation of inflammation.

Developing Palpation and Compression Techniques

Skin palpation, whether palpation of the skin's freedom of movement over underlying tissues or palpation of the quality of the skin itself, has tremendous value in NMT application. When the practitioner lifts the skin over a suspicious area and rolls it between his or her fingers and thumb (as in connective tissue massage or *bindegewebsmassage*) or when the practitioner slides the skin over the underlying fascia of a dysfunctional tissue, it is often found to be adherent or "stuck" to the underlying tissue. This lack of skin flexibility helps confirm a suspicious zone, which may be the target referral pattern of a TrP or may actually house a TrP. When the skin itself is assessed, it is often found to have increased hydrosus (sweatiness); to have a rough, coarse texture; or to have a cutaneous temperature that is hotter or cooler than the surrounding skin. These symptoms identify what Lewit[29] calls a *hyperalgesic skin zone,* the precise superficial evidence of a TrP.

Simons and colleagues[38] state the following about the adherent tissues:

In panniculosis, one finds a broad, flat thickening of the subcutaneous tissue with an increased consistency that feels coarsely granular. It is not associated with inflammation. Panniculosis is usually identified by hypersensitivity of the skin and the resistance of the subcutaneous tissue to "skin rolling." The particular, mottled, dimpled appearance of the skin in panniculosis indicates a loss of normal elasticity of the subcutaneous tissue, apparently due to turgor and congestion.

BOX 4-3

Establishing a Myofascial Pain Index

- The term *pressure threshold* is used to describe the least amount of pressure required to produce a report of pain or referred symptoms.
- It is useful to know whether the degree of pressure required to produce a report of pain is different after treatment than at the start of treatment.
- The criteria for diagnosing fibromyalgia are that 11 of 18 specific test sites must test positive (i.e., hurting severely) when 4 kilograms of pressure are applied.[1]
- An algometer (pressure meter) can be used to objectively measure the degree of pressure required to produce symptoms.
- An algometer also helps a practitioner learn how to apply a standardized degree of pressure and to judge how hard he or she is pressing.
- Belgian researchers Jonkheere and Pattyn[25] have used algometers to identify what they term the myofascial pain index (MPI).

- To measure a client's MPI, various standard locations are tested (e.g., the 18 test sites used for fibromyalgia diagnosis). The total poundage required to produce pain is divided by the number of points tested, from which the MPI is calculated.
- Although the MPI relies on the client's subjective pain reports, it is used as an objective measure.
- The calculation of the MPI determines the maximum degree of pressure that should be required to evoke pain in an active trigger point.
- If greater pressure than the MPI is needed to evoke symptoms, the point is not regarded as active.

Jonkheere and Pattyn based their approach on earlier work by Hong and colleagues,[22] who investigated pressure thresholds of trigger points and the surrounding soft tissues.

Courtesy Chaitow L, DeLany J: *Clinical application of neuromuscular techniques,* Edinburgh, 2000, Churchill Livingstone.
Note: This concept is discussed more fully in *Clinical Application of Neuromuscular Techniques,*[15] Chapter 6.

Panniculosis should be distinguished from panniculitis (inflammation of subcutaneous adipose tissue), adiposa dolorosa, and fat herniations, or lipomas. Skin rolling techniques and myofascial release should not be applied if inflammation is indicated; however, when appropriately used they often dramatically soften and loosen the skin from the underlying fascia and cause a softening of the involved muscles deep to the adherent skin.

Flat palpation (Figure 4-2) begins by sliding the whole hand, finger pads, or fingertips through the skin over the underlying fascia to assess for restriction. Pressure is increased to compress the tissue against underlying bony surfaces or against muscles that lie deep to those being assessed. Congestion, fibrotic qualities, indurations (areas of relative tissue hardness), and tone of the tissue become apparent as pressure increases. The palpating digit or hand meets tension within the tissue, and should attempt to closely match that tension while taking the slack out of the tissues. The practitioner avoids inducing excessive discomfort in the tissue by using the discomfort scale previously discussed. The fingers, thumb, or

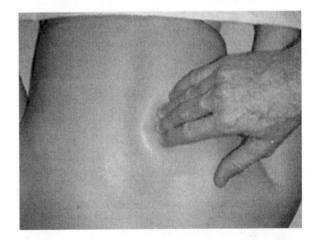

Figure 4-2 Deeply applied flat palpation evaluates deeper layers underlying the skin and superficial muscles. (Courtesy Chaitow L, DeLany J: *Clinical application of neuromuscular techniques,* vol 1, The upper body, Edinburgh, 2000, Churchill Livingstone.)

hand examines the tissue for TrP nodules (usually exquisitely tender points), congestion, fibrosis, or conditions otherwise altered from a normal, healthy tissue quality.

Flat palpation primarily is used to assess muscles that are closely adherent to the body (e.g., the rhomboids) and are difficult to lift. It may add information to that received from pincer compression techniques, revealing how wide a band has been found, for example. As pressure is applied to the tissues, particularly if the taut bands are deeply situated, the tissues may have a tendency to shift or roll away from the applied pressure; more care may be needed to precisely palpate the tissue. It is often useful to apply the pressure at an angle of approximately 45 degrees to the surface and to offer slight support to prevent the tissue from escaping the hands.

Compression techniques (Box 4-4) involve grasping and compressing the tissue between the thumb and fingers with one or both hands. With *flat compression,* a broad general compression is applied by the finger pads when they are flattened like a clothespin (Figure 4-3, *A*), whereas the more precise *pincer compression* of specific sections of the tissue is provided by the fingertips when the fingers are curved like a C-clamp (Figure 4-3, *B*). Static pressure may be applied in either of these techniques, or the tissue may be manipulated, either by holding it between thumb and fingers and then sliding the thumb across the fingers or by rolling it back and forth between the thumb and fingers.

Snapping palpation (Figure 4-4) is very difficult to apply correctly and to adequately assess. However,

when appropriately used it may elicit a local twitch response (LTR). When a tissue meets the minimal criteria for a TrP diagnosis (e.g., a nodule located in a taut band that, when properly provoked, produces a referral pattern), an LTR confirms the suspicion. However, the lack of an LTR does not rule out a TrP, especially when the level of skill necessary to correctly apply the technique is considered.

To perform snapping palpation, the fingers are placed approximately midfiber and quickly snapped transversely across the taut fibers (similar to plucking a guitar string). Because surface electromyography may be used to record the twitch response, snapping

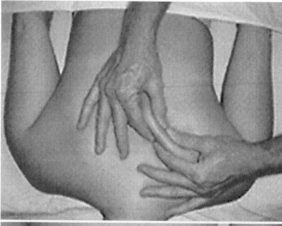

A

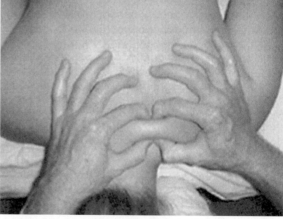

B

Figure 4-3 A broad, general release may be encouraged by applying pincer palpation with the finger pads **(A),** whereas the fingertips provide a more precise application **(B).** (Courtesy Chaitow L, DeLany J: *Clinical application of neuromuscular techniques,* vol 1, The upper body, Edinburgh, 2000, Churchill Livingstone.)

BOX 4-4

Compression Definitions

Compression techniques involve grasping and compressing the tissue between the thumb and fingers with one or both hands.
- *Flat compression* (like a clothespin) (see Figure 4-3, *A*) provides a broad general assessment and release.
- *Pincer compression* (like a C-clamp) (see Figure 4-3, *B*) compresses smaller, more specific sections of the tissue.

Courtesy Chaitow L, DeLany J: *Clinical application of neuromuscular techniques,* Edinburgh, 2000, Churchill Livingstone.

palpation is a useful skill in clinical research when precise diagnosis of a TrP location is crucial. Used repetitively, snapping palpation is a treatment technique that is often effective in reducing fibrotic adhesions.

Moving from Assessment to Treatment

There are many variations of the basic NMT techniques developed by Stanley Lief, Raymond Nimmo, and others. The choice of which techniques to use depends on particular presenting factors and personal preference. The practitioner often moves from assessment to treatment and back to assessment in almost seamless fashion, or moves from the application of one modality to another (e.g., from palpation to TrP pressure release to passive stretching or muscle energy techniques).

As the palpating digit moves from normal tissue to tense, edematous, fibrotic, or flaccid tissue, the amount of pressure needed to "meet and match" the tension found in the tissue varies. Some areas may be extremely tender, such as the doughy, textured, tender points of fibromyalgia, and thus may require very little pressure, whereas other areas may have a ropey or stringy feel and may respond favorably to increased pressure. When an area feels hard or tense, pressure should actually be lightened rather than increased during the assessment, so that the quality and density of the tissue can be evaluated. Deeper or firmer pressure may then be applied in treatment mode. Appropriate pressure is best determined after the extent of tissue involvement (e.g., the size of the involved area, degree of tenderness, a sense of the depth of tissue involvement, level of hydration) is determined.

Using Lubricants

Lubrication is not always advantageous, and at times even inhibits the practitioner's ability to lift and manipulate the tissues. However, it does provide a distinct advantage by reducing friction on the skin when the practitioner needs to glide smoothly over the skin surface. Both the European and American™ versions of NMT call for use of lubrication when applying certain techniques, although the American™ version uses it far more often than does its European counterpart.

When lubrication is used, a suitable amount of oil or lotion allows smooth passage of the palpating digit while avoiding excessive oiliness. When too much oil is applied, the essential traction by the thumb or finger is reduced and a great deal of palpatory information is lost. Certain procedures should be performed before lubrication is applied, such as those requiring friction or those in which the skin or myofascial tissues are lifted for stretch or manipulation. If the area has already been lubricated, a tissue, paper towel, or thin cloth may be placed between the palpating digit and the skin to prevent slippage, or the oil can be removed with an appropriate alcohol-based medium.

The practitioner may best locate taut bands by sliding the palpating digit transversely across the

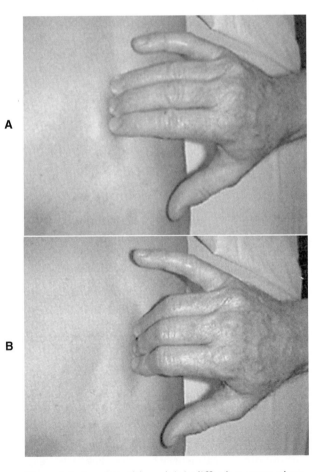

A

B

Figure 4-4 **A** and **B,** Although it is difficult to correctly apply, snapping palpation is often effective in confirming a trigger point by producing a local twitch response (LTR) in the suspicious tissue. (Courtesy Chaitow L, DeLany J: *Clinical application of neuromuscular techniques,* vol 1, The upper body, Edinburgh, 2000, Churchill Livingstone.)

fibers. Once located, the fibers may be assessed longitudinally to locate the approximate center of the fiber, where CTrPs form, and then at the attachment sites for the degree of tenderness and the possibility of inflammation. Several procedures may be incorporated as the practitioner moves from one tissue site to the next, including the following:

- A light, superficial stroke in the direction of lymphatic flow
- Direct pressure along or across taut fibers
- Direct pressure or traction on fascial tissue
- Sustained or intermittent inhibitory pressure

In the described manner, the practitioner can move from assessment to treatment and back to assessment without interruption. Once taut bands are located, reduced in size and density, and then examined, TrPs are more easily located. The TrPs may then be treated by means of compression (TrP pressure release), fiber elongation (stretching, with or without vapor coolants), heat and/or ice (when appropriate), vibration, or movement, all of which usually encourage the release of the taut fibers that house the TrP.

Palpating and Treating Trigger Points

The minimal criteria for diagnosing a CTrP is a nodule (located in a taut band) that when properly provoked produces a referral pattern. Referral patterns are usually painful, but they may also be patterns of tingling, numbness, itching, burning, and other sensations. When the client recognizes the referral pattern as common, it is said to be an *active* TrP, whereas an unfamiliar TrP is said to be *latent*.

When palpating for CTrPs, the practitioner often encounters a dense, congestive thickening in the taut fiber at approximately midfiber region. The more distinct nodule associated with the TrP may not be obvious at first because of the sometimes extensive tissue congestion. However, the nodule's distinct characteristic—exquisite tenderness—is usually felt by the client, and pressure may need to be decreased if the client reports heightened discomfort. The tissue's colloidal matrix may be softened by manipulation, gliding strokes, applications of heat (when appropriate), or elongation of the tissue; successful softening often results in more distinct palpation of the nodules and a reduction in size of the taut bands. Depending on the practitioner's ability to grasp the tissue, compression and pincer palpation may then be more easily and more precisely applied.

Once a TrP is located and confirmed by the minimal criteria and other observations (e.g., LTR; pain on contraction; a muscle testing as weak; or altered cutaneous humidity, temperature, or texture), a number of treatment choices are available. Depending on the practitioner's scope of practice (license) and prior training, he or she may choose from the following techniques:

- TrP pressure release (e.g., sustained ischemic compression)
- Chilling techniques (e.g., cryospray, ice, spray, stretch)
- Dry or wet needling (e.g., acupuncture, injections)
- Positional release methods (e.g., strain-counterstrain, facilitated positional release [see Chapter 1])
- Muscle energy (direct stretch) techniques
- Myofascial release methods
- Combination sequences (e.g., integrated neuromuscular inhibition techniques [INITs], discussed later)
- Correction of associated somatic or osseous dysfunction, possibly involving high velocity thrust adjustments or osteopathic or chiropractic techniques
- Education to correct perpetuating factors (e.g., posture, diet, stress, habits)
- Self-help strategies (e.g., stretching, hydrotherapy)

Note that regardless of the approach used, a TrP is more likely to be reactivated unless the muscle in which it lies is restored to its normal resting length following deactivating procedures. Muscle energy techniques or other appropriate stretching protocols should therefore be a part of all TrP treatment applications.

TrPs (whether central or attachment, active or latent) should be charted as to their location and referral patterns and reexamined at future sessions. TrPs ideally evidence their response to treatment with a reduction in referred phenomena and an increase in pain threshold. TrPs that do not respond to appropriate treatment may actually be satellite TrPs that lie in the target zone of a key TrP located elsewhere, thus maintaining the satellite in a reactive state. Satellite TrPs respond favorably (and often spontaneously without direct treatment) when their key TrPs are located and deactivated.[38]

Treating a Central Trigger Point

Once CTrPs have been located, the attachments are assessed for general tenderness and inflammation. (If inflammation is suspected, the stretching components of the following procedure are delayed and a precise myofascial release of the central sarcomeres is substituted for the passive or active stretches until the attachment sites improve.) The following is a basic sequence for treating CTrPs:

1. Digital pressure (i.e., pincer compression) is applied to the center of taut muscle fibers where TrP nodules are found.
2. The tissue is treated in this position or a slight stretch may be added as described later, which may increase the palpation level of the taut band and nodule.
3. As the tension becomes palpable, the pressure applied to the tissues is increased to meet and match the tension within the tissue.
4. The practitioner then slides his or her fingers longitudinally along the taut band near midfiber to assess for a palpable (myofascial) nodule or thickening of the associated myofascial tissue.
5. Spot tenderness is usually reported near or at the TrP sites.
6. Stimulation from the examination occasionally produces an LTR, especially when a transverse snapping palpation is used. When present, the LTR confirms that a TrP has been encountered.
7. When pressure is gradually increased into the core of the nodule (i.e., the CTrP), the tissue may refer sensations that the client either recognizes (indicative of an active TrP) or does not recognize (indicative of a latent TrP). Although pain is the most common sensation, other sensations may also include tingling, numbness, itching, and burning.
8. The degree of pressure should be adjusted so that the person reports a midrange number (between 5 and 7 on the discomfort scale) as the pressure is maintained.
9. The practitioner feels the tissues "melting" and softening under the sustained pressure. The client often reports the sensation that the practitioner is *reducing* the pressure on the tissue.
10. Pressure can usually be mildly increased as tissue relaxes and tension releases, provided that the discomfort scale is respected.
11. Although the length of time pressure is maintained varies, tension should ease within 8 to 12 seconds and the discomfort level should drop. If the tension does not begin to respond within 8 to 12 seconds, the amount of pressure should be adjusted accordingly (usually decreased); the angle of pressure may also need to be adjusted. An al-

ternative is to find a more precise location for the application of pressure (i.e., move a little one way and then the other to find heightened tenderness or a more distinct nodule).
12. Because the tissues are deprived of normal blood flow while pressure ischemically compresses (blanches) them, it is suggested that 20 seconds is the maximum length of time to hold the pressure.

Treating an Attachment Trigger Point

Once the taut band is located and a CTrP is suspected, the attachment sites of the taut band are assessed. ATrPs apparently form as a result of excessive, unrelieved tension on the musculotendinous or periosteal attachments (or both); these sites are often extremely sensitive and inflamed.[38] Palpation is performed cautiously and further tension is applied to the attachments. Stretching techniques applied to tissues that house ATrPs may provoke or increase an inflammatory response.

To lengthen the shortened fibers without placing undue stress on the attachments, gliding stokes may be applied from the center of the fiber toward the attachments (Figure 4-5). These strokes may be performed by gliding both thumbs simultaneously from the center to opposite ends, or one thumb may begin

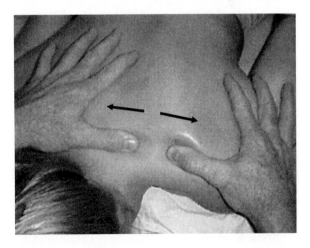

Figure 4-5 A localized myofascial release and precise traction of shortened sarcomeres may be applied by gliding the thumbs simultaneously in opposite directions. (Courtesy Chaitow L, DeLany J: *Clinical application of neuromuscular techniques,* vol 1, The upper body, Edinburgh, 2000, Churchill Livingstone.)

at the center of the fibers and glide toward one attachment, then repeat the motion from the center toward the other attachment.

Once the associated CTrP has been released, ATrPs usually respond without direct treatment. In the interim, cryotherapy (ice therapy) can be used daily on the ATrPs until the CTrPs have been successfully deactivated.

Other Trigger Point Treatment Considerations

- Taut muscle fibers may sometimes be felt more distinctly by placing them in a slightly stretched position. However, if movement produces pain or if assessment of the attachment sites reveals excessive tenderness, the practitioner exercises caution because ATrPs and inflammation may be present. These conditions may be aggravated by additional tension, strumming of the taut fibers, or frictional techniques.
- Because TrPs often occur in "nests," three to four repetitions of the TrP treatment may be required in the same area.
- If the colloidal state can be changed sufficiently, the tissue will be more porous, a better medium for diffusion to take place.[35]
- Each time digital pressure is released, blood flushes into the tissue, bringing nutrients and oxygen and removing metabolic waste. Therefore several repetitions of short-duration compression with its resultant "flush" is usually preferred over lengthy, sustained pressure.
- Treatment of a TrP is followed by several passive elongations (stretches) to the tissue's range of motion barrier. Unless contraindicated, passive stretching is then followed by at least three to four active repetitions of the stretch, which the client is encouraged to continue as "homework." Overtreatment is avoided.
- Although residual discomfort often accompanies this form of therapy, it may be reduced significantly by avoiding excessive treatment, by staying below 8 on the client's discomfort scale, and by using appropriate hydrotherapy applications during the session and at home.
- Because the elastic components of muscle and fascia are less pliable and less easily stretched when cold,[32] myofascial tissues are typically stretched

when they are warm and more liquid. If prolonged application of cold has already been used, the area may be rewarmed with a hot pack (unless contraindicated) or with mild movement before stretches are applied. Note that these precautions concern prolonged cold and do not apply to brief exposures to cold, such as spray-and-stretch or ice-stripping techniques.

DIFFERENCES BETWEEN AMERICAN AND EUROPEAN NEUROMUSCULAR THERAPY

Although European and American NMT have many similarities, there are distinct differences as well. Although a practitioner may prefer one form over the other, it is suggested that such preferences are personal and that either style, especially when highly developed, works equally well to locate and release somatic dysfunctions.

Distinctive Features of American Neuromuscular Therapy

Although the American version often uses dry-skin applications, the use of a lubricant with repetitious gliding techniques is one of its distinguishing features. These gliding procedures warm the tissues, flush lymphatic waste, and increase circulation, and simultaneously serve as assessment strokes to examine the underlying tissues for ischemia, TrPs, and areas of congestion or fibrosis. They allow the practitioner to rapidly become familiar with the individual quality, internal (muscle) tension, and degree of tenderness in the tissues being assessed. Box 4-5 is a summary of American NMT assessment protocols.

The positioning of the hands during the gliding strokes differs significantly from the European version (discussed later). In the American version, the thumbs lead and the entire hand moves with the stroke. Although the fingers usually stabilize the glide while the thumb applies the pressure, sometimes the fingers (or the palm or forearm) apply the pressurized stroke instead (Figure 4-6). Gliding repeatedly (six to eight repetitions is customary) on areas of hypertonicity accomplishes the following:

- Often changes the degree and intensity of the dysfunctional patterns

BOX 4-5

Summary of American NMT Assessment Protocols

- Glide where appropriate
- Assess for taut bands using pincer compression techniques
- Assess attachment sites for tenderness, especially where taut bands attach
- Return to taut band and find central nodules or spot tenderness
- Elongate the tissue slightly if attachment sites indicate this is appropriate, or tissue may be placed in neutral or approximated position
- Compress CTrP for 8 to 12 seconds (using pincer compression techniques or flat palpation)
- Instruct client to exhale as the pressure is applied; this often augments the release of the contracture

- Apply appropriate pressure to elicit a discomfort scale response of 5, 6, or 7
- Maintain pressure for up to 20 seconds if the tissue responds within 8 to 12 seconds
- Allow the tissue to rest for a brief time
- Adjust pressure and repeat, including application to other taut fibers
- Passively elongate the fibers
- Actively stretch the fibers
- Use appropriate hydrotherapy treatment in conjunction with the procedure, if desired
- Advise the client as to specific procedures that can be used at home to maintain the effects of therapy

Courtesy Chaitow L, DeLany J: *Clinical application of neuromuscular techniques,* Edinburgh, 2000, Churchill Livingstone.

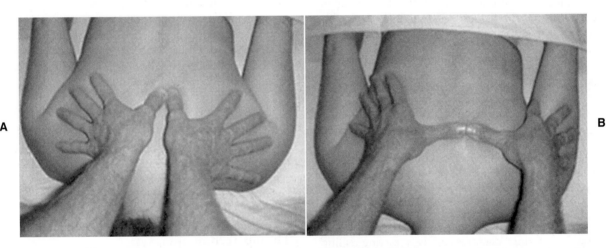

Figure 4-6 **A,** The thumbs lead the gliding strokes while the fingers offer support and enhance control. **B,** Incorrect positioning of the hands may produce stress on thumb joints. (Courtesy Chaitow L, DeLany J: *Clinical application of neuromuscular techniques,* vol 1, The upper body, Edinburgh, 2000, Churchill Livingstone.)

- Reduces the time and effort needed to modify dysfunctional patterns in subsequent treatments
- Tends to encourage the tissue to become more defined, which particularly assists in the evaluation of deeper structures
- Allows for a more precise identification of the location of taut bands and TrP nodules

- Encourages changes in hypertonic bands, which commonly become softer, smaller, and less tender than before

Occasionally taut bands become more tender after the gliding techniques, which may indicate an underlying inflammation for which applications of ice are indicated. Because heat, friction, deep gliding strokes, or aggressive stretching may aggravate inflamed tissue, these techniques are avoided when contraindicated. Applications of gentle myofascial release, cryotherapy, positional release, and lymphatic drainage are commonly applied in such instances.

Unless contraindicated by excessive tenderness, redness, heat, swelling, or other signs of inflammation, a moist hot pack placed on the tissues between repetitions further enhances the effects of gliding. When signs of inflammation are present or when heat cannot be tolerated for other reasons, applications of ice may be used instead. Cryotherapy is especially appropriate on ATrPs, where the constant concentration of muscle stress tends to provoke inflammation.[38,39]

American NMT has adopted several treatment tools that were developed by practitioners in an attempt to preserve their thumbs and hands and to more easily access attachments that lie under or between bony protrusions (e.g., in the lamina area of the vertebrae) or between bony structures (e.g., between ribs). The treatment tools that remain "tools of the trade" of neuromuscular therapy are a set of pressure bars (Figure 4-7), first introduced in the work by Dr. Raymond Nimmo[34] and associated with his receptor tonus techniques. These tools may be used in addition to (or in place of) finger or thumb pressure, unless contraindicated (e.g., at vulnerable nerve areas, near sharp protrusions, on extremely tender tissues). Tableside training with a knowledgeable instructor and subsequent practice is required to safely use the pressure bars.

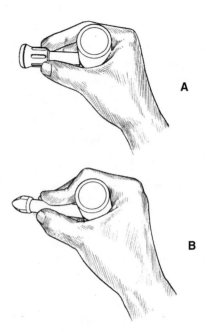

Figure 4-7 **A** and **B,** Pressure bars (such as shown here) and other tools may be carefully and properly used to reduce stress on practitioners' thumbs. (Courtesy Chaitow L, DeLany J: *Clinical application of neuromuscular techniques,* vol 1, The upper body, Edinburgh, 2000, Churchill Livingstone.)

Distinctive Features of European (Lief's) Neuromuscular Therapy

Variable ischemic compression is a distinguishing feature of European NMT. Whereas American NMT tends to apply static or increasing pressure for 8 to 12 seconds, then to rest for a time before repeating the pressure, European NMT offers a variation that applies deep pressure (sufficient to produce referred pain symptoms) for approximately 5 seconds, followed by an easing of pressure for 2 to 3 seconds. This is repeated until the local or referred pain diminishes (or, rarely, until either pain increases) or until 2 minutes have elapsed. This procedure is then followed by additional elements of an integrated sequence, INIT (described later).[14]

Pulsed ultrasound, application of hot towels (followed by effleurage), or the positional release "ease"

position for 20 to 30 seconds may further ease the hyperreactive patterns of a TrP. A final absolute requirement, regardless of the method used to release the trigger, is to stretch the tissues to help them regain their normal resting length.[38]

European Neuromuscular Therapy Thumb Techniques

The use of the thumb in European NMT differs greatly from the American version. The following main points regarding European NMT make this distinction clear:

- A light, nonoily lubricant is often used to reduce drag and facilitate easy passage of the palpating digit.
- The thumb and hand seldom impart their own muscular force except when treating small, localized contractures or fibrotic nodules.
- In contrast to American NMT, the hand and arm remain still while the thumb, applying variable pressure, moves through the tissues being assessed or treated.

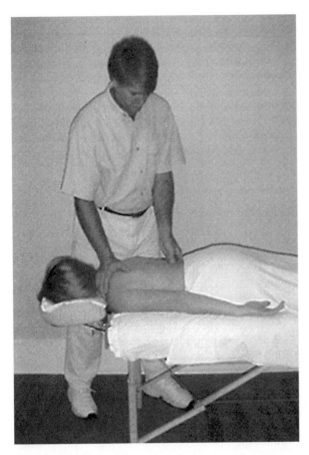

Figure 4-8 The thumb-drag method of European NMT (shown here) distinctly differs from the gliding style of American NMT. (Courtesy Chaitow L, DeLany J: *Clinical application of neuromuscular techniques,* vol 1, The upper body, Edinburgh, 2000, Churchill Livingstone.)

It is desirable to vary the amount of pressure used during strokes across and through the tissues. The degree of pressure imparted depends on the nature of the tissue being treated and is moderated by feedback from the client regarding the discomfort level. While being treated, the client may feel varying degrees of discomfort as the thumb varies its penetration of dysfunctional tissues. Although pain is seldom felt, the client is instructed to report immediately to the practitioner when the discomfort scale rises above a seven. The client's discomfort scale, coupled with the practitioner's experience with tissue response, helps the practitioner determine pressure application from moment to moment (Figure 4-8).

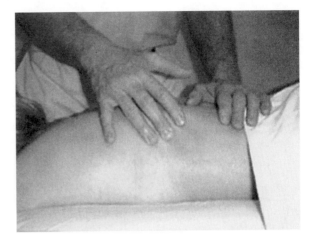

Figure 4-9 The straight-arm pressure technique uses body weight to apply force while maintaining a comfortable posture. (Courtesy Chaitow L, DeLany J: *Clinical application of neuromuscular techniques,* vol 1, The upper body, Edinburgh, 2000, Churchill Livingstone.)

Lief's Neuromuscular Therapy Finger Technique (Figure 4-9)

When the thumb's width prevents the degree of tissue penetration suitable for successful assessment or treatment, the middle or index finger can usually be substituted. This usually occurs when trying to access the intercostal musculature or when trying to penetrate beneath the scapula borders, especially in tense or fibrotic tissues. Working from the contralateral side, the finger technique is a useful approach to curved areas, such as the area above and below the iliac crest or on the lateral thigh (Figure 4-10). Sensitive areas are indicative of some degree of associated dysfunction (local or reflex), because pain is usually an indicator of abnormal physiology. Transient pain and mild discomfort are expected and recorded so that reexamination becomes part of the treatment plan for the next session.

Treating a Trigger Point—European Neuromuscular Therapy

INIT[3,13,23,27,37] is a treatment protocol for the deactivation of myofascial TrPs. The INIT protocol recommends the following sequence, described by Chaitow and DeLany[15]:

- The trigger point is identified by palpation methods after which ischemic compression is applied,

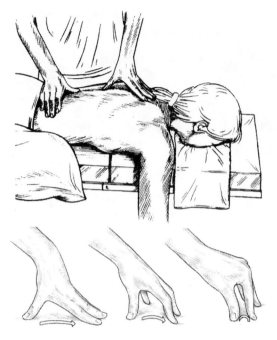

Figure 4-10 Finger technique is especially useful in curved areas, such as the intercostal region or the lateral thigh. (Courtesy Chaitow L, DeLany J: *Clinical application of neuromuscular techniques,* vol 1, The upper body, Edinburgh, 2000, Churchill Livingstone.)

sufficient for the patient to be able to report that the referred pattern of pain is being activated.

- The preferred sequence after this is for that same degree of pressure to be maintained for 5 to 6 seconds, followed by 2 to 3 seconds of release of pressure.
- This pattern is repeated for up to two minutes until the patient reports that the local or referred symptoms (pain) have reduced, or that the pain has increased (a rare but significant event) sufficient to warrant ceasing application of pressure.
- If, therefore, on reapplication of pressure during this "make-and-break" sequence, reported pain decreases or increases (or if 2 minutes elapse with neither of these changes being reported), the ischemic compression aspect of the INIT treatment ceases.
- At this time pressure is reintroduced and whatever degree of pain is noted is ascribed a value of "10," and the patient is asked to offer feedback information in the form of scores as to the pain value, as the area is repositioned according to the guidelines of positional release methodology. A position is sought which reduces reported pain to a score of 3 or less.
- This "position of ease" is held for not less than 20 seconds, to allow neurological resetting, reduc-

tion in nociceptor activity and enhanced local circulatory interchange.

- At this stage an isometric contraction focused into the musculature around the trigger point is initiated and following this the tissues are stretched both locally and where possible in a manner which involves the whole muscle.
- In some instances it is also found useful to add a re-educational activation of antagonists to the muscle housing the trigger point to complete the treatment.

Rationale for the Integrated Neuromuscular Inhibition Technique[15]

- When a trigger point is being palpated by direct finger or thumb pressure, and when the tissues in which the trigger point lies are positioned in such a way as to eliminate (most of) the pain, during positional release application, the most (dis)stressed fibers in which the trigger point is housed will be in a position of relative ease.
- At this time the trigger point has already received and is again under direct inhibitory ischemic pressure and is positioned so that the tissues housing it are relaxed (relatively or completely).
- Following a period of 30 to 60 seconds of this position of ease, the patient/client introduces an isometric contraction into the tissues and holds for 7 to 10 seconds, involving the precise fibers which had been repositioned to obtain the positional release.
- The effect is to produce (following the contraction) a reduction in tone in these tissues. These tissues can then be stretched locally or in a manner to involve the whole muscle, depending on their location, so that the specifically targeted fibers are be stretched.

A FRAMEWORK FOR ASSESSMENT

The European and American basic treatment protocols follow a set pattern. The suggested order is meant as a framework or guide; it provides a starting point and an ending point and precise steps along the way. However, each treatment session is different and the degree of therapeutic response in the areas of dysfunction depends on numerous factors.

The astute practitioner records areas of dysfunction, referral patterns, clinical findings, postural assessments, client symptoms, and all other relevant information on a case card or in a case file, along with the person's medical history and the findings of other health care professionals. Out of this substantial information base, a picture emerges from the client's whole body, and from this picture a therapeutic plan can be formed.

Training and Certification

Training for the practice of neuromuscular therapy includes a solid foundation in anatomic palpation, an understanding of myofascial physiology, and development of skills in locating TrPs. An emphasis on contraindications and areas where precautions apply is crucial in any course that teaches NMT techniques. When practicing certain techniques, tableside assistance with qualified instructors is imperative (e.g., when teaching anterior throat work); however, many of the protocols may be practiced without supervision.

The American version and the St. John method of NMT certification trainings have been successfully conducted in short course seminar events. Completion of four or five weekend courses is usually required, with a period of time allowed between each course for the trainee to practice the techniques. Once the required courses are completed, the trainee may take a certification examination, which includes a written examination and practical demonstration of NMT techniques and knowledge. Although continuing courses are not required to maintain the basic certification, advanced courses and seminars offering new developments in the field are often available.

NMT American version™ has been successfully taught in a pilot program offered by three massage schools in the United States. The NMT courses at these schools are taught by qualified NMT instructors and use the same NMT course manuals and protocols offered in the graduate level short courses. The pace of the school curriculum is slower than the short course version and students have almost daily access to instructors and assistants who can recheck the techniques learned previously. The graduating student receives NMT certification as well as the massage school diploma and is ready to enter the job market as a certified neuromuscular therapist.

A program has been specifically designed and successfully piloted in the chiropractic field that presents the NMT curriculum in weekend format exclusively for licensed chiropractors and chiropractic students.

The program, which is currently taught by a chiropractor, integrates the NMT American version's™ hands-on training with information relevant to the chiropractic approach.

The European version of NMT is taught as a module in the undergraduate program in the School of Integrative Health, University of Westminster. The NMT course involves twelve 4-hour lecture and practical classes spread over a semester. It is an elective module, available in the 3-year bachelor of science degree course in Therapeutic Bodywork offered by the university. It is available as a stand-alone course to suitably qualified manual therapists, who receive a certificate of proficiency after successfully completing the course and its knowledge and skills evaluation examinations.

Although there are no national requirements for certification or licensure to practice NMT, each state establishes requirements for a license to practice manual therapies. State licenses may restrict the practitioner's scope of practice to certain areas of the body. For instance, some states allow a massage therapist to perform intraoral protocols, whereas other states restrict this treatment to the dental profession. Conversely, a practicing dentist is usually confined to the area cephalad to the clavicles, thus limiting his or her ability to treat temporomandibular joint dysfunction, which may originate in a pelvic distortion. It is important that each practitioner understand the legal limits of his or her scope of practice. To better care for a wide variety of clients, some of whom may require treatment that is outside a practitioner's scope of practice, practitioners should build a referral network with other qualified practitioners.

The National Certification Board for Therapeutic Massage and Bodywork (NCBTMB) has successfully promoted national standards of certification within the field of general massage therapy. NCBTMB is continuing to research the feasibility of developing specialty and advanced certifications in addition to the current entry-level certification program. One of the specialties under consideration is NMT.

CONCLUSION

A thorough, whole-person approach to wellness, such as that on which NMT is founded, has quickly come to the forefront of complementary and integrative medicine. Although it is not often practical, and at times not even legal, for each practitioner to address all aspects of wellness and illness with every client, it is certainly relevant for each practitioner to bear in mind the interaction of biomechanical, biochemical, and psychosocial factors. Integrative support by the practitioner and his or her referral network offers the best possibility for a higher quality of health.

Neuromuscular techniques offer substantial promise in the areas of chronic pain management and preventive medicine. Comprehensive training and a strong knowledge base are essential factors in developing the skills for successful application of NMT. The practitioner who masters these skills touches people's lives with proficiency and confidence.

References

1. American College of Rheumatology: Criteria for the classification of fibromyalgia, *Arthritis Rheum* 33:160, 1990.
2. Athenstaedt H: Pyroelectric and piezoelectric properties of vertebrates, *Ann NY Acad Sci* 238:68, 1974.
3. Bailey M, Dick L: Nociceptive considerations in treating with counterstrain, *J Am Osteopath Assoc* 92:334, 1992.
4. Baldry P: *Acupuncture, Trigger points and musculoskeletal pain,* Edinburgh, 1993, Churchill Livingstone.
5. Barnes M: The basic science of myofascial release, *J Bodywork Movement Ther* 1(4):231, 1997.
6. Branstrom MJ: *Interactive physiology: muscular system,* Atlanta, 1996, ADAM Software, Inc. and Benjamin/Cummings Publishing.
7. Brostoff J: *Complete guide to food allergy,* London, 1992, Bloomsbury.
8. Butler D: *Mobilization of the nervous system,* Melbourne, 1991, Churchill Livingstone.
9. Cailliet R: *Soft tissue pain and disability,* ed 3, Philadelphia, 1996, FA Davis.
10. Cantu R, Grodin A: *Myofascial manipulation,* Gaithersburg, Md, 1992, Aspen Publications.
11. Chaitow B: Personal communication, 1983.
12. Chaitow L: *Acupuncture treatment of pain,* Rochester, Vt, 1990, Healing Arts Press.
13. Chaitow L: Integrated neuromuscular inhibition technique, *B J Osteop* 13:17, 1994.
14. Chaitow L: *Modern neuromuscular techniques,* New York, 1996, Churchill Livingstone.
15. Chaitow L, DeLany J: *Clinical application of neuromuscular techniques,* vol. 1 The upper body, Edinburgh, 2000, Churchill Livingstone.
16. DeLany J: Clinical perspectives: breast cancer reconstructive rehabilitation: NMT, *J Bodywork Movement Ther* 3(1):5, 1999.
17. DeLany J: *NMT course manuals: applications pack,* Saint Petersburg, 1994, NMT Center.
18. Feldenkrais M: *Awareness through movement,* New York, 1972, Harper & Row.
19. Ferraccioli G: Neuroendocrinologic findings in fibromyalgia and in other chronic rheumatic conditions, *J Rheum* 17:869, 1990.
20. Gilbert C: Hyperventilation and the body, *J Bodywork Movement Ther* 2(3):184, 1998.
21. Hanna T: *Somatics,* New York, 1988, Addison-Wesley.
22. Hong C-Z, Chen Y-N, Twehouse D et al: Pressure threshold for referred pain by compression on trigger point and adjacent area, *J Musculoskel Pain* 4(3):61, 1996.
23. Jacobson E: Shoulder pain and repetition strain injury, *J Am Osteopath Assoc* 89:1037, 1989.
24. Janda V: Introduction to functional pathology of the motor system: proceedings of the VII Commonwealth and International Conference on Sport, *Physiother Sport* 3:39, 1982.
25. Jonkheere P, Pattyn J: *Myofascial muscle chains,* Brugge, Belgium, 1998.
26. Juhan D: *Job's body: a handbook for bodywork,* ed 2, Barrytown, NY, 1998, Station Hill.
27. Korr I: Proprioceptors and somatic dysfunction, *J Am Osteopath Assoc* 74:638, 1974.
28. Latey P: Feelings, muscles and movement, *J Bodywork Movement Ther* 1(1):44, 1996.
29. Lewit K: *Manipulation in rehabilitation of the locomotor system,* London, 1992, Butterworths.
30. Lowe J: *The metabolic treatment of fibromyalgia,* Boulder, Colo, 2000, McDowell Publishing.
31. Lowe J, Honeyman-Lowe G: Facilitating the decrease in fibromyalgic pain during metabolic rehabilitation, *J Bodywork Movement Ther* 2(4):208, 1998.
32. Lowe W: Looking in depth: heat and cold therapy, *Orthopedic & sports massage reviews,* Issue #4, 1995, Orthopedic Massage Education and Research Institute, Bend, Ore.
33. Melzack R, Wall P: *The challenge of pain,* ed 2, Harmondsworth, Middlesex, Great Britain, 1988, Penguin Press.
34. Nimmo R: Receptors, affectors and tonus, *J Am Chiro Assoc* 27(11):21, 1957.
35. Oschman JL: What is healing energy? part 5: gravity, structure, and emotions, *J Bodywork Movement Ther* 1(5):307, 1997.
36. Randolph T: Stimulatory and withdrawal and the alternations of allergic manifestations. In Dickey L, editor: *Clinical ecology,* Springfield, Ill, 1976, Charles C Thomas.
37. Rathbun J, Macnab I: Microvascular pattern at the rotator cuff, *J Bone Joint Surg Br* 52:540, 1970.
38. Simons D, Travell J, Simons L: *Myofascial pain and dysfunction: the trigger point manual,* vol 1, ed 2, The upper half of body, Baltimore, 1999, Williams & Wilkins.
39. *Stedman's electronic medical dictionary,* version 4.0, Baltimore, 1998, Williams & Wilkins.
40. Ward R: *Foundations of osteopathic medicine,* Baltimore, 1997, Williams & Wilkins.

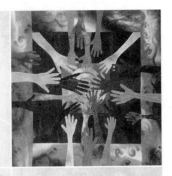

5

Cultivating the Vertical
The Rolf Method of Structural Integration

JEFFREY MAITLAND

he Rolf Method of Structural Integration was created by Ida Pauline Rolf, PhD.[9,23,24] Beginning with the insight that the human body is an upright unified structural and functional whole that stands in a unique relation to the uncompromising presence of gravity, Dr. Rolf asked this fundamental question: "What conditions must be fulfilled in order for the human body-structure to be organized and integrated in gravity so that the whole person can function in the most optimal and economical way possible?" Dr. Rolf originally named her method *Structural Integration*. This name was meant to capture her insight that long-lasting improvement in alignment, range of motion, joint integrity, and overall functioning and sense of well-being requires that the human structure be properly integrated and aligned in gravity. However, *Rolfing* was the nickname

that many clients spontaneously gave her work. After years of being identified with this nickname, *Rolfing* eventually became the trademarked name for her pioneering work.

HISTORY

Ida Rolf was born in 1896 in New York. She earned her PhD in biological chemistry in 1920 from Columbia University. Shortly thereafter she became an associate in the Rockefeller Institute's Department of Organic Chemistry, where she did research and published many articles for more than a decade. For most of her life, she was fascinated with and studied many forms of alternative healing, including homeopathy, osteopathy, and yoga.

Of all the systems of manipulation she studied, Dr. Rolf was profoundly influenced by osteopathy. She experienced the power of osteopathic manipulation when she was a young woman. During a camping trip she was kicked by a horse and developed pneumonia the next day. After receiving several sessions of osteopathic manipulation, she eventually recovered. From that time forward she remained convinced of one of the important principles of osteopathy, that structure determines function. For almost 50 years of her professional life, she studied and worked with osteopaths and chiropractors and continually refined her methods and understanding of how to integrate the body in gravity.

Dr. Rolf had an uncanny ability to perceive how gravity, misalignment, and dysfunction left their characteristic marks on both the myofascial structures and the body's inherent form of self-organization. Driven to find a solution to her own problems as well as those of her two young sons, she spent years exploring and experimenting with different systems of healing and manipulation. When she combined her discoveries with her remarkable powers of observation, Rolfing was born.

Dr. Rolf's original vision was broad and deep. She saw the need to explore her work from the points of view of philosophy, medical science, and psychology. Her life's work was devoted to the philosophic and scientific investigation into the conditions that must be fulfilled for the person as a whole to function optimally. Dr. Rolf's inspiration about the importance of fascia and the role it plays in maintaining body structure in the gravitational field was kindled by the holistic investigations of early osteopathy. Dr. Rolf was one of the first pioneers to actually develop a systematic and holistic form of fascial manipulation and movement education designed for the express purpose of integrating the body as a whole in gravity. She did so long before holism became the fashionable movement it is today. To emphasize her approach to holistic manual therapy, she often said, "Gravity is the therapist, not the Rolfer." Her relentless pursuit of how to understand and affect the impact of gravity on structure led her to develop a host of new fascial techniques, new forms of whole-body evaluation, and a powerful 10-session protocol for achieving her goal of structurally integrating the body in gravity.

To explain how we are able to remain upright, Dr. Rolf compared the body with a tent.[24] Her understanding was similar to Buckminster Fuller's tensegrity model. She compared the poles with the bones and the guy wires and tent fabric with the myofascial system. What keeps the tent up is not the poles, but the equal pull of the guy wires and the fabric across the poles. The poles act as spacers across which the guy wires and fabric can be stretched. In a similar but much more complicated fashion, our bodies are able to remain upright in gravity because the bones act as the spacers across which the myofascial network is stretched. In engineering terms, the body is more like a tensile structure than a compression structure. In this sense, it is more like a tent or suspension bridge than it is like a stack of blocks or bones.

Health and well being at every level are very much a function of the architectural integrity of the body, of the span and balance of the myofascial system within gravity. Distortions and patterns of strain within the fascial network can be expressions of injury, illness, stress, and long-standing psychological and emotional conflicts. Just as a tent is dragged down by gravity if the guy wires and fabric lose their appropriate stretch and span, the body loses its architectural integrity as some muscles and fasciae become too tight and others too flaccid.

Because the entire body is connected through its fascial network, lines of stress and strain within any section of fascia can be immediately transmitted throughout the entire fascial network. As Figure 5-1 (from Dr. Rolf's book[24]) illustrates, fascial strain can be communicated through the body in much the same way that snagging part of a sweater immediately distorts the shape of the entire sweater. These patterns of strain in the fascial network contribute to the unique form that each body displays and to unique ways of standing, sitting, and moving. Like a pair of well-worn shoes, these patterns of fascial strain display each individual's unique struggles with gravity.

Like other material structures, the body must deal with gravity. When the body is out of alignment, gravity drags it down, just as it drags down a building that has lost its architectural integrity. For whatever reason, if a body loses its architectural integrity and alignment in gravity, it loses its ability to balance and distribute weight with ease. As a result, patterns of movement become more encumbered. Gravity then becomes the invisible enemy. More fascial thickening and shortening occurs as the body struggles to move around its myofascial restrictions and tries to shore itself up against the relentless downward drag of gravity. A misaligned body is a body at war with itself and gravity.

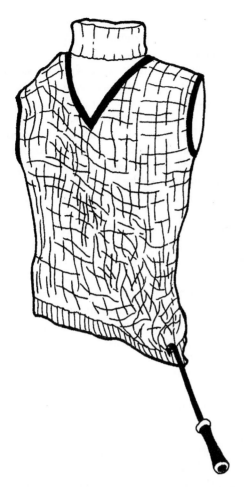

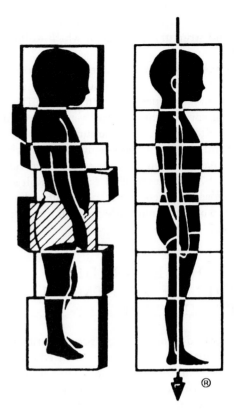

Figure 5-2 Official logo of the Rolf Institute. (Courtesy International Rolf Institute in Boulder, Colorado.)

Figure 5-1 A snag in one part of this sweater demonstrates the distortion of the whole. (From Rolf IP: *Rolfing: the integration of human structures,* Santa Monica, Calif, 1977, Dennis-Landman Publications.)

To trained eyes, the all too prevalent examples of bodily disorder—such as slouched postures with head and neck too far forward, hyper-erect structures that bow backward, knock knees or bowed legs, flat feet or high arches, excessive spinal curvature—all display complicated patterns of strain, tightness, and thickening of muscles and fasciae. These patterns, Dr. Rolf discovered, can be changed for the better by applying the techniques that she invented to release fasciae and organize the body in gravity.

To teach her work to others, Dr. Rolf created a protocol in the form of 10 sessions of fascial manipulation and movement education designed to carefully and systematically bring the body to a higher level of order and unencumbered function. Resembling a

slow form of body sculpting, Rolfers apply intelligent pressure with their fingers, knuckles, and elbows to the fascia to soften and lengthen it.[4,21,22] Depending on how the body responds, this pressure may be heavy or light.[25] As a result of Rolfing's systematic manipulation of the myofascia, the body begins to effortlessly right itself in gravity. After many years of exploration, practice, and observation, Dr. Rolf and her students realized that once a series of Rolfing treatments is completed and the inappropriate movement patterns are corrected, the body remains changed for the better: more effortlessly upright, able to move in much less encumbered ways, and better aligned in gravity.

In 1972 Dr. Rolf founded the International Rolf Institute in Boulder, Colorado. The Rolf Institute is the education and research center and professional association for Certified Rolfers worldwide. Figure 5-2 illustrates the official logo of the Rolf Institute, which is traced from actual photographs of a little boy who underwent 10 sessions of Rolfing. The logo is an excellent representation of the remarkable postural and structural changes for which Rolfing is so well known.

Because of her considerable contributions to the worldwide renaissance in holistic and manual medicine, Dr. Rolf's influence is still felt today in the many forms of somatic therapy that were inspired by her creative efforts. Recognized around the world as the leader and pioneer in whole-body alignment through fascial manipulation and movement education, she died in 1979 at the age of 83. Since Dr. Rolf's death, the philosophy, science, and art of Rolfing have continued to evolve significantly through the support of the Rolf Institute.

THE THREE-PARADIGM MODEL OF TREATMENT INTERVENTION

To better understand Dr. Rolf's contributions to holistic manual therapy and movement education, we must clearly understand the nature of a holistic practice and distinguish it from the other ways manual therapy is typically practiced. Fundamentally, there are three quite different ways of practicing any form of health care, whether we are considering psychotherapy, manual therapy, or complementary and conventional medicines. These three forms of practice can be called the *relaxation paradigm,* the *corrective paradigm,* and the *holistic* or *integrative paradigm.*[6,17]

The relaxation paradigm includes any practice that attempts to produce the relaxation response as a way to alleviate pain and other symptoms. Most forms of entry-level massage therapy are examples of a relaxation practice.

Practices that fall under the corrective paradigm aim at the symptomatic and piecemeal treatment of disease, pain, dysfunction, and structural problems. The corrective approach is most clearly represented in the crisis orientation of conventional allopathic medicine, which is capable of employing powerful and advanced life-saving measures. A great many contemporary physical and manual therapies are also practiced in the corrective mode. Corrective manual therapy treats and restores areas of the body that are considered contributing factors to the patient's pain and dysfunction. Corrective practices may use high-velocity, low-amplitude thrusting techniques or soft-tissue techniques to restore mobility to restricted joints, release local areas of myofascial strain, release muscle groups that are excessively shortened or lengthened, or restore areas that exhibit regional biomechanical misalignment.

The holistic paradigm includes practices that aim at cultivating integration, balance, and harmony for the whole person. Some examples of holistic practices are homeopathy, Chinese medicine, osteopathy as it was originally defined and practiced, and Rolfing. Rather than simply focusing on the regional release of dysfunction, the holistic manual therapist attempts to understand the effect his or her interventions have on the whole to influence and organize the whole.

Implicit in the concept of the three paradigms is a distinction between two related but different goals for any therapeutic intervention. The most commonly agreed-on therapeutic goal, and the goal to which all health care practitioners are committed, is the goal of restoring normal function. However, the goals of the holistic practitioner are more extensive. The relaxation and corrective practitioner aims only to restore normal function, whereas the holistic practitioner also aims at the enhancement of function and the whole person. The restoration of normal function is the natural result of enhancing the whole.

The three paradigms of practice are not mutually exclusive or in opposition to each other. Often patients benefit from receiving relaxation and corrective approaches before a holistic approach is initiated. However, the corrective approach is often limited by its inability to evaluate the effects of local interventions on the whole body. In contrast, holistic practitioners recognize that unless the whole person is capable of adapting to and supporting regional interventions, dysfunction will either return or be driven elsewhere in the system—or both. Holistic manual practices are capable of achieving the goals of the corrective and relaxation manual practices as a matter of course, but corrective and relaxation practices cannot achieve the goals of holistic manual therapy except by accident.

Dr. Rolf expanded the holistic approach to include the concept of *integration in gravity.* She insisted that long-lasting structural and functional change required that the body be properly organized not only with respect to itself, as all holistic therapies claim, but also with respect to gravity and the environment. She argued that the return of dysfunction or the appearance of new dysfunction after a treatment was often a result of the failure of the whole person to adapt to regional interventions. She also claimed that these unwelcome results were a result of the fact that the whole body in its relation to gravity and the environment was often unable to support the system-wide consequences of local interventions. Thus, beyond the obvious attempt to restore normal function, Rolfing has two distinct but interdependent holistic goals. One is to enhance the unique way the human body is organized with respect to itself, and the other is to organize and integrate the whole self-organizing body–person in gravity and the environment.

These interdependent goals are achieved through a variety of techniques that include but are not limited to fascial manipulation, membranous manipulation, ligamentous manipulation, energetic intervention, and movement education. Although many clients, professional athletes among them, come to Rolfing for relief from pain, soft tissue injuries, and musculoskeletal problems and the enhancement of performance, Rolfing techniques and protocols are not applied in the conventional piecemeal symptomatic fashion. The techniques are always used with an eye toward their system-wide effects on the inherent order of the whole person and how the body relates to gravity and the environment. Because Rolfing is a holistic approach that includes an understanding of the impact of gravity and the environment on structure, it is more likely than the corrective approach to achieve long-lasting change and less likely to drive strain elsewhere in the system.[6]

As a holistic practice, Rolfing has theoretically and practically investigated the impact of gravity on structure and function more thoroughly than almost any other therapy. Therefore Rolfing should not be confused with massage or bodywork, the popularized ways of releasing myofascia practiced by many manual, deep tissue, and physical therapists. Many other manual therapies have borrowed heavily from the theory and practice of Rolfing but do not work in the holistic framework that Dr. Rolf inaugurated.

NEW DEVELOPMENTS IN ROLFING THEORY AND PRACTICE

Since Dr. Rolf's death in 1979, the philosophy, science, and art of Rolfing have evolved significantly. As an expedient way to teach her work, Dr. Rolf created a 10-session formulaic protocol, which she characteristically called "The Recipe." Her recipe was astute in its conception, broad in its scope, and quite effective in its ability to benefit a wide variety of people. Every system of manipulation relies on its own version of formulaic protocols. Although Dr. Rolf's 10-session recipe is powerful and effective, it has certain obvious drawbacks common to all formulaic protocols.

Formulaic protocols by their very nature assume the existence of an ideal body or state that is assumed to constitute "normal." The theory that there is an ideal structure that every body should strive to emulate can be called *somatic idealism*. Formulism and somatic idealism go hand in hand.[15,17] Because formulaic protocols dictate the same sequence of interventions in the same order, they presuppose the same outcome for every body. Because they assume the same outcome for every body, formulaic protocols surreptitiously perpetuate somatic idealism. Unfortunately somatic idealism, whether it assumes an ideal form for the way the body should relate to gravity or an ideal notion of normality, is inappropriate for many people. In fact, treatment protocols that encourage patients to conform to these somatic ideals sometimes actually create dysfunction rather than alleviate it.

The other related drawback common to formulaic protocols is that they are sometimes incapable of attending to what is unique in each person. As a result, they are incapable of sequencing treatment strategies in the order required by each person's unique needs. Dr. Rolf understood the second drawback and did not always follow her own recipe. But she was less clear about somatic idealism and tended to use her idea of the ideal body as a standard against which to evaluate clients' bodies and the success of her work.

The Rolfing logo, pictured in Figure 5-2, can be seen as a example of the typical postural and structural changes for which Rolfing is known, or as an example of somatic idealism common to many other systems of manual therapy.[12] As an example of somatic idealism, the logo illustrates a body organized around the line of gravity. However, the belief that the weight centers of the human body can be organized around the line of gravity is problematic. It presupposes that the body is equally dense throughout. Clearly, however, the human body is not organized in gravity the way stacks of blocks or other nonliving material structures are, and it does not manifest the same density throughout, as does a stack of blocks. Thus the practice of using the line of gravity as a way to evaluate how well or how poorly a body relates to gravity has limitations.

The limitations of somatic idealism and formulism were overcome after Dr. Rolf's death through the efforts of a number of advanced teachers at the Rolf Institute.[15,17,25,26] As a result, Dr. Rolf's somatic idealism has been abandoned and a greater appreciation of how diverse psychobiologic types handle the effects of gravity has become part of the theory and practice of Rolfing.[26] Every type of soma can benefit from the work of Rolfing; but not all benefit in the same way or exhibit the same psychobiologic pattern as a result of Rolfing.

Coming to terms with somatic idealism and formulism has also led to a more appropriate and complex understanding of normality.[15,17] This developing concept of "normal" is quite different in scope and implication than the commonly accepted idea of normal—measuring up to a norm, statistical average, or standard that is imposed on the human body. *Normal,* in the sense in which Rolfing now uses it, refers to what is appropriate and optimal for each individual person. Finding "normal" for each client is not a matter of imposing a structural template by means of formulaic protocols, but is a process of discovery. Because there is no one form or pattern that can serve as the standard for what constitutes normal for all human beings, discovering what is normal for each individual in relation to his or her environment is a much more complex matter of uncovering what is natural or inherent in the being of the whole person. What constitutes normal for each client unfolds by means of careful and sensitive structural manipulation and movement education, which explores and uncovers the plasticity and limitations inherent in each person's form in relation to how he or she has adapted to the environment. Living human organisms are self-organizing, self-regulating, self-sensing systems characterized by the continuous attempt to balance, organize, harmonize, adapt, and enhance their lives. "Normal" is neither an ideal nor static state, but an evolving orthotropic achievement that is won again and again during the course of a life.

Because somatic idealism and formulism go hand in hand, it is not possible to abandon one without abandoning the other. However, if both concepts are abandoned, the question of how to plan treatment without the benefit of formulaic protocols and a somatic ideal becomes especially acute and complex. Like so many other gifted practitioners and theorists in manual therapy, Dr. Rolf intuitively understood the principles of intervention. However, because she was unable to articulate the principles, she expediently taught her ways of evaluating and manipulating structure in the form of a formulaic protocol.

When attempting to sequence clinical decisions into a treatment strategy, three simple questions must be answered: What do I do first, what do I do next, and when am I finished? Answering these questions without the benefit of a formulaic protocol and its attendant somatic idealism requires understanding of the principles of intervention.[5,19] The word *principle* can refer to a basic law, a fundamental property, or a value. But the meaning relevant to a principle-centered clinical decision-making process is that of a constitutive rule from which a chain of reasoning proceeds. Constitutive principles define the parameters of intervention and the conditions for optimal human activity. Strategies are then sequenced in accordance with these constitutive rules, analogous to the way the principle "add 2 to the last number" allows the sequence "2, 4, 6, . . ." to be completed.

All holistic paradigm approaches, including Rolfing, are based on *the holistic principle.* In its simplest form, the holistic principle states that no principle of intervention can be completely fulfilled unless all the principles are fulfilled. Because the holistic principle describes how the principles of intervention function together, it is properly called a meta-principle. There are five constitutive principles of intervention that fall under the holistic principle.

The first principle of intervention is called the *adaptability principle.* It is defined as the client's ability to adapt to and accept new options of self-perception, alignment, and motion. It recognizes that an intervention is therapeutic to the extent that the client is capable of adapting to it.

The *support principle* is a specific application of the adaptability principle and is based on Dr. Rolf's understanding of the effects of gravity on structure. The support principle states that an intervention is successful to the extent that the client is capable of supporting the change in gravity. It refers to the ability of the client to adequately adapt to gravity after the body's movement and alignment patterns have been changed through an intervention. It also refers to the ability of the client to express and maintain new shifts in perception and world view.

The *continuity principle* is also a further specification of the adaptability principle. Because a living whole is an irreducible holistic complexity, the continuity principle recognizes that restrictions at any level of the human organism are reflected at all other levels. Every intervention affects the continuity, organization, and functioning of the whole person, and the continuity, organization, and functioning of the whole person either limit or augment how any particular intervention affects the whole. Continuity manifests in living wholes as freedom from fixation. Loss of continuity can appear as joint restrictions, distortions in energetic fields, blocks to appropriate flow of energy, an overcharged or undercharged nervous system, imbalance between agonist and antagonist muscle pairs, myofascial strain patterns and scar tissue, strain patterns in the celomic sacs, loss of organ motility and mobility, emotional or psychological problems, dysfunctional movement patterns, or a dissociated world view.

The *palintonic principle* recognizes that the success of any intervention or series of interventions is a function of appropriate spatial relationships—for example, back-front, side-side, top-bottom, and inside-outside balance. The term *palintonic* is derived from the Greek word *palintonos,* meaning "unity in opposition" (literally, "stretched back and forth"). Palintonic harmony describes the spatial, somatic geometry of order, which becomes apparent as a body approaches integration. It expresses the unity of opposition that arises among all structures, spaces, volumes, and planes of an integrated soma as it moves through space. For example, a patient with an imbalance between the agonist and antagonist muscle groups of the flexors and extensors of the neck, lower back, and pelvis displays one kind of palintonic imbalance. Lack of extensor-flexor balance can also be present in inside-outside imbalance when the rectus abdominis is stronger than the psoas.

The *closure principle* recognizes that when the patient has achieved the highest level of somatic and perceptual integration possible within his or her current set of limitations, treatment should be terminated.

Answering the questions, "What do I do first, what do I do next, and when am I finished?" in accordance with a principle-centered decision-making process also requires a clearly developed and systematic evaluation process. Along these lines the advanced instructors are now developing elaborate taxonomies of assessment designed to direct the evaluation process toward a more detailed understanding of how structural, functional, and energetic dysfunction, conflicted world views, and emotional and physical trauma impact the body as it organizes itself within gravitational fields.[5,15,17] By creating a principle-centered, nonformulaic decision-making process based on empirical observations across a wide range of assessment taxonomies (Figure 5-3), Rolfing theory and practice finally freed itself from the grip of formulism and somatic idealism.

Applying the principle-centered decision-making process requires that the practitioner perform a clear evaluation that locates the client's fixations and dysfunctions in each of the taxonomies of assessment and determines what issues most interfere with the overall organization of the body with respect to itself and gravity. In evaluating the whole, the practitioner

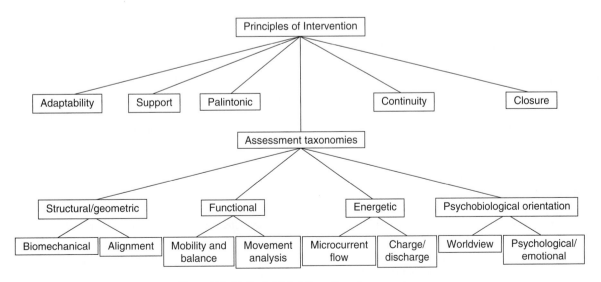

Figure 5-3 Holistic Third Paradigm Intervention.

determines which aspect or aspects of the client, if properly treated, will most benefit the whole. Then the practitioner uses the principles of intervention to determine whether the body can adapt to, support, and sustain the changes that will result from the proposed intervention strategy.

Rolfing also evolved in a number of other important ways. Rolfing began as a rather painful style of manipulation and over the years has sustained this reputation in the mind of the public. However, the techniques of Rolfing have broadened to include a softer and more discriminating sense of touch. These newer techniques are both less invasive and sometimes more precise in their ability to release and organize the body at every level. Many clients who have experienced this gentler approach are surprised to discover that their experiences with massage are actually more uncomfortable than Rolfing.

Also a host of new soft-tissue techniques have been created that can easily release restrictions in facets of the spine and other joints with as much precision as any other system of manipulation.[18] Rolfing accomplishes these results without resorting to techniques developed in other schools of manipulation, such as high-velocity, low-amplitude thrusting or muscle energy techniques. These techniques work by positioning the body to challenge the joint restriction while applying gentle but firm pressure to the small muscles and ligaments responsible for the fixation. As the strain patterns in the fascia and ligaments are eased under the intelligent pressure applied by the Rolfer, bones and other structures quietly shift their aberrant positions as motion restrictions at many levels of the body dissolve.

A number of faculty members at the Rolf Institute are also exploring the concept of biologic organization in more detail. Although Dr. Rolf understood the importance of organizing the body with respect to itself and the need for a holistic biology of form, she tended to pursue the question of bodily organization primarily in terms of how the body was organized in gravity. Although it is true that human morphology and morphogenesis cannot be understood apart from the effects of gravity, it is also true that how the body responds to gravity is a function of its unique morphology. Dr. Rolf used the analogy of a stack of blocks to understand *organization in gravity* as *organization around the line of gravity,* and she used the tent analogy to illustrate the body's tensile organiza-

tion. Both of these analogies make a useful point, but by comparing the body to inanimate material structures they divert attention from the important points that living creatures are organized differently from nonliving things and that human bodies are organized differently from animal bodies.

The analogies also occlude the important point that living creatures are not passively acted on by gravity the way material objects are. Organisms establish their biologic identity by differentiating themselves from inorganic objects, their environment, and other organisms. As a result of this self-organizing, self-sensing cognitive ability, organisms continually define themselves in opposition to gravity and their world as they are continually compelled to adapt to their ever-changing internal and external environments.[13,16,27]

Living organisms are not serially cobbled together from preshaped parts the way machines and other constructed material structures are. Living organisms are irreducible complexities. They are self-sensing, unified, seamless wholes in which no one aspect, detail, or part is any more fundamental to the make up and organization of the whole than the whole itself. Unlike a machine, a tent, or a stack of blocks, every detail of the organism, whether an organ, a bone, or a myofascial structure, is an unmistakably clear, although differently formed, expression of the same wholeness and biologic identity. Every aspect (or, to speak loosely, every part) of an organism is an expression of its self-organizing unified wholeness, every aspect of the organism exists for and by means of every other aspect, and every aspect enters into the constitution of every other aspect of the organism. Although the human form has evolved from the animal form and shares the same anatomic structures common to mammals, human morphology is quite different.[2] By vertically appropriating gravity, human morphology transforms these common animal structures and organizes them into an upright, self-directed, self-sensing, self-conscious whole.

Because corrective practices tend to overlook the significance of the orthotropic, holistic organization of the body in gravity, they tend to treat symptoms with little grasp of how local interventions impact the whole. Clearly holistic somatic practices must be more attentive to the nature of biologic organization, as Dr. Rolf insisted. By pursuing the question of what constitutes human biologic organization and morphology, the advanced faculty has continued to deepen this understanding and develop new techniques designed to enhance and integrate the body's self-sensing, self-organizing nature with respect to itself. New regional and global techniques have been developed that both take advantage of and normalize the body's inherent motility and fluid dynamics. Techniques also have been developed that address the unique internal pushes and pulls in the body's cavities and how they affect the whole. Other approaches have also been designed to enhance the organization of the body in gravity and the unique orthotropic, morphologic whole that is living to express itself in each client.

Although Dr. Rolf began her investigations by emphasizing structure, over the years the faculty of the Rolf Institute has come to realize that equal weight must also be put on understanding function, movement patterns, energy systems, and the effects of physical and emotional trauma. Rolfing now works not only with structure (myofascial strains, joint fixations, cranial, visceral, and other membranous strains) but also with unconscious patterns of holding in movement, suppressed emotions, trauma, neurologic fixations, perceptual and world-view confusions,[5,16] and blocked or distorted energy.

Although Dr. Rolf believed the functional approach was very important and although she created a form of movement education, she tended to develop her structural approach almost to the exclusion of her functional approach. Over the years the Rolf Institute faculty has significantly developed Dr. Rolf's early functional approach far past her original insights and practices. Rolfing movement work has evolved into a therapeutic exploration and education in somatic awareness and unencumbered movement.[1,10,20] Rolfing movement practitioners work with a variety of techniques ranging from verbal instruction, touch, self-awareness, and other forms of education designed to guide clients toward finding more appropriate options for movement in their everyday activities as they relate to gravity and their world.

Without attempting to make Rolfing a substitute for psychotherapy, the faculty has also developed new ways of understanding and releasing the effects of emotional and physical trauma on the body.[14] These advances in Rolfing are continually being refined as new insights and discoveries are integrated into the work.

WHAT TO EXPECT

Some Rolfers work within variations of the 10-session protocol, whereas others work in a more individualized way. The basic work of Rolfing usually requires between 8 and 12 sessions. Many clients also return for advanced sessions, which typically take place in a one-, three-, or five-session series. The client is usually clothed in underwear, shorts, or a bathing suit. To create an effective strategy for organizing the client's body, the Rolfer usually begins the session by observing and evaluating the client while standing and walking. The client receives the work while lying on a specially designed padded table and at times while sitting on a Rolfing bench. A typical Rolfing session takes between an hour to an hour and a half and includes hands-on manipulation coupled with movement analysis and corrective suggestions. Prices for a Rolfing session vary around the world. One session can cost anywhere from $80 to $150.

Training

Candidates applying to be trained in Rolfing are required to have a college degree. They must receive basic and advanced Rolfing training and a series of Rolfing movement sessions. Rolfing training is divided into basic, intermediate, and advanced phases. The basic phase is roughly equivalent to three semesters. Rolfing is taught according to the principle-centered decision-making process that requires understanding of how to apply the comprehensive taxonomies of assessment. In the early stages of the training, Rolfing is taught according to a 10-session protocol that is not only much more elaborate than Dr. Rolf's original version but is also much more sensitive to the variety of psychobiologic types. Students are taught the principles of intervention and how to vary the protocols according to the needs of the patient. After completing the basic stage of the training, students are certified by the Rolf Institute to practice Rolfing in the expanded 10-session protocol. Rolfers continue their training in the intermediate stage by taking a series of classes designed to expand their theoretic and practical skills and to prepare them for advanced training. The intermediate class consists of 18 days of training. All Rolfers are required to complete advanced training. During the 6 weeks it takes to complete the advanced level of training, Rolfers are taught how to plan their work solely according to the principles of intervention without any reliance on formulaic protocols. They are extensively trained in how to evaluate the whole person by using much more elaborate taxonomies of assessment. They are also taught how to intervene by using a more refined and discriminating sense of touch.

Although Rolfing is not a substitute for psychotherapy, Rolfing education now places more emphasis on understanding how to create the appropriate therapeutic environment and how to work with the effects of psychological and physical trauma on the body. Movement education is now integrated into the training of every Rolfer. For those who are interested in specializing in movement education, there is also a complete certification program in Rolfing Movement Education. After completing advanced training, Rolfers are certified by the Rolf Institute as Advanced Rolfers.

Research

Scientific research on Rolfing is encouraged and supported by the Rolf Institute and there is a small but growing body of research that supports many of the claims of Rolfing. Research conducted at UCLA shows that Rolfing creates a more efficient use of the muscles, allows the body to conserve energy, and creates more economical and refined patterns of movement.[11] Other recent research has demonstrated that Rolfing significantly reduces chronic stress and changes body structure for the better.[3,7,8] In these studies, Rolfing significantly reduced the spinal curvature of subjects with lordosis. Evidence also indicates that Rolfing enhances neurologic functioning. Some of this research supports the idea that holistic manual therapy based on the Rolf method not only has a more long-term effect on the body but also has a more integrative effect that in fact contributes to the long term effect. A case study indicates that a holistic approach using Rolfing and movement education shows greater promise in treating low back pain than the corrective approach.[6] Another case study combines philosophic counseling and Rolfing manual therapy for the treatment of amyotrophic lateral sclerosis.[5] In this study, an assessment protocol was used in conjunction with the principles of intervention to demonstrate how a holistic approach that is sensitive to the whole person can improve function by changing a patient's world view.

Professional Organization

The Rolf Institute is the professional membership organization for Rolfers and the international headquarters for Rolfing training and research. It is located at 205 Canyon Boulevard, Boulder, CO 80302, USA (800-530-8875). The Internet address is www.rolf.org. The Rolf Institute is the sole certifying agency for the Rolfing method of Structural Integration. Rolfing is taught at many locations in America and around the world. There are affiliated training centers in Munich, Germany, and Sao Paulo, Brazil. Inquiries should be directed to the Rolf Institute in Boulder, Colorado.

References

1. Bond M: *Rolfing movement integration: a self-help approach to balancing the body,* Rochester, Vt, 1993, Healing Arts Press.
2. Bortoft H: *The wholeness of nature: Goethe's way toward a science of conscious participation in nature,* New York, 1996, Lindisfarne Press.
3. Cottingham JT: *Effects of soft tissue mobilization on pelvic inclination angle, lumbar lordosis, and parasympathetic tone,* Bethesda, Md, 1992, National Center of Medical Rehabilitation Research of the National Institute of Health.
4. Cottingham JT: *Healing through touch: a history and review of the physiological evidence,* Boulder, Colo, 1985, Rolf Institute.
5. Cottingham JT, Maitland JA: Integrating manual and movement therapy with philosophical counseling for treatment of a patient with amyotrophic lateral sclerosis: a case study that explores the principles of holistic intervention, *Altern Ther Health Med* 6(2):120, 2000.
6. Cottingham JT, Maitland JA: Three-paradigm treatment model using soft tissue mobilization and guided movement-awareness techniques for a patient with chronic low back pain: a case study, *J Orthop Sports Phys Ther* 26:155, 1997.
7. Cottingham JT, Porges SW, Lyon T: Soft tissue mobilization (Rolfing pelvic lift) and associated changes in parasympathetic tone in two age groups, *Phys Ther* 68:352, 1988.
8. Cottingham JT, Porges SW, Richmond K: Shifts in pelvic inclination angle and parasympathetic tone produced by Rolfing soft tissue manipulation, *Phys Ther* 68:1364, 1988.

9. Feitis R: *Ida Rolf talks about Rolfing and physical reality,* New York, 1978, Harper and Row.

10. Flury H: *Die neue Leichtigkeit des Körpers: Grundlegen der normalen Bewegung Übungen und Selbsthilfe für Alltag und Freizeit.* München, 1995, Deutscher Taschenbuch Verlag GmbH & Co.

11. Hunt V, Massey W: *A study of structural integration from a neuromuscular energy field and emotional approaches,* Boulder, Colo, 1977, Rolf Institute.

12. Kendall FP, McCreary EK: *Muscles, testing and function,* ed 3, Baltimore, 1983, Williams & Wilkins.

13. Lakoff G, Johnson M: *Philosophy in the flesh: the embodied mind and its challenge to western thought,* New York, 1999, Basic Books.

14. Levine PA: *Waking the tiger—healing trauma,* Berkeley, Calif, 1997, North Atlantic Books.

15. Maitland JA: Moving toward our evolutionary potential, *Rolf Lines* 24(2):5, 1996.

16. Maitland JA: *Radical somatics and philosophical counseling.* Invited paper presented at the Annual Meetings of the Eastern Division of the American Philosophical Association, Washington, DC, December 29, 1998.

17. Maitland JA: *Spacious body: explorations in somatic ontology,* Berkeley, Calif, 1995, North Atlantic Books.

18. Maitland JA: *Spinal manipulation made simple: a manual of soft tissue techniques,* Berkeley, Calif, 2001, North Atlantic Books.

19. Maitland JA, Sultan J: Definition and principles of Rolfing, *Rolf Lines* 20(2):16, 1992.

20. Newton AC: Basic concepts in the theory of Hubert Godard, *Rolf Lines* 23(2):32, 1995.

21. Oschman JL: *Readings on the scientific basis of bodywork,* Dover, NH, 1997, Nature's Own Research Association.

22. Oschman JL: Structure and properties of ground substances, *Am Zoolog* 24:199, 1984.

23. Rolf IP: *Rolfing: the integration of human structures,* Santa Monica, Calif, 1977, Dennis-Landman Publications.

24. Rolf IP: Structural integration: a contribution to the understanding of stress, *Confin Psychiatr* 16(2):69, 1973.

25. Salveson M: *Rolfing. Groundworks: narratives of embodiment,* Berkeley, Calif, 1997, North Atlantic Books.

26. Sultan JH: *Towards a structural logic: notes on structural integration* 1:12, 1986.

27. Varela J, Thompson E, Rosch E: *The embodied mind: cognitive science and human experience,* Cambridge, Mass, 1991, MIT Press.

6

Applied Kinesiology

DAVID S. WALTHER

Applied kinesiology (AK) is a system of examination that evaluates normal and abnormal body function and helps bring together many complementary therapeutic disciplines. It deals best with functional disorders that are caused by disturbance in physiopathology rather than structural pathology in which there is an underlying anatomic or biochemical lesion causing disease. Functional conditions develop because of altered activity in the nervous and neuromuscular systems. Common clinical conditions are back and neck pain, general body pain, gastrointestinal disturbances, autoimmune conditions, fatigue and exhaustion, and anxiety and depression states. Because AK can determine what treatment will return the altered state to proper function, the optimal form of treatment can often be determined by this examination method.

AK is differentiated from kinesiology, which is *the study of the principles of mechanics and anatomy in relation to human movement.*[1-3] Coaches and athletic trainers are the primary users of academic kinesiology for enhanced function in sports. AK uses these same principles but broadens their application into the examination and treatment of health problems. Many treatment methods established outside of AK are used in this broadened treatment, and some new methods have been developed within its framework.

AK originated when George J. Goodheart Jr., DC, of Detroit, Michigan, was examining a patient's shoulder problem.[3] Structurally, the scapula flared away from the thorax. The serratus anterior muscle tested exceptionally weak although there was no muscle atrophy, and the muscle appeared to be normal with the exception of small nodules at its origin. In the process of palpating the nodules to determine their characteristics, Goodheart noticed that with continued palpation the nodules disappeared and the muscle immediately tested strong. The scapula no longer flared away from the thorax and was symmetrical with the other side. The patient's shoulder problem was eliminated, and normal muscle function persisted on follow-up examination with no further treatment. This treatment method was called the *origin and insertion technique,* and Goodheart presented it, along with specific muscle testing protocol patterned after Kendall and colleagues,[7] at the inaugural meeting of the American Chiropractic Association in 1964.

After Goodheart's presentation a small group of chiropractors added manual muscle testing to their general examination procedures. The origin and insertion technique provided dramatic relief with enough consistency to encourage continued muscle testing, but examiners performing manual muscle testing often observed dysfunction in which the muscle did not have small nodules at the origin and insertion point and thus did not respond to that technique. Over time practitioners found many therapeutic procedures from different disciplines that returned a weak muscle to a normal state. Because of this success, AK has become an interdisciplinary examination approach, drawing together the core elements of complementary therapies and creating a more unified approach to the diagnosis and treatment of functional illness.

Basic to AK is the manual muscle test, which evaluates the ability of a muscle and the nervous system to adapt to changing pressure applied by the examiner. Early in the development of AK, practitioners were able to locate muscles that tested weak in comparison with patients' other muscles. When this type of dysfunction was found the muscle was designated as "weak," a term that is still used although it is now considered inappropriate. A muscle that tests weak on manual muscle testing usually produces adequate power when tested against a dynamometer. The manual muscle test evaluates how the nervous system modifies muscle function to meet the changing demands of the examiner's timing and application of force against the muscle's resistance. The terms replacing *weak* and *strong* are *functionally inhibited* and *normally facilitated,* respectively.

Manual muscle testing (Figure 6-1) is both a science and an art. To do manual muscle testing prop-

erly, the examiner must be well trained in the scientific aspects of testing, including anatomy, physiology, and neurology of muscle function. A major objective is to isolate the muscle being tested by placing it at its greatest mechanical advantage, and concurrently placing any synergistic muscles at a disadvantage. Once the physician has sufficient knowledge of the scientific aspects of manual muscle testing, the *art* must be developed. In addition to developing the skill to perceive the muscle's function, the examiner must develop the ability to control speed, which must be reproducible from test to test. A physician does not have to be of large stature; when muscle testing is done correctly, it does not require a lot of applied force. The following factors must be carefully considered when testing muscles in clinical and research settings:

- Proper patient positioning, ensuring that the test muscle is the prime mover and synergistic muscles are at a disadvantage
- Adequate patient stabilization, ensuring that the test muscle is functioning from a stable base
- Observation of the patient's effort to change the test parameters to recruit synergistic muscles

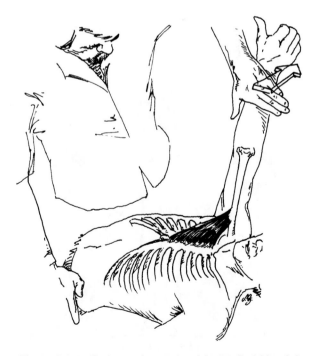

Figure 6-1 Typical muscle test used in applied kinesiology. (Courtesy Systems DC.)

- Consistent test timing, pressure, and maintenance of the test position
- Avoidance of examiner's preconceived impressions regarding the test outcome
- Avoidance of patient pain caused by the examiner's contact over bony surfaces or resulting from the patient's condition

APPLIED KINESIOLOGY LOGO AND PHILOSOPHY

The AK logo represents basic principles and some of the treatment methods used in the discipline (Figure 6-2). AK originated with the analysis of posture and movement, and it remains a primary consideration. The person standing in the center of the logo represents this analysis. The triad surrounding the man represents the *structure, chemical,* and *mental* or *spiritual* factors. AK recognizes that disturbance in any side of the triad can disturb health. Finally, there are five circles representing the initial basic treatment methods used in AK.

Structure

The first step in an examination by an applied kinesiologist is usually the evaluation of posture and movement. With proper muscle function, standing postural alignment is level when viewed from anterior to posterior; when viewed laterally, specific points of the body are in alignment with a plumb line.

Deviation from normal posture is often secondary to muscle weakness. Hypertonic-shortened muscles are often secondary to antagonist muscles that test weak on manual muscle testing (Figure 6-3). When the muscle is strengthened by whatever treatment technique is indicated, the hypertonic-shortened muscle returns to normal (Figure 6-4). This often produces dramatic relief in patients who previously were unresponsive or obtained only temporary improvement when treatment was directed to the hypertonic muscle, which was the common treatment because the hypertonic muscle manifests the pain.

AK is a receptor-based examination of the nervous system and other systems that control or influence health. Postural distortion is often caused by improper receptor (proprioceptor) stimulation from the joints or other areas of the body, causing muscle dysfunction. When postural distortion develops, it causes further improper stimulation of the receptors in joints and other areas of the body, compounding the problem.

With the increased neurologic disorganization that develops from the structural deviation, movement is disturbed. Whatmore and Kohli[20] use the term *dysponesis* to describe this type of disturbance. Dysponesis is "a reversible physiopathologic state consisting of unnoticed, misdirected neurophysio-

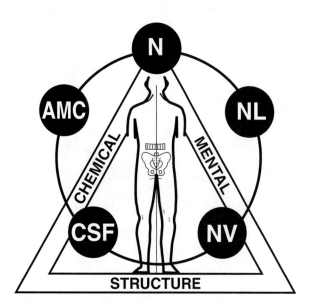

Figure 6-2 Applied kinesiology logo.

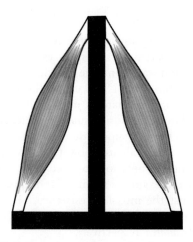

Figure 6-3 Balanced muscles maintain structural balance. (Courtesy Systems DC.)

logic reactions to various agents (environmental events, bodily sensations, emotions and thoughts) and the repercussions of these reactions throughout the organism."[1]

The initial postural analysis considers the position of the head, shoulders, arms, trunk, pelvis, legs, and feet. Is one shoulder higher or more forward than the other? Is the head level? Is one arm rotated internally more than the other? Is the pelvis level? Finally, the feet and their function during walking are evaluated.

One of the first areas evaluated is whether the head is level and whether it is in front of or behind the plumb line. Functional balance here is particularly important because the nerve receptors of the neck provide some of the most important proprioceptor information for the maintenance of equilibrium.[5] Also in the ligaments of the upper neck area are the head-on-neck reflexes that must organize with the visual righting and vestibular (inner ear) reflexes. Disorganization within these reflexes causes neurologic disorganization that can manifest as health problems almost anywhere in the body.

Another very important area of structural evaluation is the feet. The neurologic receptors in the feet are stimulated by weight bearing and facilitate the postural muscles used to stand upright.[4] The spinal cord pattern generator involved in gait also receives input from the receptors in the feet.[11] An applied kinesiologist may find that foot dysfunction is the cause of a person's shoulder pain, headache, or back

pain. Posture improves as muscle function is returned to normal, thus removing strain that may be causing improper nerve receptor stimulation almost anywhere in the body.

TRIAD OF HEALTH

The triad of health, consisting of structural, chemical, and mental or spiritual factors, is embraced by AK to explain the cause of health problems (Figure 6-5). The founder of chiropractic, D.D. Palmer,[14] and many others have described the triad. It represents aspects that influence health, which can be lost or gained through any side of the triad.

One of the problems in health care today is that, because there is so much knowledge available, physicians tend to specialize, which often limits their practice to one side of the triad.

Structural

The importance of structure in AK is emphasized by its location at the base of the triad (Figure 6-6). Doctors specializing in structure are usually orthopedists, classical osteopaths, and chiropractors. Patients often seek a structurally oriented doctor because of

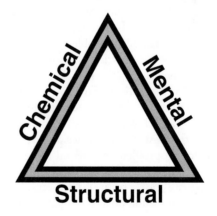

Figure 6-5 Triad of health.

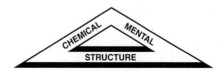

Figure 6-6 Structural emphasis.

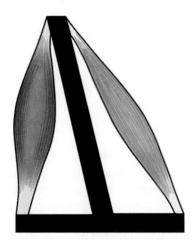

Figure 6-4 Structure deviates away from weak muscle toward the normal antagonist muscle. (Courtesy Systems DC.)

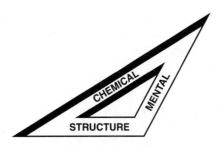

Figure 6-7 Chemical emphasis.

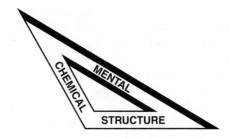

Figure 6-8 Mental emphasis.

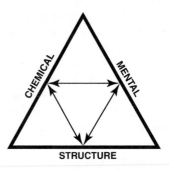

Figure 6-9 Optimal examination considers all three sides of the triad. Most chronic conditions have interplay between all sides of the triad.

trauma, such as a lifting injury, fall, or auto accident. In these acute situations, a chiropractic manipulation of the sacroiliac may rapidly return the person to normal. If there is a disc herniation, it may respond to the conservative chiropractic approach or, in some cases, may require surgical correction by an orthopedic surgeon. In chronic or unresponsive structural conditions, the answer to the problem may be found in the triad of health. For example, many people have chronic recurring sacroiliac joint dysfunction that responds only temporarily to chiropractic manipulative efforts. The applied kinesiologist may find poor function of the sartorius or gracilis muscles that provide anterior support to the innominate (pelvic bone), allowing it to rotate at the sacroiliac articulation. Manipulation may return the innominate to the normal position, but if the primary cause of muscle involvement is not corrected the patient is vulnerable to recurrence of the sacroiliac problem. AK describes an association between muscles, the soma, organs and glands, and the viscera (the muscle–organ/gland association). For example, dysfunction of the sartorius and gracilis muscles is associated with adrenal stress that may be caused by either the chemical or mental side of the triad. An applied kinesiologist may find a sugar handling problem or mental stress, either of which can cause an adrenal stress disorder; thus the underlying cause of a recurrent structural sacroiliac problem may be found on another side of the triad of health.

Chemical

Although the allopathic physician dominates the chemical side of the triad of health (Figure 6-7), nutritionists are rapidly gaining respect in this arena. The difference between the two is that the allopathic physician uses drugs to control, regulate, or otherwise overcome dysfunction, whereas the nutritionist uses natural supplements to provide raw material for the body to build tissue, produce neurotransmitters, and otherwise return to homeostasis. The nutritionist's use of mega dosages of a vitamin is similar to the allopathic physician's use of medicine. Herbs are often used as a natural form of medication.

The chemically oriented physician often attempts to control the other sides of the triad by medication, such as muscle relaxants and analgesics for structural faults or antidepressants for the triad's mental side. Such treatments don't necessarily address the root cause of the problem.

Mental

Psychiatrists, psychologists, and counselors of various types have dominated the triad's mental side (Figure 6-8). Physicians who have a strong "personality dominated" practice often influence this side of the triad.

Many conditions rooted in the mental side of the triad respond to the balanced approach of AK. An example is the child who has problems in school because of attention deficit hyperactivity disorder. The

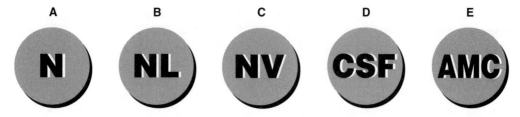

Figure 6-10 Five factors of treatment: **A,** Nerve. **B,** Neurolymphatic. **C,** Neurovascular. **D,** Cerebrospinal fluid. **E,** Acupuncture meridian system.

cause of this problem may be found in neurologic disorganization (sometimes structurally caused), food or additive sensitivity, or adrenal stress disorder, among other causes. It is important to find the cause of the problem, not merely to treat the symptoms.

Interplay Within the Triad

Although health problems usually develop on one side of the triad of health, over time the initial problem usually involves the other two sides (Figure 6-9). Although cervical trauma caused by the whiplash dynamics of a motor vehicle accident is initially a structural problem, it can ultimately affect the other sides of the triad. The trauma can disturb the relationship between the head-on-neck, visual righting, and vestibular reflexes, causing neurologic disorganization that can ultimately affect integration of movement almost any place in the body. In addition, disturbance of the craniosacral primary respiratory system (discussed later; see also Chapter 1) can lead to subtle entrapment of the vagus nerve, disturbing digestive and endocrine function and thus affecting the chemical side of the triad of health. Over time additional symptoms develop and many doctors may attend the patient. As the problems increase, the patient may become depressed and be treated with antidepressants. The condition now involves all three sides of the triad.

FIVE FACTORS OF TREATMENT

The five small circles of the AK logo represent the early treatments that Goodheart found effective for muscle dysfunction (see Figure 6-2). The integration of some of these treatments led to a muscle–organ/gland association. Because Goodheart was a chiropractor, he associated these five factors with the in-

tervertebral foramen; they are often called the *five factors of the intervertebral foramen* in AK. Although the number of techniques used by applied kinesiologists has grown during the years since Goodheart founded the practice, most of them still fall under these five factors (Figure 6-10).

Nerve

Because AK is a nerve receptor–based examination technique, the nervous system is the basis for all AK examination. The International College of Applied Kinesiology (ICAK)-USA Chapter[6] lists the following stimuli to the nervous system as among those that have been observed in clinical practice to alter the outcome of a manual muscle test:

- Transient directional force applied to the spine, pelvis, cranium, and extremities
- Stretching muscle, joint, ligament, and tendon
- The patient's digital contact over the skin of a suspect area of dysfunction, known as *therapy localization*
- Repetitive contraction of muscle or motion of a joint
- Gustatory stimulation, usually by nutritional material
- A phase of diaphragmatic respiration
- The patient's mental visualization of an emotional, motor, or sensory stressor activity
- Response to other sensory stimuli, such as touch, nociceptor, hot, cold, visual, auditory, and vestibular

All of these stimuli are mediated through the nervous system. AK is considered as examining functional neurology.

Neurolymphatic Reflexes

The *NL* circle in the logo (Figure 6-10, *B*) represents neurolymphatic reflexes. These reflexes are based on reflexes described by Frank Chapman, DO, in the 1930s.[16] He described these reflexes (now also known as *Chapman's reflexes*) as points on the body that influence lymphatic drainage of specific organs and glands and are associated with different types of health problems. Goodheart found that stimulating these reflexes often returned a weak muscle to normal. These reflexes are referred to as *neurolymphatic reflexes* in AK.

Neurovascular Reflexes

The *NV* circle in the logo (Figure 6-10, *C*) represents neurovascular reflexes. In the early 1930s, Terrence Bennett, DC, discovered locations about the head and body that he proposed influenced the vascular supply of different organs and structures. Ralph J. Martin, DC, has brought this work to print by quoting from Bennett's work[9,10] and expanding on it. During the mid-1960s Goodheart found that stimulation to these reflexes returned specific weak muscles to normal function in some cases. Most of the Bennett reflexes that Goodheart found to be associated with muscle weakness were located about the head. A specific muscle responded to only one reflex, but most reflexes influenced more than one muscle. Bennett's reflexes are referred to as *neurovascular reflexes* in AK. The association of the neurovascular reflex with muscle function appeared to relate to the ectodermal folding of the embryo and the association of the general nervous system with skin receptors. Goodheart's association of muscle dysfunction with Bennett's reflexes, along with the discovery of therapy localization (discussed later), added an objective evaluation of the reflexes that determines when treatment is necessary and whether it is effective. This enhanced both Bennett's and Goodheart's work.

Cerebrospinal Fluid

The craniosacral *primary respiratory mechanism* described by W.G. Sutherland, DO, is represented in the five factors by the *CSF* circle (Figure 6-10, *D*). *CSF* is an acronym for *cerebrospinal fluid*.[16] Many others, including Major DeJarnette, DC, in chiropractic and Harold Magoun, DO, and John Upledger, DO, in osteopathy, have discussed dysfunction of the craniosacral primary respiratory mechanism. Dysfunction within this system is thought to cause muscle dysfunction throughout the body. Movement of the cranial bones and meninges is enhanced by thoracic respiration, as objectively measured by Viola Frymann, DO.[2] In AK,

a muscle that tests weak and regains strength on a deep inspiration, expiration, or other specific phase of respiration indicates disturbance in the craniosacral primary respiratory mechanism. Examination of this system, along with general dural tension, often reveals important treatment needed in AK.

Acupuncture Meridian System

Imbalance within the acupuncture meridian system, represented by the *AMC* circle in the logo (Figure 6-10, *E*), can be responsible for muscle weakness. Balancing the Chi in the meridian system returns weak or hypertonic muscles to normal. Initially, diagnosis and treatment of the meridian system were done with standard acupuncture techniques; however, several meridian examination and treatment techniques have developed in AK.

As meridian imbalance was correlated with the results of manual muscle testing, specific muscle weakness was correlated with specific meridian imbalance. The pattern of muscle–organ/gland association of the meridians often paralleled the relation previously noted with Chapman's and Bennett's reflexes, thus enhancing the relationship. These correlations, along with clinical observation, established the muscle–organ/gland association of AK.

MUSCLE–ORGAN/GLAND ASSOCIATION

Specific muscle weakness is often an indication of an associated organ or gland disturbance. Among the associations are the tensor fascia lata muscle with the colon, pectoralis major (clavicular division) with the stomach, and quadriceps muscles with the small intestine. The muscle–organ/gland relationship of AK is clinically valuable, but is not considered absolute. It is considered "body language," indicating what *may* be taking place in the body. Muscle weakness may be considered in the same light, as an observation of paleness of the interior eyelid capillaries and a pale complexion. This observation suggests that the physician should test for anemia, but without confirming blood tests it does not mean the patient is anemic.

When the quadriceps muscles test weak, it does not necessarily mean there is a problem in the small intestine; however, it gives the physician an indication to further consider possible involvement. On the other hand, when a peptic ulcer is confirmed by a radiologic study, the pectoralis major (clavicular division) does not necessarily test weak. Further AK tests may reveal the stomach meridian is overactive as the body attempts to heal the ulcer; consequently, the associated muscle tests strong.

THERAPY LOCALIZATION

When a patient touches an area of the body where there is dysfunction, the results of manual muscle testing change. This change in the result of testing is known as *therapy localization;* it indicates something is wrong, but does not indicate what is wrong. From this point the physician must apply further muscle testing and exercise diagnostic skills. There are many therapy localization applications that determine why a muscle tests weak. For example, when the quadriceps muscles test weak the physician can ask the patient to touch the skin at the location of the associated neurolymphatic reflex; if the muscles now test strong, this indicates that the patient will benefit from stimulation of the reflex. Therapy localization can be used to determine further if the reflex has been adequately stimulated. If the now strong quadriceps muscles weaken when the patient touches the neurolymphatic reflex, further reflex stimulation is necessary. When a strong muscle becomes weak with therapy localization to the reflex, the muscle is considered subclinically weak.

The exact physiology of therapy localization is unknown. It is thought to have its effect by stimulation of cutaneous nerve receptors, but there is obviously more to it than that. It appears that energy is passed to or away from the area of therapy localization; it may be electromagnetic. If a patient holds an electrode connected to a wire that is connected to the point being localized, the results are the same as if the patient were touching the point. Polarity seems to be involved, because touching with the palmar or dorsal surface of the hands often does not give the same results. The apparent energy of therapy localization cannot pass through a thin foil of lead or certain types of ceramics, but it usually passes through several layers of natural fabric.

Therapy localization and manual muscle testing provide an extra dimension that supplements the physician's other methods of examination, especially examination of functional conditions.

INTERPRETING MANUAL MUSCLE TESTS

Many types of stimuli have the ability to alter the outcome of a manual muscle test. The muscle may test stronger or weaker, depending on the patient's condition and type of stimulation. Analysis of the change correlated with other examination findings helps identify the optimal treatment for returning the patient to homeostasis. Some of the stimuli that change muscle function are as follows[6]:

- Myofascial dysfunction (microavulsion and proprioceptive dysfunction)
- Peripheral nerve entrapment
- Spinal segmental facilitation and deafferentation
- Neurologic disorganization
- Viscerosomatic relationships (aberrant autonomic reflexes)
- Nutritional inadequacy
- Toxic chemical influences
- Dysfunction in the production and circulation of cerebrospinal fluid
- Adverse mechanical tension in the meningeal membranes
- Meridian system imbalance
- Lymphatic and vascular impairment

The AK examination is integrated with the physician's routine examination procedures. The following example elaborates on the recurrent sacroiliac problem presented previously.

A typical patient seeks help for low back pain that developed one week previously, when he stooped to pick up a box. The patient's history and review of symptoms reveal that the low back pain has occurred before. At that time he took analgesics and muscle relaxants prescribed by his physician, and rested until the pain was relieved. This time the pain is getting worse rather than diminishing, and is now radiating down the back of his leg to the knee. The patient denies other health problems. His family history includes adult onset diabetes suffered by his father, who died of a heart attack. On his mother's side there is history of alcoholism. During examination, the blood pressure is 156/92 sitting and 140/90 standing. Bechterew, Lindner seated, straight leg raise, and Bragard tests are negative for sciatic radiation, but the Bechterew and straight leg raise tests cause increased pain in the sacroiliac joint. Deep tendon reflexes and sensation are normal, and the tibialis anterior and extensor hallucis longus are strong (the AK protocol for intervertebral disc evaluation mentions other procedures that are not applicable to this case). Gaenslen and Fabere-Patrick tests cause pain in the sacroiliac joint and some increase in leg pain. Mennell's sign is positive. Additional tests fail to indicate intervertebral disc involvement or other cause for radiculopathy causing the leg pain. There is indication of a sacroiliac lesion with referred pain down the leg from the joint receptors. Further AK testing reveals that the gracilis and sartorius muscles are weak. Therapy localization to the neurolymphatic and neurovascular reflexes returns strength to the muscles on testing. Palpation of the muscles' origin and insertion reveals extreme tenderness. On observing this pain, the patient exclaims that he has had a lot of pain in that knee lately. The examiner remarks, "You said during history taking that you don't have any joint pain in your extremities." The patient replies, "I didn't think it was important for fixing my back, which is why I'm here." The examiner explains how the sartorius and gracilis muscles provide support to the innominate bone and the knee. The lack of support allows structural strain to develop in the sacroiliac and knee, causing pain. Further explanation is given about the relation of the sartorius and gracilis muscles with adrenal stress disorder. The positive findings of adrenal stress disorder, such as the blood pressure drop on standing, tenderness at the posterior eleventh rib (Rogoff's sign), pupillary response to light, and AK's ligament stretch reaction test, are explained. The patient admits to getting dizzy for a short time when rising to a standing position, and that bright light has been bothering his eyes to the extent that he wears sunglasses. Further questioning reveals that the patient has been under a lot of stress lately, drinking a lot of beer and coffee and smoking more heavily. The relation of adrenal stress disorder, hyperinsulinemia, followed by insulin resistance, and finally the cardiovascular problems of syndrome X are discussed with the patient. At this time he admits his last blood test indicated borderline diabetes and he recognizes that the series of events he is now experiencing led to his father's death.

This patient came in for relief of back pain, relief that he could not obtain from the previous approach of analgesics, muscle relaxants, and rest. The AK approach of probing into the cause of dysfunction has found involvement on all three sides of the triad of health. This has brought the patient to consider the need for correction of far more serious problems to avoid the series of events that took his father's life.

Finding the cause and correcting the adrenal stress disorder by AK examination and treatment follows a similarly structured step-by-step functional analysis of the hypothalamus-pituitary-adrenal axis. Treatment for adrenal stress disorder is not the same

for every patient. Treatment may be directed to any side of the triad of health or, as in this case, all sides. AK examination proceeds as the patient improves, and treatment is redirected as necessary.

INTERNATIONAL COLLEGE OF APPLIED KINESIOLOGY

The techniques of examination and treatment used in AK are presented in organized syllabi and individual lectures by certified teachers of the ICAK and in textbooks on the subject.[17-19] Texts on complementary therapeutic disciplines often have considerable AK information,[8] and George Goodheart, DC, continues to present his new findings at the ICAK meetings and in periodic Applied Kinesiology Workshop Procedural Manuals.

The ICAK,[6] chartered in 1976, is an organization of physicians whose main purpose is to improve and expand the scientific use of AK in determining the cause of health problems. Membership in the ICAK is open to all who have studied the subject in approved courses and are licensed as primary health care providers. There are chapters throughout most of the world. The U.S. chapter (ICAK-USA) consists mostly of chiropractors; other chapters consist of a more homogenous mixture of medical doctors, osteopaths, dentists, chiropractors, and other health care disciplines. At a recent ICAK-USA annual meeting, an orthopedic surgeon from another country related, "I am now treating conditions with AK that I used to have to do surgery on."

RESEARCH

Members of the ICAK present papers of their observations in clinical practice and on basic AK research. The clinical research papers provide stimulus for others to investigate, broaden, and solidify the discipline of AK. In this manner, AK has been able to encompass a large amount of effective treatment from complementary therapeutic disciplines into a unified, workable system.

The ICAK-USA, along with the Foundation for Allied Conservative Therapies Research, provides grants for basic research on AK. A recent literature review of AK research has been published by Motyka and Yanuck,[12] and a neurologic overview of the subject has been published by Schmitt and Yanuck.[15] Other references can be found at www.icakusa.com.

TRAINING

AK is taught by ICAK-certified teachers only to doctors licensed as primary health care providers. This is necessary because AK examination must be integrated with the standard methods of examination, including patient history and physical examination as well as laboratory and special testing and imaging analysis, when indicated. The teaching schedule of ICAK can be found at www.icak.com and www.icakusa.com, or from the organization's central office.[6]

References

1. *Dorland's illustrated medical dictionary,* ed 29, Philadelphia, 2000, WB Saunders.
2. Frymann VM: A study of the rhythmic motions of the living cranium, *J Am Osteopath Assoc* 70(9):928, 1971.
3. Goodheart GJ, Jr: *You'll be better—the story of applied kinesiology,* Geneva, Ohio, undated, AK Printing.
4. Gowitzke BA, Milner M: *Scientific bases of human movement,* ed 3, Baltimore, 1988, Williams & Wilkins.
5. Guyton AC, Hall JE: *Textbook of medical physiology,* ed 9, Philadelphia, 1996, WB Saunders.
6. International College of Applied Kinesiology–USA Chapter: *Status Statement.* Available at www.icakusa.com/status.html. [Accessed on 11/27/01.]
7. Kendall FP, McCreary EK, Provance PG: *Muscles—testing and function,* ed 4, Baltimore, 1993, Williams & Wilkins.
8. Maffetone P: *Complementary sports medicine,* Champaign, Ill, 1999, Human Kinetics.
9. Martin RJ, editor: *Dynamics of correction of abnormal function—Terrence J. Bennett lectures,* Sierra Madre, Calif, 1977, privately published.
10. Martin RJ: *The practice of correction of abnormal function—neurovascular dynamics (NVD),* Sierra Madre, Calif, 1983, privately published.
11. Miller S, Scott PD: The spinal locomotor generator, *Exp Brain Res* 30:387, 1977.
12. Motyka TM, Yanuck SF: Expanding the neurological examination using functional neurologic assessment, Part I: Methodological considerations, *Int J Neurosci* 97:61, 1999.
13. Owens C: *An endocrine interpretation of Chapman's reflexes,* ed 2, Beachwood, Ohio, 1963, Academy of Osteopathic Medicine.
14. Palmer DD: *The science, art and philosophy of chiropractic,* Portland, Ore, 1910, Portland Printing House.
15. Schmitt WH, Jr, Yanuck SF: Expanding the neurological examination using functional neurologic assessment: part II neurologic basis of applied kinesiology, *Int J Neurosci* 97:77, 1999.
16. Sutherland WG: *The cranial bowl,* Mankato, Minn, 1939, privately published.
17. Walther DS: *Applied kinesiology, vol 1, Basic procedures and muscle testing,* Pueblo, Colo, 1981, Systems DC.
18. Walther DS: *Applied kinesiology, vol 2, Head, neck, and jaw pain and dysfunction—the stomatognathic system,* Pueblo, Colo, 1983, Systems DC.
19. Walther DS: *Applied kinesiology synopsis,* ed 2, Pueblo, Colo, 2000, Systems DC.
20. Whatmore GB, Kohli DR: *The physiopathology and treatment of functional disorders,* New York, 1974, Grune & Stratton.

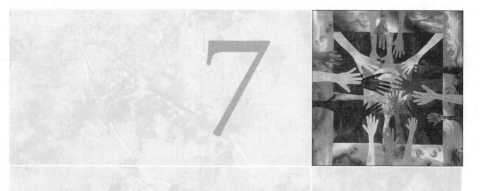

The Trager® Approach

ADRIENNE R. STONE

Medicine is not only a science, but also the art of letting our own individuality interact with the individuality of the patient.

ALBERT SCHWEITZER

HISTORY

The *Trager® Approach,* also know as *Trager Psychophysical Integration,* was developed by Milton Trager, MD, over a 70-year period of his life (1908-1997).

As a young man delivering mail for the postal service, Trager was inspired by a simple sign hanging in the post office: "Take a deep breath." He did, and later said that doing so was the beginning of his work and the first time he really felt himself intimately. It helped him to pause and shift his attention inward. He began to listen and find his internal rhythm and movement. He explored working with his body as an acrobat and later a boxer. A career in boxing never materialized, because, although he had the necessary dexterity, lightness, stamina, and strength, he never cared for the idea of beating another person.[7] However, from that experience he learned to develop a finely tuned body and created the opportunity for his evolving work to be experienced and acknowledged for the first time.

As the story goes, during his short boxing career in Chicago, Trager's trainer, Mickey Martin, gave him rubdowns after every fight. One day, Mickey looked a little tired. Trager asked Mickey to lie down on the table so he could work on him. As he worked, Mickey looked up at him and asked where he learned to do what he was doing. Trager said he was doing what Mickey usually did for him. Mickey looked at him and said, "I don't know what you're doing kid, but you sure got hands." After that experience, Trager went home and worked on his father, who had a history of sciatic pain. He was able to help his father, his first real patient, and after a few sessions was able to relieve his pain. He later quit boxing so he could better care for his hands.

Trager later moved with his family to Miami, Florida. He and his brothers practiced acrobatics on the beach. During these sessions, Trager diverged from the use of power his brothers were trying to develop. Rather than striving to jump the highest, he wanted to see "who could land the softest." This shift in thinking opened doors to new movements marked by effortlessness and a surrender of tension.[7] He also began to "play" with people on the beach who had aches and pains and with children who had polio. He taught the children to use the affected parts of their bodies without thinking about it. Soon people began to seek him out, and *Trager work* was born.

Trager soon felt that he wanted more formal training. In 1941 he received his Doctorate of Physical Medicine from the Los Angeles College of Drugless Physicians, and was certified by the California Medical Board as a Drugless Physician the same year. During World War II he worked in the Physical Therapy Department as part of his service in the Navy.[7]

It was not until Milton Trager was in his 40s that he decided to go to medical school. He very much wanted his work to be better recognized and knew that a medical degree would create greater opportunities. In spite of many obstacles, one of them being his age, he was admitted, and in 1955 he received his MD from the University Autonoma de Guadalajara in Mexico. He did his internship in Hawaii followed by a 2-year residency in psychiatry.[7]

In an interview, Dr. Trager cited one of many examples that contributed to his conclusions regarding his work. While he was doing a rotating internship at St. Francis Hospital in Honolulu, he was asked to do a history and physical examination on a very stiff 75-year-old man who was to have surgery the following day. The patient was so rigid and stiff that he couldn't turn his head, and had to turn his whole body to look in another direction. During the surgery it was necessary to turn the man, requiring several people to change his position. It wasn't that he was heavy, but extremely limp. Following surgery, Dr. Trager watched the patient while he came out of the anesthesia. By degrees he slowly came to himself, gradually returning to his original pattern of stiffness. Observing this, Trager realized that there is more to the aging process than mere changes in tissue. The pattern of aging exists more in the unconscious mind than in the tissues.

The mind is the whole thing. That is all I am interested in. I am convinced that for every physical non-yielding condition there is a psychic counterpart in the unconscious mind, corresponding exactly to the degree of the physical manifestation. . . . These patterns often develop in response to adverse circumstances such as accidents, surgery, illness, poor posture, emotional trauma, stresses of daily living, or poor movement habits. The purpose of my work is to break up these sensory and mental patterns which inhibit free movement and cause pain and disruption of normal function.[6]

As a physician, Dr. Trager had a general medical practice in Honolulu. He began his day doing one Trager session, giving his special treatment to patients who needed it.

It was not until the mid-1970s that he gave the first public demonstration of his work to a group at the Esalen Institute in California. There he met Betty Fuller, who later became his first student and the founder of The Trager Institute. Before meeting Fuller, he was uncertain that he would ever be able to teach his methods. With her encouragement he found a way to make his ideas available for others to learn.

PRINCIPLES, PHILOSOPHY, AND DIAGNOSIS

Dr. Trager's work, the Trager Approach, is a unique method of movement reeducation. It is a sensitive feeling approach that brings the client and the practitioner into a rapport that is of great benefit to each of them. This is accomplished using the language of refined touch and movement to influence psychophysical patterns in the mind and body. The purpose is to break up deep-seated patterns and resulting psychophysical compensations that inhibit free-flowing movements, cause pain, and disrupt normal function in affected areas. When blocks are released at the source (the mind), the client can experience long-lasting release and relief from these fixed patterns. The result is general functional improvement.[16]

It should be noted that the recipient of the session is referred to here as a *client* rather than a *patient* to remove any suggestion that the person receiving the work is necessarily ill.

In our society, from the time we are young children, we are taught by parents and teachers alike to try our hardest, push through obstacles, do the most we can. In the Trager Approach, things are viewed quite differently. It is about *not* trying. It is about coming back to the essential concept that "less is more," and even asking the rhetorical question, "What is nothing?" For many, it is an unlearning of many years of life's teachings. The Trager Approach is a simple concept that is totally foreign to many. It is a different way to approach life and the body. It is a wonderful alternative, often used when more traditional approaches have failed. It is training in "letting go," leading the body and mind in a new direction rather than continuing in the direction of tightening. It is about surrender.

The client is viewed as a whole being with the focus on how this person, this body-being, can be better than he or she is (without judgment). This is not about *trying* to make the person different. It is a thoughtful, feeling process. How would it be to move more freely and more effortlessly? The practitioner uses information gathered through observation and touch to make verbal and tactile (proprioceptive) suggestions to the client. The client-practitioner relationship is one of partnership. There is no *fixing;* the client must want and be willing to take responsibility for his or her health and well being.

It is important for the practitioner to consider any and all past injuries, any disease processes, and current status of the client. This information, and any other information that the client may wish to volunteer, is obtained through inquiry before a session. There is much verbal, visual, and tactile observation and evaluation. The practitioner may compare the size and weight of limbs and the feel and temperature of tissue, make observations regarding alignment, and note the client's passive (and at times active or active-assisted) mobility. This is usually done on the treatment table as part of the session. There is a "getting acquainted" period. During this initial contact there is much gentle, subtle inquiring, getting to

know where the body "holds," where it moves well, where the tissue is soft and where it is not. The areas of holding (restriction) and increased tissue density are the focus of the session. The client's reactions are monitored during this introductory phase and throughout the entire session.

Before beginning a session, the practitioner asks the client to describe any pain or discomfort that may occur during a session and any other needs he or she may have. Establishing a safe, comfortable working environment and relationship are of the utmost importance for this and any other therapeutic relationship.

During the session, the mode of working is one of exploration, nonjudgment, and grace. The Trager Approach is about offering movement suggestions to the body via pleasurable feeling messages to the unconscious mind.

This approach does not make demands or require the client to go through barriers. It is about going up to the proverbial door and knocking, waiting to be let in. This is done with a soft, exquisite touch with quality that is able to capture the attention of the unconscious mind, bringing new information to the tissues, *allowing* them to change. Dr. Trager (Figure 7-1) often spoke of it as a transmission from his mind, through his hands to the patient's tissue and then to their mind. "At that moment, unbeknownst to him, he [the patient] became the therapist and sent the message to his tissue."[16] As areas of holding, tightness, and limitation are found (if present), increased attention is paid and these problems are addressed. Compensations from these holding patterns are included in the focus of the session.

One of the great benefits of this work is the experience of a sense of deep relaxation and peace that can be achieved during a session. This state is often referred to as the *byproduct* of this work. It is not something that is actively sought, but something that happens. What is so wonderful about this is that relaxation is not something that one can ever work to achieve! With so many other techniques one must go through many types of mind-engaged activities. Dr. Trager often spoke about relaxation. "Don't try! Trying is effort! To try is to fail. If there is effort we can't relax!"[14]

The noninvasive qualities of this work and the trust that is established between the client and practitioner apparently create the environment that allows this state of relaxation to emerge. It is during this state of deep relaxation and peace that healing

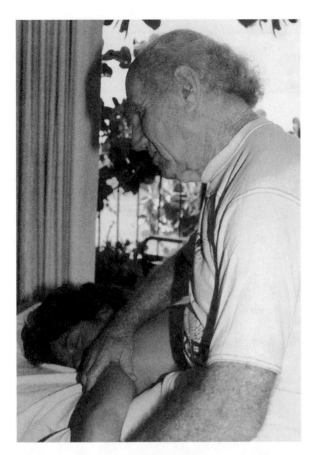

Figure 7-1 Milton Trager, MD, working on the shoulder of the contributor, during a 1983 training session in Hawaii. (From the contributor's private collection.)

occurs. It is also in this state that our immune system can be affected in a positive manner. Dr. Trager often said, "It is a feeling beyond relaxation!" When experiencing deep relaxation, people can reconnect with their own inner beings without trying. It is also an opportunity for the clients to take this experience into their being and know that it is now a part of them, available for recall any time it is desired. Dr. Trager often expressed that it was this need for reconnection with the self that was often lacking in traditional healing methods. The patient may have been given a proper diagnosis and the right medications, but without the reconnection with the self that is often lost during illness, the person cannot return to a state of good health. R.N. Remen writes,

It is only recently that illness and healing have been defined in terms of the body. At the beginning of medicine,

the shamans, or medicine men, defined illness not in terms of pathology but in terms of soul. According to these ancients, illness was "soul loss," a loss of direction, purpose, meaning, mystery and awe. Healing involved not only recovery of the body but the recovery of the soul.[11]

Recall is a very important adjunct of the Trager Approach. Once the relaxed state or the feeling of a movement is in the experience of the individual, it is part of him or her. It is then available for that person to draw upon from the unconscious, accessible at any time. Thus each session is a building block, a lesson.

The road to this peaceful experience comes from the mode of being with which the practitioner connects during a session. Dr. Trager referred to this state as *hook up*. It is a quiet, peaceful, almost meditative state that allows full sensitivity and alertness in the connection between the practitioner and the client (Figure 7-2). Trager wrote that "hook up is a state of being. It is a hook up of this power that you are surrounded by. It is a life-giving, life-regulating force that has always been there and will always be there."[15]

There are many ways to describe this state. It can be compared with looking out the window and seeing beautiful cloud formations; some may relate the feeling to remembering the first time they saw and held a newborn baby. It is the connection we see between ice-dancing couples that glide with ease in unison. For the practitioner, it is a way of being mindful that allows for focused attention and being fully present with the client. It is the role of the practitioner to help bring the client into this state. The greater the development of the practitioner the better able he or she will be to give a deeper, more integrated session.[14]

Dr. Trager discussed this essential theory regarding his approach:

The success I have had with low back pain is not because the tissues in the lumbo-sacral area were manipulated in a special way. It has come because I have succeeded in reaching the psycho-physiological components. I never tell my hands what to do. I hook up and I go. My job is to impart to my patient what it is like to be right in the sense of a functionally integrated body-mind. This is transmitted, I feel, through the autonomic nervous system from the therapist's mind, through his hands, to the involved areas. This feeling is picked up by the patient's mind because of the manner in which the tissues are worked, creating the feeling of relaxation. In this way, the sensory feedback, which maintains the psychic component of

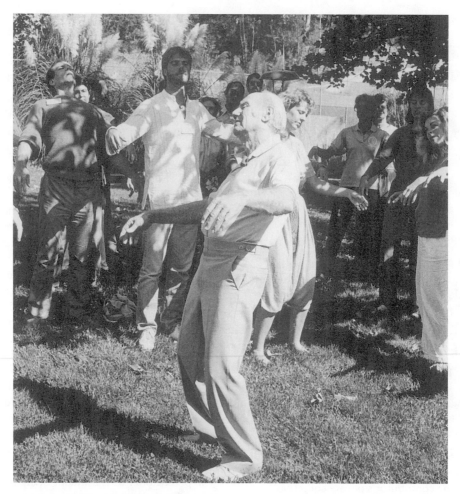

Figure 7-2 Milton Trager, MD, practicing Mentastics with his students, with deep sense of hook up. (From the contibutor's private collection.)

muscle spasm, is broken. Until this feeling reaches the patient, no lasting results can be expected. It is the manner in which I work, not necessarily the technique that I use, which brings about the change. Every move, every pressure of my hands, every thought, is directed towards bringing new feeling experiences to the unconscious mind of how the affected area should feel. The holding pattern is then broken.[14]

It is the beginning of a change in the direction of loosening and freedom of movement rather than continuing in the direction of tightness and dysfunction.

In the Trager Approach, diagnosis is not separate from the treatment. During a Trager session there is an ongoing interaction between the client and the practitioner. Information obtained during the ses-

sion provides the practitioner with the information needed to develop a diagnostic impression at the end of the session. Although some Trager practitioners have additional training and may use other diagnostic examinations that help guide their Trager sessions, such examinations are not an integral part of the Trager session or the Trager training.

Trager work provides a context in which the client may learn to recognize and release deep-seated unconscious, physical, or emotional holding patterns that may have developed as the result of accident, injury, poor postural habits, or trauma. Goals of Trager work include decreased muscular tightness, increased mobility and flexibility, greater resiliency and ease of being, improved alignment, enhanced conscious awareness, the experience of total relaxation and peace, and a sense of a functionally integrated body and mind. This process involves sending many positive feeling experiences to the unconscious mind to offset the negative, allowing the positive to take over.

PRACTICES, TECHNIQUES, AND TREATMENT

There is no actual technique with Trager work, no set formulas. It is an approach to being with the body. There is a basic design of moves that is a suggested order to working with the body. This is open to modifications as necessary. The client's body guides the practitioner with the component of hook up. An average session lasts between 60 and 90 minutes. The following components may be included.

Components of a Trager Session

Table Work

Most of the session takes place on a padded treatment table. The client is comfortably dressed in loose fitting clothing or underwear. What is most important is that the client feels safe and at ease. It is important to remember that the practitioner is addressing the unconscious mind. From the very beginning, all input must be congruent, reinforcing safety and comfort.

No oils or lotions are used. Using "soft hands" to guide a series of gentle, noninvasive motions of joints and muscles, the body is moved through its full available (pain free) range of movement. This gentle motion uses the weight of the body to help it treat itself, set in motion by the practitioner. The rhythm of movement is derived from the client and picked up by the practitioner as he or she takes that individual body through its available excursion of motion through hook up. The softness of touch is primary, because it is the vehicle at the beginning of the feedback loop between the mind and the muscles. Every touch relays information. Any hardness of touch gives the wrong message. It is essential to avoid the need for the client to clench or tighten. Softness and quality touch help avoid tightening and help capture the attention of the unconscious mind.

With a combination of gentle shaking, rocking, jiggling, oscillations, and shimmering, the joints and tissues are explored. The practitioner looks for areas of guarding, tightness, and increased tissue density. These areas, when found, are the focus of the session. There is a quality of working with the unconscious in a mode that almost teases. With the aforementioned actions, including repetition and slight variation of motions made as adjustments to the changing status of the tissue that are too complex for the client to figure out, the body and mind will begin to surrender. Movements and gestures are used to coax and suggest softness and freedom of movement to the unconscious.

These messages to the unconscious mind differ from those of many other modalities—instead of emphasizing tightness, they seek to remind the body and mind what it might have felt like before it got tight. Because the body tends to shorten and pull inward with increased tension or stress, the session includes many movements and suggestions of lengthening, widening, and fluffing. The experience of being moved and touched in this manner is very unique. It is usually experienced as pleasurable and nurturing. The gentle rocking is often reminiscent of being rocked as an infant or young child. All of this contributes to the deep level of relaxation often achieved in a session. The benefits of the sessions are cumulative. A series of sessions with follow up reminder sessions is often recommended.

Mentastics®

Mentastics, a very significant, *active* component of Trager work, consists of mind-guided movements. Dr. Trager and his wife Emily coined the word *Mentastics* many years ago to mean "mental gymnastics." These movements are best described as light, effortless, pain-free motions that originate in the mind and are designed to help release tension from the body. Some of them resemble movements that Olympic swimmers use before an event when they "shake out" to relieve tension in their bodies so they can perform more optimally. Mentastics can be performed as an adjunct to the work begun on the table, either in a session or independently. They have the potential to enhance what was begun in a session and are a practical tool that can be integrated into daily activities.

As a practitioner of the work, I find these movements are critical to help maintain a free, comfortable body. In that way it is easier to give quality sessions with the proper attitude of softness and freedom of movement, and the sessions are more effective. These motions can be fun and easy to do, can be done any time you chose, and can be personally modified to suit almost all needs. This is true even for those in chronic pain.[13] Asking the self and discovering the correct amount of movement for the individual body without increasing pain or discomfort and perhaps relieving symptoms is the primary concept. Mentastics can be a very empowering tool for the client.

Differing from but still resembling exercise, these movements offer an initiation of motion and a release followed intermittently with a pause. This makes it somewhat different than the constant and repetitive motion of exercise. In addition, how free and effortlessly one can move (see Figure 7-2) guides the Mentastics practice, rather than concepts such as how much weight, how many repetitions, or how long a session, which are often the focus of traditional exercise. It is also an opportunity to turn the attention inward. If only for a moment, in the midst of a busy day the client can pause and "feel in" to the body. To be mindful can make a great difference.

Reflex-Response

Reflex-response is the link between relaxation and function. In this aspect of the work an *active* response is desired from the client, and may be achieved voluntarily or reflexively. It is integrated into the table work in a manner that stimulates responses without fatigue.

Follow-up work of this nature may be continued off the table as well. Instructions may also be given for a home program. A reflex-response program is indicated in cases of muscle imbalances, weakness, paralysis (without total spinal cord lesion), and balance problems. Its principles are similar to those of basic Trager work, which includes giving a feeling experience to the client that he or she is doing or performing a certain motor task and reinforcing that feeling. With this aspect of the work there is often evidence of increased strength, endurance, and improved balance.

INDICATIONS AND CONTRAINDICATIONS

Although only a few clinical studies have been published, systematic recordings of clinical experience has shown the broad application of the work, as discussed below. This approach allows for its effectiveness in such a wide variety of situations because it responds to imbalances throughout the body.[13]

Trager work has been used effectively with both acute and chronic musculoskeletal injuries and conditions, including those of the back,[17] neck, shoulder, foot, and knee. This method has been used to help people increase their body awareness and improve posture. There is potential benefit to persons with such diverse conditions as arthritis,[12] scoliosis, headaches (including migraine), frozen shoulder, temporomandibular joint, and myofascial problems. The gentle noninvasive quality of this work has been found extremely helpful in cases in which involuntary muscle-guarding patterns have developed.

Neuromuscular disorders such as cerebral palsy,[19] polio, stroke, multiple sclerosis,[5] muscular dystrophy,[8] Parkinson's disease,[10] and incomplete spinal cord lesions have been successfully addressed by experienced practitioners. Reduced spasticity and rigidity have been reported, leading to improved function. With many neuromuscular conditions there is focus on improving muscle tone (when there is too much or not enough) and then strengthening the connections between mind and muscle, which leads to greater motor function. The client is taught to recognize the correct amount of exertion. For example, in cases of central nervous system involvement, such as stroke, the practitioner may explore the importance of moderation with the client, who may otherwise exert full effort to achieve a task.

For those interested in improved general well being or for athletes wanting to enhance their performance, this work may be extremely helpful. Athletes have reported a reduction of injuries and faster recovery when injured. The work has led to smoother, more relaxed performance. In addition to providing physical benefits, Trager work has been documented as helpful in releasing the untapped potential of the mind and providing an important competitive advantage. Trager work allows clients to do the most with the least effort and offers ways to optimize mental and physical performance in daily life, not only for athletes but also for average people.[1]

Pulmonary problems such as asthma and emphysema are indications for intervention with Trager work. Increased compliance of the rib cage has been reported. In cases of sexual and physical abuse, the Trager Approach has been used to decrease pain and help clients become more comfortable in their bodies again.[4,13]

It is important to note that the Trager Approach is a very valuable tool for many types of disabilities and dysfunction. The great value of this work for personal growth and general stress reduction should be underscored. There is always room to be better.

Contraindications are few and need to be specifically modified to the individual client. These are all relative contraindications and the experienced practitioner may successfully adapt the Trager Approach to work under such conditions. Generally, the work should be avoided in acute flare-ups of arthritis; over severe varicose veins; following recent surgery (generally less than 6 to 8 weeks); fractures; and muscle, ligament, or tendon tears. During pregnancy, especially in the later stages, Trager work may be most helpful when modified by an experienced practitioner, because certain moves are best avoided.

TRAINING AND CERTIFICATION

The International Trager Association sponsors a training program that trains and certifies individuals to become Trager practitioners. Training consists of a series of classes and fieldwork, including supervised practice sessions, independent practice, and personal Trager sessions. Trager instructors are located throughout the world and provide training in many different locations.

The training program, which was revised in July 2001, requires a total of 409 hours. The program now includes two 6-day training sessions, one 5-day training session, one 6-day anatomy class, and 24 hours of Mentastics training. There is a designated period for fieldwork and evaluation.

Fieldwork requires the student to provide 90 sessions without charge and receive at least 30 sessions. A minimum of nine tutorials is also required. These are individualized, private lessons with a tutor who is trained to assess the student's progress, provide feedback, and recommend additional steps as necessary. The fieldwork is conducted according to a specific outline and schedule. Senior Practitioner status can be achieved with additional training. Additional information can be obtained through the U.S. and International Trager Associations.

RESEARCH

There have been numerous case studies to support the effectiveness of the Trager Approach. Many years ago, Dr. Thelma Moss carried out some of the first documented research regarding Trager work at UCLA. Dr. Trager was invited to be tested with Kirlian photography as he gave a session. The energy field of Dr. Trager's thumb was photographed three times. The first photograph was taken before beginning a session and showed a fully vibrant field. The second, taken 20 minutes into a short session, showed some depletion of the field. The last was taken at the end of the session, after pausing and going into hook up for 45 seconds. This photograph showed that the vibrancy of the field had returned, verifying for Trager the efficacy of hook up.[16]

In 1985, in a study done to determine the effect of Trager Psychophysical Integration on patients with documented chronic lung disease, significant changes were observed in forced vital capacity, respiratory rate, and chest expansion. Trager work was also shown to have a positive effect on the restrictive component of lung disease.[18]

A case report from 1989 reveals substantial improvement in increasing trunk and lower extremity range of motion, limited by soft tissue tightness in a 13-year-old with severe spastic diplegia.[19]

Mentastics has been studied, comparing it with traditional active relaxation exercises (AREs) using surface electromyogram electrodes. Mentastics was found at least as effective as AREs and appeared less likely to exacerbate muscle tension levels. This study demonstrated that Trager Mentastics can be a useful tool in the therapist's repertoire.[3]

Recent research in the field of psychoneuroimmunology has shown that neuropeptides and their receptors are the biochemical correlates of emotions. They mediate intercellular communication throughout the brain and the body. In theory, then, it may be possible for a certain state to affect the immune system in a positive manner, which may explain some of the beneficial affects seen with the use of the Trager Approach.[2,9] Committees are currently working to conduct further research on the Trager Approach.

References

1. Butler M: The Trager athlete, *Trager J* II:6-8, 1987.
2. Cousins N: *Head first: the biology of hope*, New York, 1989, EP Dutton.
3. Grossman L, Mascolo R, Stone A: *The effect of Trager Mentastics on upper trapezius EMG in a cervical/thoracic pain patient group*, *L*, Pain Management Center, Saint John's Hospital and Health Center, Santa Monica, CA. Poster presentation at the Sixth Annual Meeting of the American Pain Society, Washington, DC, Nov. 6-9, 1986.

4. Hoch M: Practice support, In *The Trager handbook,* Mill Valley, Calif, 1999, Trager Institute.

5. Juhan D: *Multiple sclerosis: the Trager approach.* Available at www.trager.com/articles/Multiple%20Sclerosis.htm.

6. Juhan D: The Trager approach: psychophysical integration and mentastics. In Dury N: *The bodywork book,* Dorset, England, 1984, Prism Alpha.

7. Liskin J: *Moving medicine: the life and work of Milton Trager, MD,* Barrytown, NY, 1995, Station Hill Press.

8. Molatore T, English J: Trager applied to muscular dystrophy, *Trager J* I:4-6, 1982.

9. Moyers B: *Healing and the mind,* New York, 1993, Doubleday.

10. Partridge M: *The Trager approach as an adjunct therapy to Parkinson's disease,* Presentation to Mount Sinai Hospital Department of Movement Disorders, New York, 1997.

11. Remen RN: *My grandfather's blessings,* New York, 2000, The Berkeley Publishing Group.

12. Savage FL: *Osteoarthritis: a step-by step success story to show others they can help themselves,* Barrytown, NY, 1990, Station Hill Press.

13. Stone AR: The Trager approach. In Davis CM: *Complementary therapies in rehabilitation,* Thorofare, NJ, 1997, Slack.

14. Trager M: Personal communication.

15. Trager M: *The Trager handbook,* Mill Valley, Calif, 1999, The Trager Institute.

16. Trager M: Trager psychophysical integration and Mentastics, *Trager J* I:5-9, 1982.

17. Witt P: Trager psychophysical integration: an additional tool in the treatment of chronic spinal pain and dysfunction, *Whirlpool,* 24-26, Summer 1986.

18. Witt PL, MacKinnon J: Trager psychophysical integration, a method to improve chest mobility of patients with chronic lung disease, *Phys Ther* 66(2):214-216, 1986.

19. Witt PL, Parr CA: Effectiveness of Trager psychophysical integration in promoting trunk mobility in a child with cerebral palsy: a case report, *Phys Occup Ther Pediatr* 8(4):75-94, 1988.

Supplementary Readings

Juhan D: *Job's body,* Tarrytown, NY, 1987, Station Hill Press.

Trager M: *Trager mentastics: movement as a way to agelessness,* Tarrytown, NY, 1987, Station Hill Press.

Watrous IS: The Trager approach: an effective tool for physical therapy, *Phys Ther Forum* April:10, 1992.

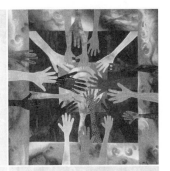

8

Feldenkrais Method

CARLA REED
JAMES STEPHENS

How did you learn to drive a car? I remember being in the car with my father, who was very impatient with mistakes, trying to master the multiple demands of operating a manual transmission automobile. While coordinating my feet on the clutch and accelerator pedals in our Volkswagen Beetle, I would look down at the gearshift to see which direction to move it. When I looked up again, I would find myself swerving off the road and my father yelling.

Now I drive my five-speed Honda Accord while I tune the radio, eat a snack, listen to a tape, talk with a passenger, and/or speak on my cell phone. However, when my teenage daughter recently got her learner's permit, I found I didn't really know how to explain what I do when I'm driving.

The *Feldenkrais Method* (FM)* is an organic learning process. The FM helps a person to spontaneously move more easily in fundamental human movements like rolling, turning, speaking, writing, and walking. It also occasions significant changes in the person's sense of self as the person is able to move more easily than he or she thought possible. The FM can be applied to basic functional issues such as how to get up and down more easily while gardening; athletic performance issues such as improving skiing skills or tennis swing; recovery from limitations acquired from an

*The terms *Feldenkrais®, Feldenkrais Method®, Awareness Through Movement®,* and *Functional Integration®* are registered service marks of *The Feldenkrais Guild®* of North America (FGNA). *Guild Certified Feldenkrais Practitioner*CM is a certification mark of FGNA.

119

accident or stroke; facilitation of basic developmental learning such as in clients with Down syndrome or cerebral palsy; communication and cognitive learning issues such as in the aftermath of closed head injury or with children known as autistic; and improvement of seemingly physiologic functions such as vision, hearing, circulation, and blood pressure.

HISTORY

Origins and Education

Moshe Feldenkrais (Figure 8-1) was born in Baranovitz, Russia, in 1904 and moved to the British Mandatory territory of Palestine in his adolescence. He studied mathematics and was a surveyor in Palestine for several years until he went to Paris to complete a degree in me-

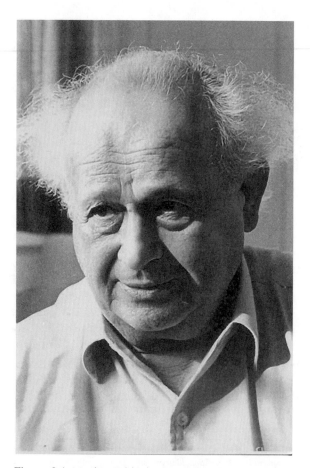

Figure 8-1 Moshe Feldenkrais, 1904-1984. (Courtesy Feldenkrais Institute, Tel Aviv, Israel.)

chanics and engineering. He read for his doctorate at the Sorbonne, where he was attached to the laboratory of Joliet-Curie. During this time, he studied judo with its creator, Professor Kano, and his pupils, gained his judo black belt, and started the Judo Club de France. He escaped to England from the Nazi occupation of France and spent the rest of World War II as a scientific officer with the British Admiralty in the antisubmarine establishment.[13]

Knee Injury and Self-Study

During his nearly 20 years in Europe, Feldenkrais exacerbated a knee injury originally incurred while playing soccer in his youth. It interfered with his walking, and surgeons at that time offered him no better than a 50% chance of recovery from an operation. He rejected those odds as scientifically unreliable and began experimenting with his own movement to determine, on the basis of his experience, how to move comfortably. This triggered the beginning of an expansive self-directed study of how people learn self-direction; this study was built on the foundation of 20 years of teaching judo and 30 years working as an engineer and physicist.[13]

Scientific Mentors

Feldenkrais was a man of enormous intellectual curiosity. He researched and integrated aspects of the existing scientific disciplines of psychology, human development, biology, evolution, and cybernetics. In his writings, Feldenkrais refers to the work of innumerable other scientists, including Salvador Luria, Ivan Pavlov, Sir Charles Sherrington, A.D. Speransky, Sigmund Freud, Paul Schilder, Sir Arthur Keith, Ernest Starling, Charles Darwin, Henri LeChatelier, Heinrich Jacoby, Jacques Monod, Konrad Lorentz, J.Z. Young, and Milton Erickson.

Russian Influence

Because his first language was Russian, Feldenkrais could access the original writings of Russian scientists unavailable or inaccessible to other Western scientists until the recent dissolution of the Union of Soviet Socialist Republics. It is interesting to speculate what perspectives existed in the Russian social and scientific milieu that may have affected the development of Feldenkrais' ideas. The concept of *disability,* for example, is often viewed in the United States as synonymous with *deficiency,* with the derogatory implication of *lack of capacity.* In the Russian literature, disabilities are referred to as *deficits,* implying impediments or obstacles to function. Russian psychologist Lev Vygotsky, for example, describes *impediment,* or *defect,* as a condition that causes a child to develop differently. This conception of disability permits people who have deficits or impediments to be viewed in much the same way any growing, living, organic entity—a tree or a plant, for instance—that must overcome an impediment to grow is viewed. If the plant cannot grow in one direction, it grows around the impediment in another direction.[7]

Asian Influence

In addition to a Russian influence, there was clearly an Eastern, or Asian, influence on Feldenkrais, resulting from his deep involvement in the study and teaching of the Japanese martial art of judo (Figure 8-2). Judo was the topic of his first two books: *Judo*[8] and *Practical Unarmed Combat,*[10] and his fourth book, *Higher Judo.*[9] Feldenkrais also investigated numerous Eastern healing practices, including acupuncture and reflexology.

THE FELDENKRAIS METHOD

Feldenkrais' first book about his evolving theories on human self-direction, *Body and Mature Behavior,*[12] was published in England in 1949, after which he returned to what was then Palestine to be the first director of the Electronic Department of the Defense Forces. He gradually ceased work as a physicist and engineer and devoted all his time to teaching individuals and groups his emerging method. His first "students" were professional peers, including Professor J.D. Bernal; Lord Boyd-Orr, first president of the World Health Organization; Professor Aaron Katzir, Director of the Weitzman Institute; and David Ben-Gurion, first Prime Minister of the State of Israel.[11] Feldenkrais taught group classes in Tel Aviv several times every week for more than 20 years, for which he

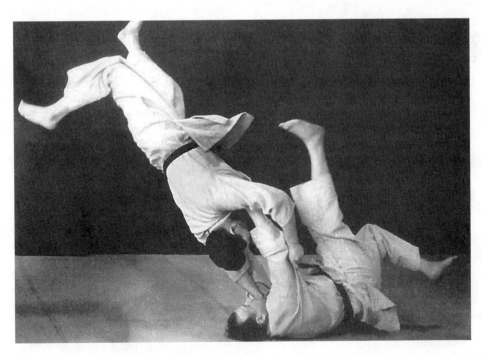

Figure 8-2 Feldenkrais at the Jiu-Jitsu Club, circa 1935. (Courtesy Feldenkrais Institute, Tel Aviv, Israel.)

created and recorded hundreds of lessons that are gradually being transcribed through agreements with his estate.

Professional Influences

In the 1970s Feldenkrais was invited to teach at the Esalen Institute in the San Francisco Bay area, where he connected with Jean Houston and others in the Human Potential movement. He developed close relationships with some of the bright minds of his time such as Margaret Mead, Karl Pribram, and Ida Rolf, and made acquaintance with other important peers such as F.M. Alexander and Milton Erickson (Figure 8-3).

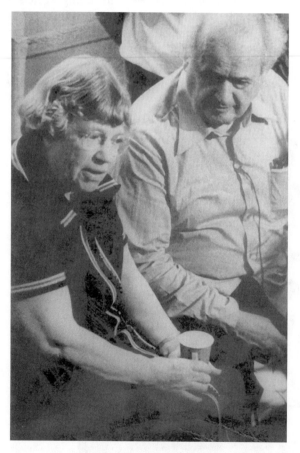

Figure 8-3 Feldenkrais with Margaret Mead, circa 1970. (Courtesy Feldenkrais Institute, Tel Aviv, Israel.)

Feldenkrais Begins to Teach His Method

The first training offered by Feldenkrais was to an apprentice group of students in Israel in the early 1970s. He taught the first North American Feldenkrais Professional Training Program (FPTP) in San Francisco from 1974 through 1977. Another FPTP was initiated in 1980 in Amherst, Massachusetts, but his senior Israeli assistants taught the program during the last 2 years of Feldenkrais' illness. Since Feldenkrais' death in 1984, training sessions have been taught by trainers authorized by The Feldenkrais Guild, which he established in 1977.

RATIONALE

An Accidental Revelation

In Feldenkrais' search for ways to function better with his damaged knees, he discovered that the role of the nervous system was enormously more significant in determining function than even the integrity of the structure. A personal experience had a profound effect on the foundations of his work, as he explained in the following passage from *The Elusive Obvious*:

I badly injured a knee while playing soccer . . . and I was incapacitated for many months. The healthy leg had to work overtime and lost much of its former flexibility and nimbleness. . . . I slipped on an oily patch on the pavement while hopping on the only leg that functioned. . . . Gradually I felt my good leg stiffen and thicken with synovial waters. My original injured knee was . . . sufficiently painful to prevent me standing on the foot. I hopped around, therefore, on the leg which I had nearly sprained. . . . I fell asleep. . . .

When I woke up . . . I could actually stand on the foot which I had been unable to use since the original troubles. The trauma of the good knee had somehow made the injured leg more usable than before. . . . How could a leg with a knee that had prevented me standing on it for several months suddenly become usable and nearly painless? . . . When the quadriceps of the leg had nearly vanished, as is usual in severe injury of the meniscus, and the thigh was visibly thinner . . . the vanished quadriceps had become suddenly toneful enough to allow me to stand on the foot . . . when physical anatomical abnormalities were clearly to be seen on the X-ray pictures. . . . The old injured leg would not straighten completely, and I leaned on the toes rather than the heel, but there was no doubt that it supported the bulk of my weight. . . .

Many years later, on reading Professor Speransky's book, *A Basis for the Theory of Medicine*,[27] it dawned on me that changes like the one I had experienced can be understood only by referring to the nervous system. . . . Inhibition of one part of the motor cortex can alter the neighboring symmetrical point even to excitation, or reduce its inhibition. . . . It seemed . . . possible to effect a change in an anatomical structure through an alteration in the functioning of the brain, which involves negligible energy, compared with one in the skeleton. Later I gathered stories of many similar happenings with other people. . . . Professor Speransky . . . gathered from medical doctors all over Russia stories of similar phenomena to the ones he observed himself. . . . He found no explanation possible outside of one involving the nervous system.[11]

Habits, Images, and Spontaneity

Thus began Feldenkrais' exploration of the nonlinear workings of the human nervous system. Structural issues seemed to operate by simple cause-and-effect rules, but the nervous system occasioned profound changes in surprising ways not explainable by the logic used to explain structures. He realized that living systems were governed by cybernetic rules in which the nervous system managed the complex interrelationships of the many parts of the self.

Furthermore, nervous reorganization occurs spontaneously to recreate a workable homeostasis that adapts to the present circumstances. A person's action pattern is activated by his or her internal image of an action (e.g., standing up, reaching for a glass of water, seeing the traffic to the rear) rather than by the specific components of that action. Each person stores images of repeatedly initiated actions, and these images become that person's database of habits. By accessing this database the person initiates often-repeated actions, such as driving a car, so spontaneously that the person is no longer aware of what he or she is actually doing or how. One of Feldenkrais' assistants, Ruthy Alon, refers to these habits as the *grammar of spontaneity*.[1] Feldenkrais said, "If you know 'what' you are doing, and even more important, 'how'

you use yourself to act, you will be able to do things the way you want."[11]

Brain Created by Experience

Feldenkrais researched biology and evolution to clarify human potential for learning. All nonhuman animals are born with their brains almost fully developed. There is very little difference between the size of most animals' brains at birth and at maturity. However, in humans the brain at birth is only a fraction of its adult size. Similarly, other animal species are born with most of their self-direction wired in—that is, inherited from the phylogenetic evolution of their kind. Most mammals get up on their legs and follow their mothers within minutes or hours of their emergence from the birth canal. However, in humans only the basic physiologic activities that sustain life, such as the beating of the heart, circulation of body fluids, breathing, and digestion, operate spontaneously at birth; other activities develop only with individual experience. In contrast with other animals, human self-direction—the ability to move the self through space in the gravitational field and effect change in the environment—is almost absent at birth; its development requires a long period of dependence while it is learned by trial and error. Feldenkrais saw this dependence during the formation of individual patterns of self-direction as the source of many of the difficulties humans encounter.[13] However, he saw enormous untapped potential in the fact that all patterns of human self-direction are learned through experience.

Organic Learning

Feldenkrais differentiated the kind of learning to which he was referring from academic training. Academic education is often designed to transmit a fixed body of information from one person to another by memorization or imitation, on a timeline defined by the instructor. However, Feldenkrais was most interested in the learning that occurred within an individual on the basis of his or her own sensory experience, which he termed *organic learning*. He noticed that the most creative people in their professions were those who continued to use organic learning to create their own ways of doing the art or skill they had chosen to pursue. Furthermore, he found that organic learning occurred in time intervals defined by the interest and attention of the learner.

Individuality of the Human Homunculus

The human brain is a reflection of the individual's experience. In his study of neurophysiologic research, Feldenkrais saw evidence that the very growth of the brain's cellular structure is strongly influenced by the experience of the person. The individuality of our ontogenetic organic learning is reflected in the homunculus. Although there is some commonality regarding where on the human cortex different body parts are represented, the actual representation in any given person is a reflection of the ways and frequency with which those parts have been moved in the life experience of that person. Feldenkrais understood the individuality of a person's homunculus to be a complex image of the self, created by interactions with the environment experienced from birth. Therefore a person's abilities are not limited by genetically endowed structure or musculoskeletal biomechanics, but can be changed by shifting the internal representation of self as the person engages in focused organic learning at any age. Feldenkrais' method was developed to occasion such organic learning, making it possible for anyone to reshape the brain's architecture and, with it, the patterns of self-direction.

Individuality of Human Movement Patterns

Organic learning occurs spontaneously during infancy as the baby creates his or her own patterns of self-direction from the sensory experience of and responses to his or her unique internal and external environment. Because the overall set of movement skills is similar from one average human to another, the individuality of learning is often overlooked. Although every average baby learns to sit up, creep on all fours, walk, and talk, the actual pattern of those actions is as individual as a fingerprint. The pattern of a person's action is not only the representation of identity to that person but also the representation of that person to others, ev-

idenced by the fact that you can recognize a person from whom you have been separated for years by his or her walk or the sound of his or her voice.

Self-Image

Feldenkrais observed how human infants experimented with variations of movement and patterns of behavior to develop a coherent and functional self-image. From a Feldenkrais perspective, self-image includes (1) the totality of the person's kinesthetic and proprioceptive sensations concerning the experienced interrelationship of all physical body parts, and (2) the experience throughout life of the ability to effect change in the environment. Therefore self-image includes beliefs about what can or cannot be done effectively; for example, "I am a person who can (or cannot)" sing, jump, succeed in relationships, or dance.

Excluded Parts of the Self

Feldenkrais was aware of the self-imposed limits of self-image and skill development that emerge in the course of growing up. This awareness was demonstrated even in his early writings, such as in the following excerpt from *Higher Judo:*

In a perfectly matured body, which has grown without great emotional disturbances, movements tend gradually to conform to the mechanical requirements of the surrounding world. The nervous system has evolved under the influence of these laws and is fitted to them. However, in our society we do, by the promise of great reward or intense punishment, so distort the even development of the system, that many acts become excluded or restricted. The result is that we have to provide special conditions for furthering adult maturation of many arrested functions. The majority of people have to be taught not only the special movements of our repertoire, but also to reform patterns of motion and attitudes that should never have been excluded or neglected.[9]

Infant Learning Model

Learning the "special movements of our repertoire" is what typical infants do so beautifully in the first year of life, and then undo in unconsciously learned habits of muscular tension as they experience "promise of great reward or intense punishment" through accidents or social interactions later in life. Initially, infants are fully attentive to the sensations of their movement and the sensations of the results of their actions and spontaneously adopt the most pleasurable experience available. With the FM, the practitioner's touch and words are carefully orchestrated to bring attention to the self with the same quality presumed to have existed in the magnificent rapid-learning period of human infancy.

Movement as the Avenue to Self-Improvement

Feldenkrais found that human movement included simultaneous thinking, feeling, sensing, and acting. He saw sensing and acting (moving, self-direction) as the clearest avenues for change and improvement: "On the sensory level communication is more direct with the unconscious and is more effective and less distorted than at the verbal level."[11]

A person's body is the primary vehicle for learning about the developing self, and movement is an inclusive language of expression for the self. Because of the enormous effect that movement has on the organization of neural structures and their change over time, Feldenkrais chose movement as the most effective avenue for improving self-direction.

Attention and Discrimination

Feldenkrais observed that the human nervous system creates order in a person's experience with the same attention to detail defined in the scientific method. Four processes can be identified for the sake of discussion: attention, discrimination, differentiation, and integration. These processes are inherently interconnected and overlapping in the human experience. *Attention,* which is a person's alertness to his or her own sensory experience, presumes discrimination. *Discrimination* is the spontaneous function within the human nervous system that compares the current sensory experience with all others previously experienced to determine whether the information is the same or different. Very large differences from past pleasant experiences or similarities to past unpleasant experiences may be judged as dangerous and stimulate so-called *fight-or-flight* arousal, which includes increased heart rate, respiration, and muscle tone. Small differences stimulate a quiet and relaxed alertness, evoking awareness and a curiosity to further explore the meaning of the differences. To Feldenkrais, these qualities of awareness and curiosity were such important conditions for learning that he intended to stimulate them in people of all ages who came to him for help.

Differentiation and Integration

Differentiation and integration also overlap. *Differentiation* occurs when a person's nervous system separates the sensation of one part of the body from another. *Integration* occurs when recognition of the separateness or the relatedness among different parts of the body occasions a new movement configuration and skill. Skills develop through a progression of integrating undifferentiated and differentiated movement patterns. For example, an infant first learns how to coordinate different body parts to achieve a single action, such as lifting the legs while rounding the spine to bring the feet toward the face. This action integrates the undifferentiated movements of flexion in coordination with inhibition of extension. Later, an infant learns how to differentiate between the two sides of the body—to flex one side while extending the other to roll over easily, for example. When the infant achieves this action, he or she has integrated a differentiated relationship of the parts of the body. With ongoing differentiation, infants develop an ordered self-image of how their body parts interrelate and how they can most effectively create desired results in their environments.

Integration is the final process of initiating a new skill or action that creates a different outcome in a person's sensory experience. Feldenkrais recognized that when the learning conditions of infancy are recreated, learning can occur at any time of life with the same awesome quality that is observed in early infancy. He invented ways of touching that trigger attention and discrimination to reawaken previously learned differentiations and integrations to reclaim and refine old skills lost to later habits, injury, or disease process. Alternatively, in individuals who experienced congenital or very early postcongenital interference with these neurologic processes, such as neonatal brain trauma or embryologic disturbance, a differentiation never before experienced may be occasioned, allowing for the integration of a new skill.

Act-ure as Biologic Necessity

Although the human upright position in relationship to the gravitational field is usually called *posture,* Feldenkrais sometimes referred to it as *act-ure* to focus attention on neurologic readiness for action. The networking of vision and the other proprioceptors with muscle tone throughout the body is necessary to the organism's ability to respond to external threat with immediate movement. Readiness for movement in the cardinal directions of up and down, right and left, and forward and backward is an important survival skill. Without this skill humans could not reach maturity and therefore could not reproduce. Therefore Feldenkrais said there is no ideal static *posture,* but rather that *act-ure* is a biologic necessity.

Skeletal Conductivity of Movement

Feldenkrais' development of ways to use a person's sensory experience of the skeleton for neurologic learning is a unique contribution to the field of sensory-motor learning. He explored the physics of the human skeleton in great detail. He found that the skeleton was designed to support the upright position extremely well when allowed to assume optimal alignment in relationship to gravity. The ligaments and muscles provide backup support for when the body is not being used in the most efficient way possible or when extreme vector forces are encountered. A vector of movement introduced anywhere on the skeleton by internally generated movement or externally applied force ideally conducts through the entire skeleton, much like the ripple on a body of water into which a pebble is thrown. A ripple continues in water, dissipating only very gradually unless it is interrupted by a structure that prevents the water from flowing, the boundaries of the body of water or a dam, for example. The "ripple" in the skeleton is the conduction of the movement through successively distant parts, which is evidenced by their movement until or unless it is interrupted, or "dammed," by excessive muscle contractions. Muscle contractions are excessive when they are ongoing commitments of habit that interfere with a person's intention for action. Feldenkrais referred to such excessive muscle contractions as *parasitic.*

Skeletal Support, Muscle Tension, Stability, and Flexibility

With the FM, a reciprocal relationship is presumed between the experience of skeletal support and the mobilization of muscle tension. This reciprocity is reflected in the reciprocal relationship between stability and flexibility. When a person responds to life experience with habits of unnecessary muscle tension, his or her excess muscle tension interferes with the flow of vector forces through the skeletal structure. This in turn interferes with the experience of skeletal support and contributes to even more tension as the body adjusts in an attempt to feel stable. This cyclic increase in muscle tension tips the balance of the reciprocal relationship between stability and flexibility in the direction of stability; it interferes with flexibility because the muscular system is overmobilized and preoccupied with trying to perform the skeletal role of stability. Conversely, when skeletal support is adequate, a person feels stability throughout the body. The application of the Feldenkrais practitioner's hands to the client is designed to recreate that experience of stability through the skeleton. When a person feels more stable through the skeleton, he or she spontaneously releases the excessive muscular mobilization from the task of maintaining posture. This release increases flexibility because muscles that were previously engaged in limiting joint mobility to achieve stability are now available for action.

STRATEGIES OF PRACTICE

The Feldenkrais practitioner's role is to create the conditions for learning for the individual who seeks improvement. Each session is called a *lesson* because it is intended to create learning conditions similar to those that exist in the natural explorations of a healthy human infant. Feldenkrais said, "In saying that I work with people I mean that I am 'dancing' with them. I bring about a state in which they learn to do something without my teaching them."[9] He was clear that his contact with the person was not intended to correct directly, but to communicate information to the person's nervous system. "My touching a person with my hands has no therapeutic or healing value. Though people improve through it, I think that what happens to them is *learning.*"[11]

The FM is applied in two different forms. The hands-on practice called *Functional Integration (FI)* is a one-on-one lesson and can be verbal, nonverbal (with touch as the only form of communication), or a mixture of the two (Figure 8-4). Verbally guided group lessons called *Awareness Through Movement (ATM)* offer a more affordable alternative. In both forms of the FM, the practitioner's primary intention is to create conditions for learning in which the client's attention is focused on excluded or neglected parts of the body, and to facilitate a process of discovery in which each person uses these lost parts in a new way (Figure 8-5). ATM and FI are identical in intent and rationale. In ATM, the whole learning process is mediated through language. The practitioner verbally guides attention to how different parts of the body move and relate to one another and to feel changes as they occur. Movement sequences are introduced with gentle and slow elements to improve participants' ability to discriminate fine differences. The participants' movements focus their sensory attention in the same way the practitioner's touch does with an individual during an FI. The directions are given in common language with a self-referential orientation for the cardinal directions. This orientation remains constant regardless of how the person is positioned; for example, *up* always means the direction the top of the head is facing, regardless of whether the person is lying or sitting.

Excerpts from an abridged example of an ATM lesson[10a] are presented here.* These excerpts provide a sampler of common strategies employed in ATM and FI. Each lesson excerpt is followed by an explanation of the strategy demonstrated by that instruction.

Find yourself a nice chair. . . . Sit at the front edge of that chair so both feet are squarely on the floor and you can sit easily.

In ATM and FI, every attempt is made to begin from a position of comfort to increase receptivity to new information. Discomfort perpetuates the client's focus on whatever trouble sustains the current habits of tension. A horizontal position relieves the demand for the habitual muscular response to gravity and makes it easier to explore other movement options. To focus on specific functions or accommodate the client's current abilities, the practitioner may use positions other than prone, supine, or side-lying. This se-

*Transcription and excerpts of "ATM Lesson for the Elder Citizen," by Moshe Feldenkrais, is courtesy of Feldenkrais® Resources, Berkeley, Calif.

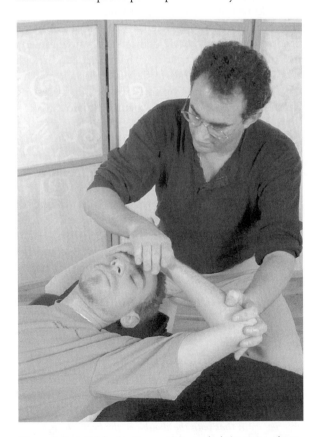

Figure 8-4 A Feldenkrais practitioner helping a student roll his head with his hand. (Courtesy Feldenkrais Guild of North America.)

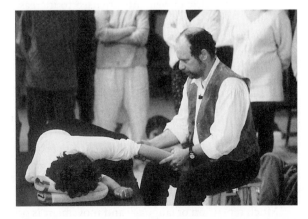

Figure 8-5 David Zemach-Bersin, Feldenkrais trainer, demonstrating Functional Integration at his training program. (Courtesy David Zemach-Bersin.)

ries began with a lesson in sitting to benefit elders or those with marked movement limitations who don't currently know an easy way to get down to the floor. Therefore another strategy demonstrated here is to focus attention on what a person can already easily do and on improving that function as the first step. Relationships are established between the client and practitioner and between the client and himself or herself; these relationships respect and affirm the client's abilities rather than *dis*abilities. Learning begins where the foundation is strongest and can then be expanded to build other skills upon that foundation.

Now, very slowly, put your hands on your knees and move your right knee a little bit forward.

A constraint is introduced—the anchoring of one body part on another. Constraints are instructions designed to focus the person's attention on the role of a particular part of the body. Anchoring one part on another focuses attention on the coordinated use of many parts of the body in an undifferentiated movement. In more complex or challenging lessons, a constraint can eliminate other movement possibilities to create a demand for a neglected part to move. Touching one part of the body with another also amplifies sensory information by bringing it into the nervous system through two or more body parts simultaneously.

Do this as small and as easy a movement as you can. Do it as simply as you can . . . just a tiny little movement forward.

Small and gentle movements are used to increase the ability to discriminate small changes. Each client is encouraged to move only in the range that is comfortable and to follow internal authority regarding where to stop. Small and gentle movements also tend to focus the client's sensory attention, just as a person tends to screen out distracting input to hear a whisper.

You are sitting at the front edge of the chair with both feet squarely on the floor and moving your right knee a tiny bit forward, and back again. Do this several times, slowly.

Much repetition of language and movement is offered to provide repeated opportunities for clients to compare and contrast the experience of how they are moving (ATM) or are being moved (FI) and to explore slight variations.

You have both hands on your knees. Pay attention to your hip. You will note that when the right knee goes forward, your right hip joint also goes forward, too. In fact, it is the hip joint that moves the knee. Also, as you are doing this, the whole body turns a tiny little bit to the left . . . the shoulders, the spine, the head, the chest, everything. Keep on doing the movement, moving the right hip joint forward . . . so that both shoulders, the chest, the head, the eyes move the tiniest little bit to the left. Observe this and continue doing the movement back and forth.

Here Feldenkrais explicitly brings the students' attention to the conduction of movement through the skeleton. The movement is simply a medium, a small vector of one part of the skeleton, used to introduce conduction through the skeleton. When the arms and legs are anchored to one another, any intention to move the leg mobilizes musculature around the pelvis and is conducted directly to the vertebrae. Feldenkrais is not asking them to *make* it happen that way, but is bringing their sensory attention to the relationship that exists. He demonstrates how moving just one side begins a turning that conducts through the individual vertebrae. In FI, a practitioner may focus a client's attention on this relationship by resting his or her fingertips on the client's individual vertebrae while moving the leg a tiny bit.

Observe the place on the wall you see as your eyes turn to the left.

A common strategy is to introduce a reference movement early in the lesson, such as having the person move (ATM) or moving the person (FI) in a simple way that will be repeated later in the lesson for comparison. The sensory experience of this movement begins to focus the attention of the client and practitioner on how the client is currently organizing himself or herself in relationship to the movement function. The movement is also placed in the functional context of looking.

Don't strain. Don't hold your breath. Do nothing extraordinary, just this simple movement. Move your right knee and hip joint forward and back, and, as you move them forward, observe again that both the shoulders, the head, the eyes and the spine, move a tiny little bit to the left.

Attention is focused on the quality of the movement, suspending any goal during the learning.

Stop. Rest. Pay attention to the sensations in your body.

Frequent pauses in ATM and FI allow clients to process information that has been introduced (i.e., to observe changes).

Now move your right hip joint backward towards the direction of the chair. Both hands are still on the knees. Observe that the body moves a tiny bit to the right as you do this movement . . . both shoulders, the chest, the eyes . . . the hip joint is going backward, the knee is going backward.

A different direction of movement with the same relationship among the parts introduces a different image of action. Maintaining the same relationship in a changing context provides more generalization of the movement relationships.

This time move your right hip forward and the body twists to the left. Then [continue the motion and] move your right hip backward and the body twists to the right. Very slowly, at your ease, keep on doing it.

Sensory attention is focused on the turning of the vertebrae, which is induced as the small vector of movement introduced at the hip turns the pelvis, which turns the vertebrae.

If, by any chance, your right hip joint or your right knee ache and you can't do this movement, don't worry, do this part of the movement in your mind. . . . Just imagine yourself moving the right hip joint forward and backward and imagine your body twisting to the left as you move your right hip joint forward and twisting to the right as you move your right hip joint backward.

When the body faces a demand for increased effort or speed, habitual patterns of tension are triggered to meet the demand. The smaller the movement, the less the mobilization of habitual patterns. If the person simply imagines the feeling of the movement without actually doing it, the person can create the image of the relationships and the sensory experience without increasing the tension associated with fear of discomfort or ambition to achieve. In FI, with hands on the student at two locations, if the practitioner makes a tiny movement of his or her own body or only imagines the movement, that movement relationship is communicated to the student. FI is like dancing in

that the touch and movement of the practitioner is a connection between the practitioner's and student's nervous systems. The movements are not passive even though they are initiated by the practitioner. Movement is introduced slowly and gently by the practitioner so that the student can feel how he or she participates or cooperates with the intention of the movement.

You will see that, if you have pain or arthritis of the hip or knee, if you imagine the movement, the body mobilizes itself just as if it were doing the movement and after a few trials you will be surprised to find that some movement becomes possible, and over time, this will go on progressing and improving.

Feldenkrais explains how imagination works and introduces positive suggestions of improvement.

Now rest, lean back in the chair. Sense your right side and your left side . . . notice if there is any difference in how they feel. Maybe the difference is tiny, maybe you don't feel it just now . . . by the end of the lesson you will know that difference very clearly.

Again there is a pause to allow the participants to discriminate differences. Feldenkrais verbally brings the participants' conscious attention to any differences and begins training them to be more aware of differences. He affirms the validity of whatever they feel and again offers positive suggestions for the future.

Observe that you breathe freely; that means . . . don't do anything special with your breathing, just let it happen. Don't take deep breaths, don't breathe "nicely" or correctly.

The relationship of movement to ease of breathing is important feedback for both the participant and the practitioner. Unnecessary muscular tension interferes with easy breathing.

And now sit again forward on the chair, your hands on your knees and again move your right hip forward/your right knee forward. But only move the shoulders to the left; keep the eyes and head stable looking toward the front like before.

Keeping the eyes and head still when turning is usually a nonhabitual pattern of interrelationship among body parts, because we habitually initiate movement by orienting with our eyes. Because our movements are guided by images of movement previously experienced, introducing a nonhabitual pattern of relationship opens a window for novel use of the body. One analogy is shuffling a deck of cards. The cards are stacked in one pattern. When shuffled, the individual cards are the same but now are arranged in a different relationship to one another. When a person initiates movement with the head and eyes held still, the previous images of movement don't apply; thus there is an opportunity to invent a novel movement.

———————————

Again move the right hip joint forward and. . . . This time turn the whole body . . . both shoulders, head, eyes to the left and observe that you are seeing so much farther to the left than when you began.

———————————

Feldenkrais returns to the undifferentiated movement of turning the whole self, allowing the participant to learn how much more effectively all the parts move together.

———————————

Now . . . stay looking to the left while you move your right hip joint backward. When the right hip joint moves backward, the shoulders move to the front, but your eyes and head keep on looking to the left. Move the right hip joint forward and the head and shoulders and eyes move even more to the left, and now keep your eyes and head to the left, as you move your right hip joint backward and forward again; the eyes and head stay looking to the left while the rest of the body turns . . . to face front and . . . as the body twists to the left . . . you are twisting each time a few degrees more to the left.

———————————

With the head and eyes held turned to the left, moving the hip backward is another variation of nonhabitual movement and differentiation. When the right hip is moved forward, the undifferentiated movement of the whole self to the left adds further turning without any additional strain.

———————————

Now turn to the front, sit back in the chair and rest. Sense the back of the chair, sense your bottom . . . the way you are sitting on it. Observe the differences between your right and left sides. Now twist your head to the left . . . look to the left and look to the right and see if there is a difference . . . is it easier to move the head toward one side than the other?

———————————

The reference movement (turning the head to look right and left) is repeated, allowing the client to experience how much change has taken place.

———————————

Move forward again to the front of the chair, both hands on your knees, and slowly move your left hip joint forward together with the left knee, and of course, your body will twist slightly to the right, both head and shoulders . . . eyes too. Your whole body twists gently to the right with the small movement of the hip joint and the left knee forward. That means that the left knee becomes a little longer than the right, and back again; move the left knee and left hip joint back and of course, the body will twist to the left and again, slowly forward, again twisting to the right.

———————————

The attention is shifted to the other side to afford an opportunity to compare and generalize what was learned about the movement from the original side. Although logic would seem to suggest that turning to the left side was already involved in the backward movements of the right side, experience proves otherwise. More and more basic scientific research shows that we move according to internalized images of movement triggered by our intentions. Turning to the other side is a different intention and thus a different image of movement.

———————————

Keep on twisting to the right as your knee goes forward. Move also your head and eyes to the right, and back again to face front. And when you move your hip joint back, move to the left and back to the front . . . and the knee forward/back to the right. And slowly make the movement a little bit easier so that you can, with the knee moving forward, look to the right, turn to the right ever so gently, and when the hip joint goes backward, let the whole body go back to the left . . . turn left, look left . . . each time easier, simpler. And breathe easily.

Bring your head and eyes to the front and keep them there; keep looking to the front while your right knee goes forward and twists your body to the left . . . the eyes and head still facing front. And then the left knee and left hip joint go forward; the body, shoulders twisted right while you still look forward with your eyes and head.

———————————

Another differentiation of the head and eyes is introduced.

———————————

Now move your right knee forward and, this time, keep your shoulders and body to the left and turn your eyes and head more to the left together with the body and see whether you can see even further than before. And now move the left hip forward, the left knee forward and let your body, eyes and head twist to the right. And again, note whether you can see a little bit more to the right than before.

———————————

Undifferentiated movement is repeated with the reference movement.

And now just sit still and move only the body, shoulders, head and eyes, leaving the hip joints as quiet and motionless as you can ... and now move your shoulders, body, head, and eyes to the left ... look around and observe. When you look to the left like that, your right hip joint will move in spite of your decision not to move. Look to the left, well to the left, with your eyes, shoulders and head.

The reference movement is repeated, demonstrating how the learning has been integrated into spontaneous, automatic function.

An understanding of ATM is fundamental to understanding the relationship between the practitioner and client in FI. ATM is the primary organic learning process through which practitioners learn the method. The changes in organization experienced by the practitioner during professional training are the infrastructure on which the practitioner later draws to create ATM and FI lessons.

The quality of the verbal exchange between the client and the Feldenkrais practitioner is considered an essential part of any lesson. The client is approached with the inquiry of how this person recovers from shock or stress. The medical diagnosis is of much less importance than the sensory description of the client's experience. Often a client describes a presenting difficulty by naming a diagnosis or reporting medical tests or data. The practitioner questions the client to elicit a personal description of sensory experience in relationship to the presenting issue. The practitioner is interested in the client's habits and how those habits relate to the difficulty being experienced. For example, a client may say that he or she has spinal stenosis or sciatica. The practitioner may ask the following questions: "What do you feel in your body that gets your attention?" "Where do you feel this sensation?" "During what activities do you notice this sensation?" "What activities intensify the sensation?" "What have you discovered that relieves the sensation?" The practitioner is interested in the client's intentions in relationship to the environment, and therefore may also ask, "What would you do differently if you felt as you want to feel?"

These questions are examples. The questions asked are at the discretion of the practitioner. Obviously the exchange would change dramatically if the presenting issue involved athletic or artistic perform-

ance or a movement limitation such as those seen with cerebral palsy or stroke sequelae.

The practitioner's intention is to identify the pivotal aspect of the client's self image around which the dysfunctional habit seems to be perpetuated. Commonly, but not always, this pivotal aspect is a part of the body that is being habitually restricted by habits of muscular tension. In FI, the practitioner's touch is a means of bringing renewed attention to different aspects of the self. The practitioner touches the client to bring sensory and neurologic attention to parts of the self that seem to be absent or distorted in the client's self-image and actions. Many strategies are used by the Feldenkrais practitioner to this end. A Feldenkrais practitioner uses the client's sensation of the skeleton to focus attention on different parts of the body and the relationships of one part to other parts.

The aspects of action identified by Feldenkrais—orientation, timing, intention, and manipulation—are the same variables that govern the quality of the practitioner's touch. The term *manipulation* was used by Feldenkrais in a very different way than it is used in the manual medicine traditions of osteopathy, chiropractic, or physical therapy. Feldenkrais was referring to any movement of the body. The practitioner may simply rest his or her fingertips on individual spinous processes and wait while the client's attention is focused on that place during the ongoing underlying movement of his or her breath. Timing is paced discreetly to focus the client's attention on the internal experience rather than alert the sympathetic nervous system to any risk from outside interference. Touch may be applied very gradually and removed just as slowly. The effect for the client is often a lingering attention to the area and its relationship to the rest of the self that persists for some time after the touch is withdrawn. The person's breathing and muscle tone are observed visually and through the practitioner's sensory anchor of touch to monitor the sympathetic state of the client in receiving the sensations offered. The practitioner constantly adjusts his or her touch to ensure an optimal sympathetic state and receptivity to learning.

The client is usually supported with whatever pads or rollers are necessary to allow him or her to rest fully and feel safe and comfortable; these feelings promote a receptive sympathetic state and allow the client to receive new information. For comfort's sake, the client remains in street clothes; thus any changes that occur during the session are related to his or her usual identity by the anchor of the clothes.

Another strategy is to introduce a movement vector to communicate to the client on a sensory level through the skeleton. When the light pressure of a vector is gently introduced and withdrawn repeatedly, the effect is an oscillating movement that is intended to conduct through the skeleton like the "pebble" image mentioned above. When a vector is introduced footward from the seventh cervical vertebra's transverse processes or headward from the feet, movement is ideally conducted without interference, creating a visible rocking movement of the pelvis, which moves through the vertebrae, eventually rocking the head or feet as well. Both the practitioner and the client receive sensory information regarding where the client's habitual muscular contractions interfere with the movement initiated by the vector. The client focuses on the natural interrelationship of the skeletal parts with the introduction of deliberate and precise movement vectors.

Many strategies contribute to the nonjudgmental and noninvasive qualities of the practitioner–client interaction. One strategy is demonstrated when the practitioner moves a client in ways that exaggerate a habitual action. When movement feels restricted across a joint, the practitioner often moves the client in the direction of the restriction rather than against the restriction. Neurologically, this occasions a relaxation of the muscular tension that previously maintained the restriction because the action of the habitual contraction has been taken over by the practitioner. In terms of body image, this strategy also validates the client's current identity rather than opposing or negating it. In terms of learning, exaggerating the habitual direction allows the client to experience how to move in the opposite direction from his or her habit. For example, a client who has experienced a cerebrovascular accident (stroke) may show excessive flexion of the fingers on the affected side and may no longer know how to extend the fingers. Exaggerating the flexion of the fingers into an even tighter fist and then gradually letting go of the exaggeration allows the client to experience the sensation of the fingers returning to the habitual degree of flexing by moving in the direction of opening or extension.

The practitioner often moves two different parts simultaneously to refine their relationship, for example, the hip and shoulder on the same side in the sidelying position. The two parts are moved simultaneously to focus attention on the role of the muscles of the torso in coordinating the movements of the hip and shoulder. The movement therefore brings attention to the role of vertebral movement in directing and empowering the limbs. Similarly, two such parts may be moved passively in opposite directions to clarify the differentiation of how the two parts can move separately from one another.

Two body parts are often attached to one another to clarify how the movement of one part can be refined by the movement of another. For example, many people develop the habit of moving the head excessively with the cervical vertebrae while restricting movement from other vertebrae with habitual muscular tension in the torso. Rolling a client's head with the palm of his or her own hand redistributes the turning to include participation of the thoracic spine.

Movements that are introduced to the client are carefully sequenced to build relationships among various parts. Other strategies may be improvised by necessity with clients who present novel challenges.

Risk and Safety

Because the nature of a Feldenkrais lesson is gentle and conservative, there is very little risk involved. In Awarenss Through Movement group classes, participants are encouraged to move within the range that is comfortable and easy. However, because struggle and competition are part of many people's habitual experience and expectation, individuals may overdo while they are learning to rediscover what comfort and ease feel like.

Any of the following "warning signs" reported by a client or discovered during Functional Integration or Awareness Through Movement lessons warrant referral to a physician for further investigation:

1. pain at night;
2. pain that doesn't change;
3. sudden onset of disabling pain, with numbness as a precipitating factor;
4. loss of conciousness;
5. pain that consistently increases after lessons;
6. lumps in muscles not consistent with muscle tone;
7. something unusual and noticeable, such as, dizziness, swelling, color or temperature changes, vomiting, sweating in one extremity or part of the body;
8. significant weight change;
9. loss of muscle or sphincter control.[2a]

TRAINING AND CERTIFICATION

Feldenkrais Professional Training Programs

Students in an FPTP usually attend a training program for 40 days a year for 4 years. Participants learn experientially through ATM lessons, which are a major part of the curriculum throughout the training program (Figure 8-6). Through the sensory experience of their own learning in the ATMs, the students learn FM strategies and their effects through the changes they experience in their own organization. Feldenkrais did not teach techniques, per se, but created opportunities for his students to experience many strategies through their own learning. Practitioners observe various strategies when they watch senior practitioners conduct lessons. The most important learning for student practitioners occurs when they experience strategies directly by participating in ATMs and FIs during and after training. Students learn anatomy in a functional context and experience the impact of the variables of orientation, timing, intention, and manipulation, and the effect of those elements. With this wealth of experience gained in training, practitioners are able to improvise new strategies in the moment to meet the learning needs of a particular student.

As the training progresses, students begin to work in pairs. In this work they begin to apply strategies learned in their own movement explorations as they apply touch to their peers. Through their work in pairs, the students learn about the factors affecting learning from the perspective of practitioner and teacher and from the perspective of client and student. A minimum of 12 FI lessons are offered to each FPTP student as part of training. The FIs are provided by trainers, assistant trainers, or other practitioners or teachers under the supervision of the Educational Director (Figure 8-7).

Training Accreditation Board

The Training Accreditation Board (TAB) of The Feldenkrais Guild of North America (FGNA) is com-

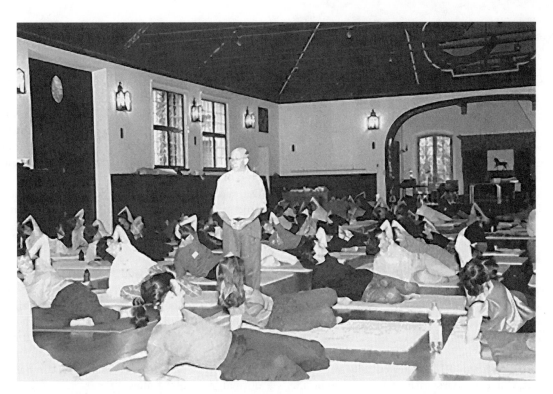

Figure 8-6 Paul Rubin, Feldenkrais Trainer, teaching Awareness Through Movement to the students at his professional training program. (Courtesy Paul Rubin.)

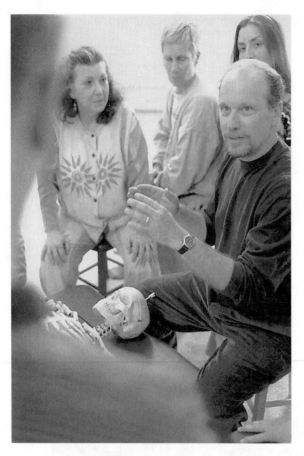

Figure 8-7 David Zemach-Bersin, Feldenkrais Trainer, teaching in his professional training program. (Courtesy David Zemach-Bersin.)

posed of volunteers from among the Feldenkrais practitioner community and Feldenkrais trainers. The TAB reviews proposals for FPTPs from approved educational directors or trainers and determines whether the proposals meet the criteria for a certified FPTP. The TAB also reviews applications from Feldenkrais practitioners requesting certification as educational directors, trainers, or assistant trainers, and awards those titles at its discretion.

Certification

Criteria for a certified FPTP are periodically revised by the FGNA. Current criteria include at least 800 hours of training lasting at least 160 days spread over at least 36 months. The distribution of training hours is at the discretion of the educational director. Because there are so many styles of practice among FM practitioners, TAB criteria also require that students be exposed to at least four different trainers. More than 50 accredited trainings in various stages are being conducted in cities across the United States, Canada, Austria, Belgium, France, Germany, Switzerland, Italy, the Netherlands, the United Kingdom, Israel, Mexico, Argentina, New Zealand, Japan, and Australia. Students who graduate from their FPTP are certified for 2 years. Every 2 years thereafter practitioners are required to participate in at least 40 hours of advanced training to renew their certification.

RESEARCH

Because the FM has such a wide range of effects, a wide range of outcomes have been observed and reported. Most clinical studies to date have involved a very small number of subjects (six or fewer). Some larger studies have used control group designs.

Pain Management

Lake[20] and Panarello-Black[23] published case studies describing the resolution of chronic back pain following the failure of other methods to ameliorate the problems they hoped to solve. A retrospective study of 34 patients using FM as an adjunct to treatment in a chronic pain management clinic showed that FM helped reduce pain and improve function and was used independently by patients 2 years after discharge. Dennenberg[6] showed decreased pain and increased functional mobility using FM as a component of treatment for 15 pain patients. A study using a group ATM intervention with five fibromyalgia patients showed significant decrease in pain and improved posture, gait, sleep, and body awareness.[4] Lake[20] showed changes in posture in patients with chronic back pain following FM. Chinn and colleagues[3] showed improvements in functional reach in symptomatic subjects. Idebergs[17] showed significant changes in pelvic rotation and pelvic obliquity during rapid walking in 10 patients with back pain, compared with normal controls, following a series of FI lessons. Narula[22] provided 6 weeks of ATM lessons to several

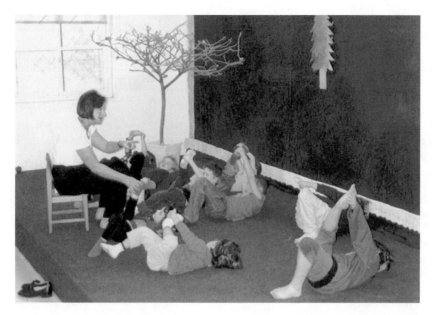

Figure 8-8 Chava Shelhav-Silverbush, Feldenkrais Trainer, teaching Awareness Through Movement with learning-disabled children in Heidelberg, Germany. (Courtesy Chava Shelhav-Silverbush.)

people with rheumatoid arthritis. Results showed decreased pain and improved function, including improved biomechanic efficiency, measured by motion analysis, in a sit-to-stand transfer from a chair.

Functional Performance and Motor Control

Four women with multiple sclerosis reported improvements in balance in daily activities and improved walking and transfers, as assessed by video motion analysis.[29] Shenkman[26] described improvements in posture in clients with Parkinson's disease when FM was part of the intervention strategy. Shelhav-Silverbush[24] reported case studies of two children with cerebral palsy who made major functional gains during several years of FM work (Figure 8-8). Ginsburg[15] anecdotally described functional and motor control improvements in young people with spinal cord injuries who were involved in the "Shake a Leg" program. Gilman[14] reported improved control of stuttering in two patients.

Evidence of FM leading to improved athletic function is mostly anecdotal information related to skiing

and kayaking. Jackson-Wyatt[18] reported a case study of improved jumping following a Feldenkrais intervention.

Other studies include changes in function of trunk and cervical muscles reflected by changes in electromyelogram (EMG) activity, muscle function and posture related to improvements in abdominal breathing, and body image or scheme. Narula[22] reported increases in EMG activity in clients with low back pain whose painful muscles had apparently become inactive. It may be that reintegrating these muscles into normal movement patterns stimulates blood flow and thus a normal healing process.

Psychologic Effects

In an interesting study using analysis of clay figures, Deig[5] described expansion in the detail and form of body image after a series of ATM lessons. Shelhav-Silverbush[25] reported improvements in mobility skills, social function, and intelligence quotient in a class of learning-impaired children. Recently, in a matched control group study of 30 children with eating disorders, Laumer[21] concluded

TABLE 8-1

Effectiveness of the Feldenkrais Method

Number of cases	Area of dysfunction	Percentage of subjects who reached various percentages of the goals established at initial visit by the time of discharge			
		100%	75%-90%	50%-75%	<50%
35	Back pain	77%	14%	8%	2%
20	Osteoarthritis	80%	15%	5%	
17	Primary diagnosis neck pain	76%	12%	12%	
13	Shoulder diagnoses	69%	23%		
6	Fibromyalgia	83%	17%		
14	Tendonitis/bursitis or other hip/knee diagnoses	85%	7%	7%	
8	Back/leg pain with spinal stenosis or spondylolisthesis	63%	12%	25%	
3	Temporomandibular joint cases	66%	33%		
7	Scoliosis	71%	14%	14%	
37	Neurologic cases:	46%	38%	11%	5%
6	Multiple sclerosis				
10	Cerebrolvascular accident or stroke (hemiplegia)				
8	Cerebral palsy				
2	Spinal cord injury				
4	Traumatic brain injury				
2	Parkinson's disease				
2	Postpolio				
3	Other				

that a course of ATM facilitated an acceptance of the body and self, decreased feelings of helplessness and dependence, increased self-confidence, and aided a general process of maturation of the whole personality. Using the Index of Well-Being, improvements in vitality and mental health were measured by the SF-36, a psychometric instrument measuring quality of life (see http://www.mcw.edu/midas/health/SF-36.html) in a group of women with multiple sclerosis.[28]

Basic Science

Dynamic systems theory as described by Thelen[31] and Kelso[19] best fits the observed processes of the FM. This theory accounts for the processes of skill acquisition, functional development, and organization change resulting from changes in posture and coordination. It relies on an understanding of the body as having a modifiable internal representation of body scheme that includes the shape of the body surface, limb length, sequence of linkage, and position in space. The processes of skill acquisition, coordination change, and functional or motor development are driven by active exploration involving awareness.

Quality of Life

Gutman[16] found a trend toward improvement in overall perception of health status in a well elderly population. This finding has been corroborated in another well elderly population by improvements in vitality and mental health as measured by the SF-36.[31] Well being was reported to be improved in a controlled study of 50 participants with multiple sclerosis (MS)[2] and in a group of 4 women with MS using the Index of Well Being.[29]

Effectiveness

Stephens[30] reports on using FM as part of a rehabilitation process with 166 clients over 5 years in his private practice. Outcome has been judged on percentage of the original goals, established at the initial visit, which were achieved by the time of discharge (Table 8-1). Four levels of outcome were used: (1) 100% achieved; (2) 75% to 90% achieved; (3) 50% to 75% achieved; (4) less than 50% achieved. Orthopedic cases made up 84% and neurologic cases 16% of the population. Age range was 8 to 84; most subject were between 30 and 60 years of age.

References

1. Alon R: *Mindful spontaneity, moving in tune with nature: lessons in the Feldenkrais Method,* Calgary, Alberta, Canada, 1990, Prism Press.
2. Bost H, Burges S, Russell R et al: *Feldstudie zur wiiksamkeit der Feldenkrais-methode bei MS—betroffenen,* Saarbrucken, Germany, 1994, Deutsche Multiple Sklerose Gesellschaft.
2a. Bowes D: *Meeting the medical model: professional considerations for the Feldenkrais practitioner,* Video Presentation, Baltimore, Md, 2001, Feldenkrais Resources.
3. Chinn J et al: Effect of a Feldenkrais intervention on symptomatic subjects performing a functional reach. *Isokinetics Exerc Sci* 4(4):131-136, 1994.
4. Dean JR, Yuen SA, Barrows SA: *Effects of a Feldenkrais ATM sequence on fibromyalgia patients.* Study reported to the California Physical Therapy Association, 1997 and the annual conference of the Feldenkrais Guild of America, August 1997.
5. Deig D: *Self image in relationship to Feldenkrais Awareness Through Movement classes,* independent study project, Indianapolis, 1994, University of Indianapolis, Krannert Graduate School of Physical Therapy.
6. Dennenberg N, Reeves GD: *Changes in health locus of control and activities of daily living in a physical therapy clinic using the Feldenkrais Method of sensory motor education.* Master's Thesis, Rochester, Mich, 1995, Oakland University, Program in Physical Therapy.
7. Donnellan AM, Leary MR: *Movement differences and diversity in autism/mental retardation: appreciating and accommodating people with communication and behavioral challenges,* Madison, Wis, 1995, DRI Press.
8. Feldenkrais M: *Judo,* ed 8, London, 1941, Frederick Warne.
9. Feldenkrais M: *Higher judo (ground work),* ed 3, London, 1952, Frederick Warne.
10. Feldenkrais M: *Practical unarmed combat,* ed 3, Tel Aviv, 1964, The Feldenkrais Institute.
10a. Feldenkrais M: *Awareness through movement: health exercises for personal growth,* San Francisco, 1990, Harper Collins.
11. Feldenkrais M: *The elusive obvious,* Cupertino, Calif, 1981, Meta Publications.
12. Feldenkrais M: *Body and mature behavior: a study of anxiety, sex, gravitation and learning,* Tel-Aviv, Israel, 1988, Alef Ltd.
13. Feldenkrais M: *The potent self,* New York, 1992, Harper Collins.
14. Gilman M: *Reduction of tension in stuttering through somatic re-education.* Master's Thesis, Evanston, Ill, 1997, Northwestern University, Department of Communication Sciences and Disorders.
15. Ginsburg C: The shake-a-leg body awareness training program: dealing with spinal injury and recovery in a new setting, *Somatics* Spring/Summer:31-42, 1986.
16. Gutman G, Herbert C, Brown S: Feldenkrais vs conventional exercise for the elderly, *J Gerontol* 32(5):562-572, 1977.
17. Ideberg G, Werner M: *Gait assessment by three dimensional motion analysis in subjects with chronic low back pain treated according to Feldenkrais principles: an exploratory study.* Unpublished manuscript, 1995.
18. Jackson-Wyatt O et al: Effects of Feldenkrais practitioner training program on motor ability: a videoanalysis, *Phys Ther* 72(suppl.):S86, 1992.
19. Kelso JAS: *Dynamic patterns: the self-organization of brain and behavior,* Cambridge, Mass, 1995, MIT Press.
20. Lake B: Photoanalysis of standing posture in controls and low back pain: effects of kinesthetic processing (*Feldenkrais Method*). In Woollocott M, Horak F, editors: *Posture and gait: control mechanisms,* ed 7, Eugene, 1992, U of Oregon Press.
21. Laumer U et al: Therapeutic effects of Feldenkrais method "Awareness Through Movement" in patients with eating disorders, *Psychother Psychosom Med Psychol* 47(5):170-180, 1997 (English abstract).
22. Narula M, Jackson O, Kulig K: The effects of six week Feldenkrais method on selected functional parameters in a subject with rheumatoid arthritis, *Phys Ther* 72(suppl.):S86, 1992.
23. Panarello-Black D: PT's own back pain leads her to start Feldenkrais training, *PT Bull* p 9, April 8, 1992.
24. Shelhav-Silverbush C: *The Feldenkrais method for children with cerebral palsy.* Masters Thesis, Boston, 1988, Boston University School of Education.
25. Shelhav-Silverbush C: *Movement and learning: the Feldenkrais method as a learning model.* Doctoral Dissertation, Heidelberg, Germany, 1988, Heidelberg University.
26. Shenkman M et al: Management of individuals with Parkinson's disease: rationale and case studies, *Phys Ther* 69:944-955, 1989.

27. Speransky A: *A basis for the theory of medicine,* New York, 1943, International Publishers.

28. Stephens JL et al: *Changes in coordination, economy of movement and well being resulting from a 2-day workshop in Awareness Through Movement.* Presentation at APTA, Combined Sections Meeting, Boston, 1998.

29. Stephens JL: Responses to ten Feldenkrais Awareness Through Movement lessons by four women with multiple sclerosis: improved quality of life. *Phys Ther Case Rep* 2(2):58-69, 1999.

30. Stephens JL: Feldenkrais method: background, research and orthopedic case studies. Orthopedic Physical Therapy Clinics of North America, *Comple Med* 9(3):375-394, 2000.

31. Thelen E, Smith L: *A dynamic systems approach to the development of cognition and action,* Cambridge, Mass, 1994, MIT Press.

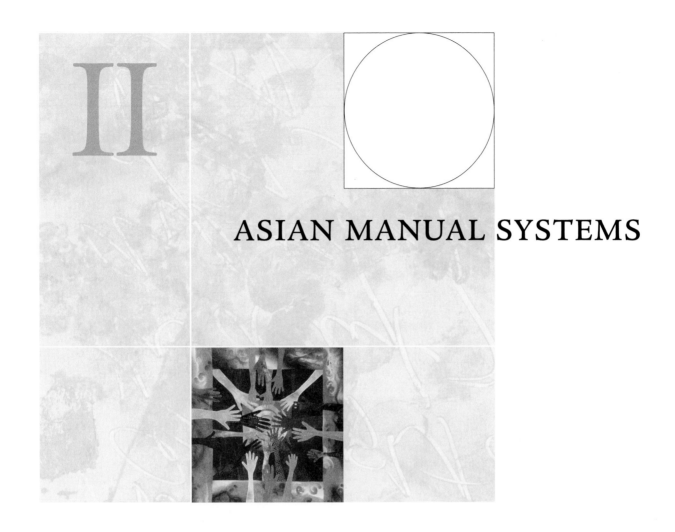

II

ASIAN MANUAL SYSTEMS

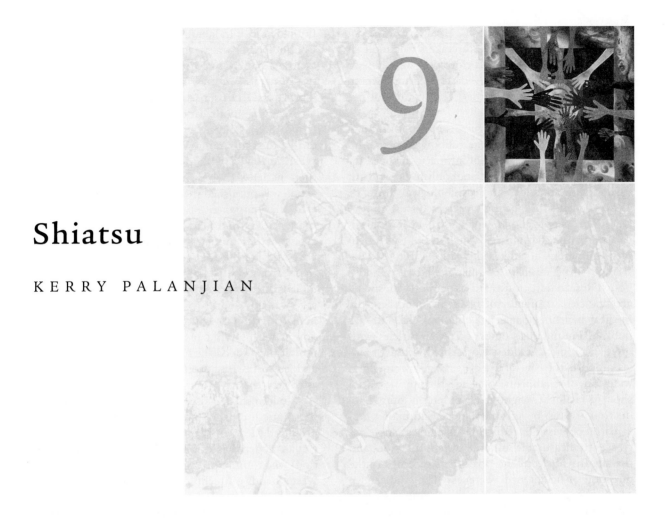

Shiatsu

KERRY PALANJIAN

Simple yet profound, the experience with shiatsu, whether a single session or an ongoing therapeutic relationship between therapist and client, brings the wisdom of ancient civilizations to our Western model of life, thought, and medicine. Shiatsu, which is reinforced by Western and Eastern clinical research and receives official Japanese government sanction, is regarded by many as a life-changing experience.

HISTORY

The literal meaning of the Japanese word *shiatsu* (she AAHT sue) is *finger pressure* or *thumb pressure*. Over the centuries Asian medicine, massage therapy, and twentieth century advancements have combined to yield "modern" shiatsu.

The word *massage* comes from the Arabic word for *stroke*. The practice of massage dates back 3000 years to China. A tomb found in modern Egypt, determined to be from 2200 BC, depicts a man receiving a foot massage. In the fourth century BC, Hippocrates, known as the father of modern medicine, wrote that "the physician must be experienced in many things, but most assuredly in rubbing."[3] Further support for the use of touch and massage as healing tools is noted in ancient Egyptian, Greek, Persian, Roman, and Asian manuscripts.[16]

During the Middle Ages, there was decreased visibility of massage as a healing tool in the West, principally because of the position of the Church, which viewed the manipulation of the body to be the work of the devil. Massage was often depicted as a tool of prostitution, a prejudice that still lingers today among the uninformed. In the thirteenth century the

142 PRINCIPLES AND PRACTICE OF MANUAL THERAPEUTICS

German emperor Frederick II seized a number of newborns and did not allow caretakers to cuddle or talk to the infants. All died before they were able to talk. The historian Salimbene described this "experiment" in 1248 when he wrote, "They could not live without petting."[3]

People instinctively recognize the need for human touch and contact. From the rubbing of a painful shoulder to the physical act of intimacy, the need for connection and human touch not only feels good but yields many physical and psychological benefits. These benefits are gaining increased recognition among lay people and are enjoying a substantial increase in support from scientific studies that document numerous broad-based positive effects (see Research). The University of Miami Medical School's Touch Research Institute (TRI) is gaining widespread acceptance as a pioneer of research supporting the medical benefits of massage therapy. The TRI has published numerous studies and review articles, with more in progress.[3] Evidence presented in these studies supports the clinical use of massage therapy for a wide range of ailments. Massage therapy has been show to facilitate weight-gain in preterm infants, reduction of stress hormone levels, alleviation of symptoms of depression, reduction in pain, positive increases in measurable immune system function, and the altering of electroencephalogram readings in the direction of heightened awareness. The studies also suggest benefits for patients with conditions such as Alzheimer's disease, arthritis, depression, fibromyalgia, job stress, and premenstrual syndrome, and for women in labor (see Research, or go to http://www.miami.edu/touch-research).[3]

Shiatsu's history lies within the antecedents of Asian medicine, as was clearly stated 2000 years ago in *The Yellow Emperor's Classic of Internal Medicine,* a text discussed in Oliver Cowmeadow's *The Art of Shiatsu.*[4] Others suggest that Chinese medical practice was derived from techniques originally developed in India and adapted to China.

Shiatsu has evolved within the genre of touch and massage therapies, as well as within Asian medicine's juxtaposition to ancient and modern Japanese culture. As a healing art or treatment it grew from earlier forms of *Anma* in Japan (*Anmo* or *Tuina* in China).[10] *An* denotes *pressure* and *nonpressure,* and *ma* means *rubbing.*[16] This method, which was well known 1000 years ago in China, found its way to Japan and was recognized as the safest and easiest way to treat the human body.[12] In Japan, shiatsu was used and taught by blind practitioners who relied on their hands to diagnose a patient's condition.[4] Anma was recognized by the medical authorities in Japan in the Nara period (AD 710-784), but subsequently lost its popularity before gaining more widespread use in the Edo era (1603-1868),[16] during which doctors were actually required to study Anma. During the Edo period, most practitioners were blind and provided treatments in their patients' homes. An extensive handbook on Anma was published in 1793, and Anma was considered one component of the Asian healing arts, a reputation it enjoys today. Anma's "understanding and assessment of human structure and meridian lines" were and are believed to be important distinctions that separate shiatsu therapy from other healing models and massage therapies.[16] When Western massage was introduced to Japan in the late 1880s, the many vocational schools that taught Anma were dominated by blind instructors. However, this very limitation stopped the further development of Anma and led to the evolution of what we recognize today as shiatsu therapy.[16]

Modern shiatsu, as noted previously, is a product of twentieth century refinements and evolution that produced the form of therapy used today. Shiatsu began its modern evolution in the 1920s (the Taisho period) when Anma practitioners adopted some of the West's hands-on techniques, including those of chiropractic and occupational therapy.[16]

The practice of shiatsu received a big boost from studies conducted after World War II, as described in the following quotation from Saito.

After World-War II, U.S.-General Douglas McArthur directed the Japanese Health Ministry. There were more than 300 unregulated therapies in Japan at that time. McArthur ordered all 300 to be researched by scientists at the Universities, to document which ones had scientific proof of merit; and which did not.

At the end of eight years, the Universities reported back; and "Shiatsu" was the only one therapeutic practice, which received scientific approval.[13]

In 1955 the Japanese parliament adopted a bill on "revised Anma," which gave shiatsu official government endorsement. This endorsement allowed shiatsu to be legally taught in schools throughout Japan.[16] Shiatsu received further official Japanese government recognition as a therapy in 1964.[10] In the early 1970s shiatsu began spreading to the West and rapidly gained widespread acceptance.[4] Although shiatsu and its distant cousin acupuncture are considered medically sound and are "accepted methods of treatment for over one-quarter of the world's population," the United States and many other Western nations consider both techniques experimental.[16] This is interesting, considering that these "experiments" have been conducted successfully for more than 2500 years.[4] However, several U.S. hospitals now allow the use of acupuncture, and medical students are taught the theories and practice of acupuncture, shiatsu, and macrobiotics. These gains suggest that an environment has been established for rapid, ongoing change in the West. There is a growing acceptance and use of these practices among Western-trained physicians and health care providers. Shiatsu can be described as a synthesis of Eastern and Western medicine, quickly gaining recognition for its success as an adjunctive healing therapy. Yamamoto and McCarty write, "The foundations for modern ideas and techniques in the healing realm come from ancient civilizations. In the West it was Greece and Rome. And in the East it was China, India, and Persia. These foundations are the basis of present scientific methods [of healing]."[16] Shiatsu's foundations, and therefore shiatsu itself, are a part of the growing trend and movement toward integrative medicine.

PRINCIPLES AND PHILOSOPHY

Many followers of Eastern traditions believe that the natural state of humanity is to be healthy. Yamamoto and McCarty describe it this way:

With observation we can see that there is a definite and distinct order in nature. Nature's power guides all things. When we do not follow nature's order we can become sick. We are often reminded of nature's order by the presence of sickness. Sickness can be our teacher. From a traditional point of view the specific name of an illness is not so important. Physical ailments such as headache, gallbladder pain, emotional states such as anger, depression, irritability; and mental conditions such as paranoia, lack of concentration, and forgetfulness; are all various states of disequilibrium or dis-ease. Theoretically there is no disease that is incurable, if we are able to change the way we think eat, and live. Of course this is easier said than done.[16]

They also write, "The simple understanding that humans are equipped to heal themselves and that

[they] can also help others, [forms] the underlying foundation of Shiatsu. Shiatsu [simply] acts like a spark or catalyst to the human body [and] the combination of treatment and way of life suggestions form the basis of total care."[16]

The major underlying principle of shiatsu, derived from the tenets of Asian medicine, is actually a reflection of scientific thought. Simply stated, "Everything is energy." When considered in the context of molecular structure, all matter is a manifestation of energy. Shiatsu interacts directly with this energy, and therefore with life itself.

From the perspective of classic Asian medicine, energy moves along 14 distinct pathways in the body; these pathways are called *meridians* or *channels* (*kieraku* in Japanese, *jing* in Chinese).[16] The meridians were discovered by accident when certain acu-points (specific locations along the meridians) were stimulated and beneficial results were observed. For example, asthmalike symptoms caused by certain types of battle wounds were relieved when the corresponding acu-point was touched, and menstrual pain was reduced when a heated rock from a fireplace accidentally brushed against a point on the inner thigh.[16] Although many in the West attempt to deny or discount the existence of the meridian network, modern research conducted by biophysicists in Japan, China, and France has documented its existence. Yamamoto and McCarty describe some of this research in the following excerpt from *Whole Health Shiatsu*.

Many studies have been conducted by biophysicists in Japan, China, and France. They postulated that a measurement of acu-point electricity would be a biophysical index that would illustrate the objective existence of the meridian system. They discovered that acu-points have a lower skin resistance. When an electrical current is passed through a classical acu-point, it has a higher electrical conductance which is a lower resistance, than the surrounding area. They also discovered that when disease or illness is present, pathological changes take place in the body while changes are found in the resistance of relevant meridians and acu-points. Similar internal changes are also reflected by the acu-points. In other words, imbalance in the organs affect the acu-points, imbalance in the acu-points affect the organs. Researchers also found that the external environment such as temperature, season, and time of day, changed the resistance of acu-points.

In the Lanzhou Medical College in China a test of the acu-points of the Stomach meridian showed significant variations in conductance when the stomach lining was stimulated by cold or hot water, either before or after eating. In Beijing, ear acu-point research learned that low resistance points on the outer rim of the ear were elevated either in the presence of disease or following long-term stimulation of a corresponding internal organ.[16]

In addition to the scientific support developed thus far, the benefits of shiatsu are supported by the experiences of clients and practitioners alike. Asthmatic clients experience volatility (pain and sensitivity) along their lung meridian. Clients with lower digestive track symptoms such as constipation experience this same sensitivity along their large intestine meridians. When clients experience this connection, which is common in shiatsu, they are quick to convert to the principles of Asian medicine and to accept the validity of the meridian network. Not only has research documented scientific evidence to support the theory behind shiatsu, but the body's own level of pain along related organ meridian lines makes a client's enlightenment regarding the existence of meridians, based on their own personal experience with shiatsu therapy, hard to deny.

It is believed that meridians evolved from energy centers in the body called *chakras* (SHOCK-ras) and that our organ systems subsequently evolved from the meridian network. There are 10 meridians directly related to internal organs, 2 indirectly related, and 2 related to systems not recognized by Western medicine.

Along the meridian lines are points called *tsubos* (SUE-bows), or *acupuncture points.* Yamamoto and McCarty describe tsubos in the following excerpt from *Whole Health Shiatsu.*

The word *Tsubo* or *acu-point* derives from the Oriental characters meaning hole or orifice, and position—the position of the hole. Traditionally, the word hole was combined with other terms such as hollow, passageway, transport, and Ki [Key, or energy]. This suggests that the holes on the surface of the body were regarded as routes of access to the body's internal cavities. The acu-points are spots where Ki comes out.

There are three phases in the historical development of the concept of these holes or acu-points. In the earliest phase people would use any body location that was painful or uncomfortable. Because there were no specific locations for the points, they had no names.

In the second phase, after a long period of practice and experience, certain points became identified with specific diseases. The ability of distinct points to affect and be affected by local or distant pain and disease became predictable. . . .

In the final phase, many previously localized points, each with a singular function, became integrated into a larger system that related and grouped diverse points systematically according to similar functions. This integration is called the *meridian* or *channel system.*[16]

Although the analogy is not completely accurate, shiatsu is often called "acupuncture without needles." To alter a client's internal energy system or pattern, an acupuncturist inserts needles in tsubos used by a shiatsu practitioner. The most significant difference between the two disciplines is that whereas acupuncture is invasive and is performed by extensively trained doctors, shiatsu is noninvasive and can be practiced by either a professional therapist or a lay person. Shiatsu is also a whole-body technique versus one that is limited to the insertion of needles at specific Tsubos. Acupuncture is considered more symptom-oriented in that people are unlikely to go to an acupuncturist without a specific complaint, whereas clients often equate shiatsu with health maintenance and go for treatments without particular "problems." Although some consider shiatsu a cousin to acupuncture, others suggest a "distant cousin" relationship. The distinctions between the two disciplines are worth noting (Table 9-1). It is also important to note here that simple shiatsu can be practiced with little or no understanding of the underlying principles. The practitioner does not have to agree with the principles or understand them to provide shiatsu; however, the techniques are part of a more complicated healing system that, when adhered to and studied, provides more effective results.

A simple and accurate analogy for understanding the meridian pathways and tsubos in relation to the body's internal organ systems is that tsubos are very similar to a system of volcanoes on the earth's surface. We know that a volcano's real energy is not at the surface, but is found deep inside the earth. A volcano is a superficial manifestation of the underlying energy. In similar fashion, a tsubo can be thought of as a manifestation of the underlying energy of the organ system. This does not imply that the therapist should ignore the area of pain a shiatsu client may describe. However, a classically trained shiatsu practitioner looks past sore shoulders, ligaments, and tendons (unless the cause of the pain is trauma to these structures), and focuses on the related organ system via the meridian network. Philosophically, shiatsu practitioners relate health to the condition of the related "vital" organs (i.e., those associated with the

TABLE 9-1

Distinctions Between Shiatsu and Acupuncture[3]

Category	Shiatsu	Acupuncture
Movement	Free flowing	Systematic
Focus	Intuitive	Adheres to laws
Theoretic inclination	Taoist	Confucian
Quality	Feminine	Masculine
Tools	Practitioner's body	Needles
Treatment goal	Balance by becoming whole	Balance by alleviating symptoms
Patient interacts with treater	Yes	No
Encourages independence	Yes— immediately	Yes—after treatment series
Physically strengthens:		
Receiver	Yes	Sometimes
Treater	Yes	No

Although not all acupuncturists agree with all of these distinctions, they form a basis for comparison. All shiatsu practitioners and acupuncturists practice according to their own interpretations and belief systems, so this chart should not be interpreted as a rigid, fixed framework.

TABLE 9-2

Five Elements of Asian Medicine

Element	Yin	Yang
Wood (tree)	Gallbladder	Liver
Fire	Small intestine	Heart
Earth (soil)	Stomach	Spleen
Metal	Larger intestine	Lungs
Water	Bladder	Kidney

meridian system). Although shiatsu is noninvasive and appears to deal with external or surface pain, according to shiatsu theory and the experience of those who practice and receive the art it stimulates, sedates, and balances energy *inside* the body as a way to address the root causes of surface and bodily discomfort.

The principles of Asian medicine evident in shiatsu theory and practice state that two types of energies exist in the universe. These two types of energy, called *yin* and *yang*, exist side by side and are considered both complementary and opposing (see Chapter 11). Unlike Western medicine, which uses more dualistic terms such as "good and bad," Eastern or Asian medicine looks at health more as a manifestation of balance between yin and yang and how an imbalance may *allow* infection or disease to manifest. An effective way to comprehend this internally is to apply the principles of yin and yang to diet through macrobi-

otics. When a person's health and metabolism adjust to what Eastern medicine and macrobiotic practitioners consider universal guidelines, natural harmony occurs from the inside out. Varying states of yin and yang are experienced by the body but are not necessarily comprehended by the mind. This experience can be made manifest by dedication (not necessarily life long) to the practice of using food according to the various energetic principles long understood by the Chinese, Japanese, and followers of macrobiotic theory.

In defining yin and yang, bear in mind that a continuum exists between the extremes of each. In shiatsu major organs are paired together under one of the five major elements. Each pair has both a yang and yin organ. One organ is more compact and tighter (yang), whereas the other is more open and vessel-like (yin). The five elements—wood (tree), fire, earth (soil), metal, and water—proceed in a clockwise manner within the five-element wheel used in Asian medicine (Table 9-2).

According to shiatsu principles, an organ is fed by its opposite energy. For the shiatsu practitioner, pressing and rubbing movements proceed in the direction energy travels along each respective meridian. Shiatsu texts often use the term *structure* to describe an organ, whereas acupuncture texts may describe the same organ in terms of the energy that *feeds* it through the meridian. A yang organ is fed by yin energy. A shiatsu practitioner generally describes the compact kidney as yang because of its *structure* (compared with its paired, more hollow and open yin organ, the bladder). A classically trained acupuncturist generally describes the kidney as yin because it is *fed by* yin energy that flows *up* the body on the kidney meridian. Such differences between the two disciplines in terms of descriptive language can be confusing, although little if any differences in application of goals, practice, or theory really exists.

Another major principle applied to the practice of shiatsu involves the concepts of *kyo* (KEY-o) and *jitsu* (JIT-sue). Kyo is considered empty or vacant, whereas jitsu is considered full, excessive, or overflowing. A jitsu condition along the gallbladder meridian may be a manifestation of a gallbladder imbalance, resulting perhaps from recent consumption of a large pizza and two dishes of ice cream. A kyo or empty condition along the lung meridian (and within the lung itself) may exist in an individual who doesn't exercise and rarely expands his or her chest cavity or heart. Understanding and finding these energy manifestations is critical to diagnosis in shiatsu practice and is an ongoing, lifelong learning experience for the serious shiatsu practitioner. Although it is generally easy to find jitsu, or excess, it is much harder to find emptiness or vacancy (kyo) within the meridian network. One of the keys to doing highly successful or refined shiatsu is the ability to find specific kyo within the body or the organ's meridian network and then to manipulate it effectively.

Shiatsu practitioners may follow the practice of macrobiotics, a set of universal dietary and spiritual guidelines originally brought to the attention of the modern world by George Ohsawa. David Sergel writes, "The ultimate goal of macrobiotic practice is the attainment of absolute freedom. The compass to reach this goal is an intimate understanding of the forces of Yin and Yang; a comprehension of an order common to all aspects of the infinite universe. The foundation of this freedom lies in our daily diet."[15] He also writes, "Since the same cultural soil gave form to both shiatsu and macrobiotics, we might expect to see strong possibilities of a harmonious integration between the two. In fact as we delve deeper, we see evidence that shiatsu arose from a macrobiotic mind and is thus according to this view, from its foundation, a macrobiotic practice."[15] It would be more accurate to state that shiatsu developed out of a society whose dietary pattern reflected the modern day perspective and application of macrobiotics. Shiatsu evolved as a result of day to day living and thinking in terms of yin and yang, as did nearly everything else in these earlier Asian societies, for example Feng Shui, art, and even politics.

Macrobiotics is a philosophic practice that incorporates the universal guidelines of yin and yang into daily life. With diet as its cornerstone, macrobiotic theory posits that these guidelines can be applied to all people, subject to their condition, constitution, lifestyle, and environment, and, most notably, the latitude at which they live. Food choices are governed by season. Macrobiotics is *not* a diet; it is a philosophy that advocates cooked whole grains as the predominant staple food, to be supplemented by other yang foods such as root vegetables and occasional fish, and yin foods such as leafy greens and occasional seasonal fruit. Extreme yin foods include white sugar, honey, caffeine, most drugs, and alcohol. Examples of extreme yang foods are animal proteins such as red meat, chicken, tuna, and shellfish. Dietary choices are adjusted according to an individual's constitution, environment, work, lifestyle, season, and location. When used indiscriminately, extreme yin and yang foods are more difficult to balance and affect energy as manifested along the meridian network. For example, eating tropical fruit in Pennsylvania in January when the temperature is 10°F may be seen as eating out of balance. Macrobiotic philosophy therefore relies on nature, from which it finds ample support. Although we are able to ship foods thousands of miles from where they are grown, nature may not have intended us to regularly consume such foods in an environment that does not support their growth or cultivation. When applied in this way, the philosophies of shiatsu and macrobiotics touch on and address what is viewed as human arrogance by suggesting that when clear-cut guidelines presented by nature are ignored, health consequences can result. Nature demonstrates that the foods that grow and *can* grow in the latitudes where we live are the foods that support our health most fully. This philosophy also states that consumption of root vegetables (i.e., those that produce more heat in the body) is important in the winter, whereas leafy greens and occasional fruit (foods that cool the body) are needed in summer. Interestingly enough, we intuitively follow this practice to some extent. People who live in locations where the climate varies from season to season tend to eat more salads and fruit in the summer and more cooked and salty foods in the winter. However, macrobiotic philosophy examines this practice more closely.

Shiatsu incorporates macrobiotic philosophy into its theory and philosophy regarding the movement of energy along the meridian pathways. A simple explanation of shiatsu philosophy states that the meridians can be seen as circulatory or plumbing channels. As long as energy moves freely (i.e., is not too weak or too strong and is not stagnated) health is maintained. If there is a blockage along the channel, the resulting disturbance can lead to minor aches and pains or a major health imbalance. It is possible to observe imbalances of energy flow in specific meridian lines and acupuncture points or tsubos. By applying pressure to a blocked meridian line or tsubo, an overactive or underactive organ system can be directly sedated or stimulated.

Shiatsu massage is not viewed by its practitioners as a panacea. Shiatsu philosophy is very clear in reinforcing the need for dietary and lifestyle guidance and changes to complement and support a shiatsu session (or series of sessions). The choices made by the recipients of treatment are theirs. Many recipients are content to stay at the level at which shiatsu is simply used for pain reduction and for producing a "calmed sense of revitalization." However, others who are open to the underpinnings of shiatsu philosophy may be willing to take additional steps suggested by a classically trained shiatsu practitioner regarding diet and behavior modification.

With sufficient training, the shiatsu practitioner learns to view the energy manifesting at major tsubos on the surface of the skin as indicative of the underlying condition of the organ to which the tsubo is related and connected. For instance, a client may think shoulder pain is caused by how he or she sleeps or sits at a desk. A classically trained shiatsu practitioner does not ignore these factors, but looks *past* them to the underlying organ system and the foods that affect that organ system. The practitioner attempts to change the energy pattern not just by working at the proximate points of client complaint and distress but also along the entire meridian (or set of meridians). Dietary suggestions are not uncommon. If the concept that everything is energy can be accepted, it may be possible to accept that the specific energies of foods can have an effect not only on organ systems and ultimately on health, but that this effect can produce effects thought unrelated to the internal metabolic state.

Shiatsu training touches on the principles of Asian medicine because the nature of the organ systems and their related energy should be understood for effective treatment to occur, although, as mentioned previously, this knowledge is not an absolute requirement to practice shiatsu. How far this education goes, particularly in relation to the underlying effects of specific foods and their yin and yang effects on various organs and the body as a whole, depends on the quality of the school, the knowledge of the instructor, and the interest of the students.

The Japanese Ministry of Health and Welfare demonstrated its support of shiatsu's efficacy when it stated, "Shiatsu therapy is a form of manipulation administered by the thumbs, fingers, and palms, without the use of any instrument, mechanical or otherwise, to apply pressure to the human skin, correct internal malfunctioning, promote and maintain health, and treat specific diseases."[12]

DIAGNOSIS

The art of Asian diagnosis is a lifelong learning process in the practice of shiatsu. Subtle yet specific, Asian diagnosis is an ongoing and evolving pursuit, which a practitioner is continually mastering and learning again from scratch. Modern diagnostic techniques are a relatively recent development in the history of medicine. Powerful, precise, and accurate to a large extent, their contribution to the improvement of the human condition cannot be denied. However, diagnostic procedures in Western medicine use a disease-oriented model and tend to focus on parts (e.g., cells, tissues, organs) rather than on the whole organism. For example, Louis Pasteur (1822-1895) believed that microbes were the primary cause of disease. Although this theory has proved correct and is applicable to a large number of cases, germs are not the sole cause of disease. Although Asian diagnosis has been practiced for thousands of years, Western medicine has largely ignored its value. However, this is changing with the increased integration of Eastern and Western diagnostic methods.

In Asian medicine and shiatsu, there are two underlying levels of diagnosing human beings: constitutional and conditional. Simply stated, an individual's *constitution* is what he or she was born with. Along with inherited traits, the quality of life, energy, and food intake experienced by the mother while a person is in utero are all considered factors that make up a person's constitution. A person's *condition* is the sum of his or her experience, which includes diet. In classical shiatsu diagnosis, both constitution and condition are assessed according to the methods listed in the following.

The following four methods of observing "phenomena" are used in Asian medicine[12]:

1. *Bo-shin:* diagnosis through observation
2. *Bun-shin:* diagnosis through sound
3. *Mon-shin:* diagnosis through questioning
4. *Set su-shin:* diagnosis through touch

Each day, whether we realize it or not, we use the first three methods of observation extensively in our interactions with others and the environment. We all have experienced a funny feeling in our stomachs when we enter a room that has recently been the site of some tension related to human interaction. We choose partners based on some innate sense of energy recognition we find compatible with our own. Although we are unaware that we use aspects of Asian diagnosis in our everyday lives, we nonetheless make assessments and judgments based on these principles. Without these "diagnostic skills" we would not survive. Shiatsu uses the first three methods liberally, and also relies heavily on the fourth.

In a traditional shiatsu session, diagnosis begins with the first contact between client and practitioner, whether in person or on the telephone. The client's tone of voice, speed of delivery, and choice of words give clues to the trained ear regarding the condition and constitution of the shiatsu client.

On meeting a client for the first time, constitutional and conditional assessments are made. How did the client enter the room? Did she walk upright? Did he smile or frown? Was her handshake strong or weak? Was his hand wet, damp, dry, hot, cold? The client is often unaware that a classically trained shiatsu therapist begins work with the first contact and continues the assessment the minute a face-to-face meeting begins. Visual diagnosis and verbal questioning continue as the first meeting between client and therapist proceeds.

To arrive at a constitutional diagnosis, the therapist looks at various physical attributes. No single factor observed gives a total picture, but a *macro* assessment takes the various *micro* elements into account. Size of ears, shape and size of head, distance between the eyes, size of mouth, and size of hands are fundamental observations made in constitutional diagnosis before any physical treatment begins.

Factors considered in conditional assessment are slightly different but work in tandem with the overall assessment. The stated reason for the visit is a factor. In addition, tone and volume of the client's voice, pupil size, eye color, color and condition of the tongue, condition of the nails, and response to palpation along specific points on the hands and arms may be used. Pulse diagnosis (the act of reading distinctly differently levels of heartbeats near the wrists on both hands) may be used, depending on the practitioner's level of training. Generally speaking, pulse diagnosis is more the tool of an acupuncturist, but it has been

and can be used by a properly trained shiatsu provider.

The four diagnostic methods (observation, sound, questioning, and touch) are used to develop a singular yin-yang analysis.[3] At its basic level, Asian diagnosis sets out to determine whether a person is *vibrationally*, or *energetically*, more yin or more yang because these two opposing but complementary states of energy affect each of us.

The diagnostic assessment process continues along specific lines, as described by Yamamoto and McCarty in *Whole Health Shiatsu:*

Yang diagnosis: Excess body heat and desire for coolness; great thirst and desire for fluids; constipation and hard stools; scanty, hot, dark urine.
    Yin diagnosis: Cold feeling and desire for warmth; lack of thirst and preference for hot drinks; loose stools; profuse, clear urine; flat taste in mouth; poor appetite.[16]

The key is not in being able to see the yin and yang extremes described in the excerpt. The key is in determining not only what tendency within an individual may be contributing to his or her state but also the particular organ or organs that have a jitsu or kyo condition, and then working those organs' meridians to change that state. This is the point at which the movement from external or initial diagnosis of constitution and condition ends and treatment begins.

At this point, the practitioner's hands become the primary diagnostic tools. Although diagnosis is an ongoing process during treatment, traditional shiatsu first assesses by palpation the major organs located in the client's *hara,* or abdomen. Alternatively, some styles of shiatsu begin a treatment session with touch diagnosis on the upper back, an area that also yields a vast amount of information regarding a person's condition. Assessment and diagnosis include palpatory observations that describe the following physical properties: tightness or looseness, fullness or emptiness, hot or cold, dry or wet, resistant or open, stiff or flexible.

Diagnosis in a shiatsu session does not cease after an initial assessment. Diagnosis is an ongoing process of observation, listening, feeling, and changing focus based on continuously revealed information. The ability to quickly make an accurate diagnosis can be extremely helpful to a practitioner and client in their mutual attempt to create energetic change for the receiving partner. However, shiatsu can be effective in the hands of a relatively unskilled diagnostician. By following the simple concept of paying attention to what is going on underneath one's hands, a lay person, with relatively little training, can provide an effective, relaxing, and enjoyable shiatsu treatment for family and friends in a nonprofessional setting.

PRACTICES, TECHNIQUES, AND TREATMENT

Unlike some disciplines, shiatsu is easy to learn. It is not possible for a lay person to practice chiropractic, acupuncture, or osteopathy, because medical professionals need not only training but also time and continuing education to master techniques and improve skills. Shiatsu also requires a disciplined approach, constant practice, and continuing study to develop in-depth understanding. However, the *basic* practice remains simple, effective, and safe. Shiatsu techniques can be learned and safely applied by anyone, typically resulting in positive effects for both the recipient and provider. It can be performed anywhere, takes place fully clothed, and requires no special tools, machines, or oils.

Sergel states, "While ki may indeed emanate from the giver's fingertips it may not be in this way or only in this way that shiatsu works. Masunaga's approach is to emphasize another side, that the healing ki of *shiatsu lies within the quality or spirit of the touch in itself,* as compared with the idea of some invisible current that emanates from the touch.[15] More than 150 years ago Shinsai Ota, in a book on Ampuku (hara, or abdominal) shiatsu, emphasized that "honest, sincere, and simple Shiatsu is much better than merely technique-oriented professional Shiatsu."[12] Indeed, shiatsu training often emphasizes that the most important element is to be in touch with what is going on *under one's hands.* Experts agree, indicating that when a practitioner applies pressure and stimulation, he or she should then react and follow up based on an intuitive sense of and reaction to internal changes within the recipient.[16] A traditionally trained shiatsu practitioner, knowledgeable in the food energy fundamentals of yin and yang and applying those principles in his or her life, is arguably better suited to respond intuitively to the client. It is believed that intuition is enhanced by being in harmony with nature, a condition achieved by following the guidelines of living within nature's principles—earth's rhythms of yin and yang. Harmony in the body is achieved by being in harmony with the universe. Eating large amounts of animal protein and simple carbohydrates, which in their cultivation and processing exploit and pollute the earth, does not yield a calm and focused mind that can easily tap into human intuition. If a person is not in harmony with the natural order, the theory goes, he or she is less likely to be able to tap into his or her intuition and tune in to another person's needs and internal energies.[15] Experienced shiatsu practitioners agree.

Although a successful shiatsu session may be based more on intuition than technical understanding, it still is necessary to outline the techniques and preparation needed for a successful shiatsu treatment. Shiatsu recipients are fully clothed. Although shiatsu techniques can be adapted to other massage styles and may be performed on bare skin, traditional shiatsu is applied to a fully clothed person. Clients should be dressed in loose-fitting cotton fiber clothing. Blends containing polyester or other synthetics are thought to block or interrupt the natural transmission of energy between the caregiver and the recipient. Static electricity builds up around synthetic fibers. Because, from an Asian perspective, *everything is energy,* nonnatural fibers, which may produce unnatural energies, should not be worn during a shiatsu session.

Because shiatsu requires no special tools or environment, it can be performed anywhere at any time. However, traditional shiatsu is generally performed on a cotton floor futon or shiatsu mat. Shiatsu techniques may be adapted to a table, but this is considered a deviation from the classical perspective. Although shiatsu can take place at any time of day, because the energetic effects of shiatsu differ dramatically in many ways from other methods, practitioners may encourage new clients to schedule a session early in the day, preferably before noon. Because shiatsu can yield a "calmed sense of revitalization," the combination of being relaxed *and* energized is an experience that should be savored throughout the day. Americans often equate "calm and relaxed" with an *inactive* state. Although shiatsu yields different results for different people, one of the most unique effects experienced by most clients is indeed this "calmed sense of revitalization." It is not uncommon for a new shiatsu client to report, when treated by a competent practitioner, that he or she has "never felt this way before."

One reason for the difference in the energetic effects of shiatsu as opposed to other techniques (usually called *regular massage* by the general public) is easy to explain. In many forms of therapeutic massage a technique described as *effleurage* or *stroking* (sweeping the skin with the hands) is used. The benefits of this type of movement on the skin are many, including stimulation of blood flow and the movement of lymph. Although this technique is beneficial, one of its effects is often a feeling of lethargy. Because the effects of shiatsu are realized more on the underlying blockage of energy related to the body's organ systems than on the lymphatic system, a shiatsu session can yield a feeling of increased short and long-term energy. This is why chair massage using shiatsu techniques is so appropriate, and considered by many superior to other techniques in the corporate setting. Employees do not experience the short-term negative energetic effects (lethargy) of effleurage, but rather the energetic boost, the *calmed sense of revitalization* so often associated with effective shiatsu technique. Masunaga and Ohashi described this difference in the following way:

> Anma and European massage directly stimulate blood circulation, emphasizing the release of stagnated blood in the skin and muscles and tension and stiffness resulting from circulatory congestion. On the other hand, Shiatsu emphasizes correction and maintenance of bone structure, joints, tendons, muscles, and meridian lines whose malfunctioning distort the body's energy and autonomic nervous system causing disease.[12]

Shiatsu, like other methods, is best received with an empty stomach. This may not always be possible, and recent food consumption is certainly no bar to receiving shiatsu. However, practitioners and recipients should bear in mind that when the body's energies are focused *inward* toward digestion, a shiatsu session, with its attempt to change the body's energies, is compromised and less effective.

In some ways the beginning of a shiatsu session is similar to other massage styles. The room used should be simple, clean, and quiet. A thorough history of the client and his or her concerns should be taken. Questions regarding sleep patterns, lifestyle, eating habits, and work history are not uncommon. A high level of trust should be established quickly. Often a client is seated in a chair or on a floor mat as the shiatsu practitioner observes and asks questions regarding the client's expectations and level of understanding. Diagnostic techniques to determine the client's constitution and condition are undertaken.

The hands, eyes, tongue, and coloration along the upper and lower limbs may be examined. Several deep breaths to begin the process may be suggested. A well-trained shiatsu practitioner obtains a complete history to uncover any risk factors affecting the appropriateness of shiatsu treatment. Clinical experience and training, coupled with good references regarding a therapist's skills and practice, should be the determining factors in selecting a shiatsu practitioner.

A shiatsu session usually begins in one of two ways. In classical shiatsu, the practitioner may use hara, or abdominal massage, to determine which organ or organ system meridians may require treatment. Because this type of probing may not be appropriate or well received by many new shiatsu clients, some practitioners start with the client seated in a chair or on a floor mat and make an initial assessment of the client's energies from the upper back and shoulder region. This does two things. It gives the practitioner some immediate feedback on the client's condition and helps the client relax. Most people are aware of tension in their upper back, shoulder, and neck, and respond rather quickly to the process of relaxation so necessary for successful shiatsu.

These early assessments of client condition, coupled with a practitioner's best understanding and synthesis of the client's overall constitution, dictates the direction in which the therapist moves. Classical shiatsu texts state that "kyo and jitsu must first be found in the meridian lines by touching or kneading" to allow the direction of the shiatsu to be most effective.[12] However, even when kyo or jitsu are not accurately determined at the outset, effective treatment may still be provided; these conditions can be addressed during the session without any specific perception or awareness of these qualities.

Whether treatment begins in a chair or on a floor mat, most of the session takes place with the client lying down. Applying various techniques along the meridian network, an attempt is made to create a better energy balance for the shiatsu recipient. Techniques used include rocking, tapotement (pounding), rubbing, and stretching. A shiatsu practitioner employs his or her entire body to apply pressure. Feet, elbows, knees, fingers, and palms are used as appropriate. A client may be face down or up, or may lie on the side as directed or moved by the practitioner.

Although certain techniques such as rubbing and kneading may be used at this point and throughout a shiatsu session, the application of more stationary pressure via the palms, thumbs, forearms, and elbows usually begins early in a session. The muscles at the base of the occiput may be kneaded with the fingers and thumbs. Often the head is rotated with one hand while maintaining a stationary base of support at the neck with the other hand. Although shiatsu providers generally use similar methods, every practitioner is different.

When the techniques applied to the upper back, shoulders, and neck are completed, the client generally reclines to the floor mat in a position the therapist deems most beneficial. This may be prone, supine, or side position. Certain individuals may use the side position exclusively because of size, pregnancy, or specific issues.

If placed in a prone position, it is not uncommon for the therapist to use his or her feet to rock the client's hips or to apply graduated pressure to the legs and feet. This "barefoot shiatsu" technique is used extensively by Shizuko Yamamoto and is a very powerful adjunct to the use of the hands, knees, elbows, and forearms. The stretching of the arms and legs and their rotation at the shoulders and hips, respectively, is not uncommon.

Depending on their relative sizes, the practitioner may also walk on the client. Caution is clearly in order when using this rarely practiced technique, but it is sometimes appropriate and beneficial.

Shiatsu sessions typically take place with the provider on his or her knees next to the client. Pressure is applied along distinct meridian lines with the palms and thumbs. Knees, elbows, and forearms may also be used along these specific channels. To access the energy of the various organs through their respective meridians, the client's position changes to side or supine as the session proceeds.

Generally speaking, conversation is minimized or absent during a shiatsu treatment. Music may be played based on the joint needs and desires of giver and receiver. Blood pressure and breathing rates generally go down during a session. It is not uncommon for a shiatsu recipient to feel some cold sensations as he or she begins to relax, a natural reaction of the body's autonomic nervous system. Shiatsu can be performed through a cotton blanket, which most practitioners have available. A shiatsu session can be of any length, although a 60-minute duration is very common. Sessions often end where they began, at the base of the client's neck or head with gentle kneading or massaging of neck or facial muscles. Shiatsu recipients are generally asked to remain quiet and still for several minutes after a session.

Most people can receive shiatsu. People with sprains and sports injuries who are seeking *direct* treatment of specific areas of trauma are best referred to massage therapists. However, gentle and focused shiatsu for these types of injuries can be applied to areas not directly related to the affected area to produce positive results by removing pressure and tension that the body may have created by compensating for the injury. Shiatsu can be used during pregnancy if provided by a practitioner trained in the specific meridians and tsubo points that should be *avoided* during a session. Shiatsu is very effective during pregnancy as long as common sense and the specific training and experience of the therapist are taken into account.

Because stationary and perhaps deeper application of pressure is a major part of shiatsu technique, caution should be exercised when treating people who bruise easily, have high white blood cell counts, or suffer from leukemia, lymphoma, or extensive skin or other cancers. Clients who have an acute or chronic cystic condition must clearly communicate their complete history to reduce any potential risk. Although burn victims have benefited from massage therapy, the application of shiatsu at or near a burn site is not appropriate. However, shiatsu should not, in theory or in practice, be considered a painful massage therapy; quite the opposite is the norm.

The foregoing description of a shiatsu session should be considered generic in nature. There are many variations to the basic techniques, and numerous schools that teach specific shiatsu practices offer more distinct focus to the underlying themes presented above. The American Organization of Body Therapies of Asia (AOBTA) notes 12 specific areas of Asian technique. The six major schools of Asian practice generally regarded as shiatsu are described in the following sections, as shown on the AOBTA web site.

Acupressure

Acupressure is a system of balancing the body's energy by applying pressure to specific acupoints to release tension and increase circulation. The many hands-on methods of stimulating the acupressure points can strengthen weaknesses, relieve common ailments, prevent health disorders and restore the body's vital life force.

Five Element Shiatsu

The primary emphasis of Five Element Shiatsu is to identify a pattern of disharmony through use of the four examinations and to harmonize that pattern with an appropriate treatment plan. Hands on techniques and preferences for assessment varies with the practitioner, depending on their individual background and training. The radial pulse usually provides the most critical and detailed information. Palpation of the back and/or abdomen and a detailed verbal history serve to confirm the assessment. Considerations of the client's lifestyle, emotional and psychological factors are all considered important. Although this approach uses the paradigm of the five elements to tonify, sedate or control patterns of disharmony, practitioners of this style also consider hot or cold; internal or external symptoms and signs.

Japanese Shiatsu

Shiatsu literally means finger (Shi) pressure (Atsu) and although Shiatsu is primarily pressure, usually applied with the thumbs along the meridian lines; extensive soft tissue manipulation and both active and passive exercise and stretching may be part of the treatments. Extensive use of cutaneovisceral reflexes in the abdomen and on the back are also characteristics of Shiatsu. The emphasis of Shiatsu is the treatment of the whole meridian; however, effective points are also used. The therapist assesses the condition of the patient's body as treatment progresses. Therapy and diagnosis are one.

Macrobiotic Shiatsu

Founded by Shizuko Yamamoto and based on George Ohsawa's philosophy that each individual is an integral part of nature, Macrobiotic Shiatsu supports a natural lifestyle and heightened instincts for improving health. Assessments are through visual, verbal, and touch techniques (including pulses) and the Five Transformations.

Treatment involves non-invasive touch and pressure using hand and barefoot techniques and stretches to facilitate the flow of Qi and to strengthen the body-mind. Dietary guidance, medicinal plant foods, breathing techniques and home remedies are emphasized, corrective exercises, postural rebalancing, palm healing, self shiatsu and Qigong are included in Macrobiotic Shiatsu.

Shiatsu Anma Therapy

Shiatsu Anma Therapy utilizes a unique blending of two of the most popular Asian bodywork forms practiced in Japan. Dr. Kaneko introduces traditional Anma Massage Therapy based on the energetic system of Traditional Chinese Medicine in long form and contemporary pressure therapy which is based on neuro-musculo-skeletal system in short form. Ampuku, abdominal massage therapy, is another foundation of Anma Massage Therapy in his school.

Zen Shiatsu

Zen Shiatsu is characterized by the theory of Kyo-Jitsu, its physical and psychological manifestations, and its application to abdominal diagnosis. Zen Shiatsu theory is based on an extended meridian system that includes as well as expands the location of the traditional acupuncture meridians. The focus of a Zen Shiatsu session is on the use of meridian lines rather than on specific points. In addition, Zen Shiatsu does not adhere to a fixed sequence or set of methods that are applied to all. It utilizes appropriate methods for the unique pattern of each individual. Zen Shiatsu was developed by Shizuto Masunaga.

The extended meridian network described and taught by Masunaga is a highly regarded part of shiatsu education. It is taught in quality schools as an integral part of shiatsu theory, diagnosis, and style. It is common for a practitioner to learn the extended meridian network toward the end of his or her shiatsu education as an *extension* to the classical meridian network, in the same manner that Master Masunaga explored this expansion in shiatsu thinking, theory, and practice.[1]

TRAINING AND CERTIFICATION

There are currently no federal regulatory standards in the United States for shiatsu practitioners or any massage therapists per se. The American Massage Therapy Association cites 30 states that have regulations governing massage therapy. There are nearly 100,000 credentialed practitioners at this writing.

Numerous schools of massage offer certificate programs in shiatsu or more broad-based programs that include shiatsu massage. These programs may be weekend seminars of 1 or 2 days, or may provide 600 or more hours of training particular to shiatsu. It is not uncommon for schools to offer 350 to 500 hours of training in classical shiatsu with an additional 150 hours in anatomy and physiology. There appears to be a growing trend for internships in all schools of massage.

The American Organization for Bodywork Therapies of Asia (formerly the American Asian Body Therapy Association) is the largest and most prevalent organization particular to the practice of shiatsu. Certified Practitioner applicants must complete a 500-hour program, preferably at a school or institution recognized by AOBTA.

The American Massage Therapy Association (AMTA) is a general association of massage practitioners; it does not actively focus on shiatsu therapy. It is a highly respected association that meets regularly with the AOBTA as a federated massage-supporting organization. The AMTA's mission is to develop and advance the art, science, and practice of massage therapy in a caring, professional, and ethical manner to promote the health and welfare of humanity.

The American Bodywork and Massage Professionals (ABMP) is another highly respected association of massage professionals. Unlike the AOBTA and the AMTA, the ABMP is a for-profit organization.

The National Certification Board for Therapeutic Massage and Bodywork (NCBTMB) is a nationally recognized credentialing body formed to set high standards for those who practice therapeutic massage and bodywork. It accomplishes this through a nationally recognized certification program that evaluates the competency of its practitioners. Since 1992, more than 40,000 massage therapists and bodyworkers have received their certification. The NCBTMB examination is now legally recognized in more than 20 states and in many municipalities. The NCBTMB represents a diverse group of massage therapists, not just shiatsu practitioners. A minimum of 500 hours of formal massage education and successful completion of a written exam are the basic requirements for certification. Practitioners must be recertified every four years.

A person considering the use of any massage therapy as an adjunct to health maintenance should carefully select the provider of that therapy. In addition to personal references, it is important to evaluate the practitioner's training, experience, professional affiliations, and certification.

RESEARCH

The results of a number of randomized, controlled trials have recently been published. What follows is a brief listing of these studies, grouped by category.

Cardiovascular

- A blind, randomized control study in a university-affiliated hospital documented a decrease in systolic, diastolic, and mean arterial pressure, as well as heart rate and skin blood flow, when acu-points were stimulated by pressure. Researchers concluded that acupressure can significantly and positively influence the cardiovascular system.[1]
- A single-blind, pretest–posttest, cross-over design study in which patients were taught how to self-administer acupressure concluded that real acupressure was more effective than sham acupressure for reducing dyspnea, and was minimally effective for relieving decathxis.[7]

Nausea with Breast Cancer Chemotherapy

- Finger pressure applied bilaterally to two "major" acupressure points during the first 10 days of a chemotherapy cycle reduced the intensity and experience of nausea among women undergoing therapy.[11]

Nausea and Vomiting

- The use of acupressure at the P6 acu-point was shown to reduce the incidence of nausea and vomiting within 24 hours of anesthesia from 42% to 19% compared with placebo.[5]
- The use of acupressure at the P6 point was shown to reduce the incidence of nausea and vomiting after Caesarean section compared with placebo.[8]
- Acupressure bands placed at the P6 points on subjects receiving general anesthesia for ambulatory surgery experienced less nausea (23%) versus the control group (41%), suggesting this method as an alternative to conventional antiemetic treatment.[9]
- The incidence of postoperative vomiting in children was significantly lower (20%) than in the

placebo group (68%) when stationary acupressure was applied to the Korean K-K9 point for 30 minutes before and 24 hours after undergoing strabismus surgery.[6]

- The stimulation of the P6 (Neiguan) acu-point was determined to prevent nausea and vomiting in adults, although no antiemetic effects were noted in children undergoing strabismus surgery. However, it was determined that prophylactic use of bilateral acuplaster in children reduced the incidence of vomiting from 35.5% to 14.7% in the early emesis phase, 58.1% to 23.5% in the late emesis phase, and 64.5% to 29.4% overall. Researchers concluded that the use of acuplaster reduced vomiting in children undergoing strabismus correction.[14]

References

1. American Organization for Body Therapies of Asia: *General definition and scope of practice.* Available at www.aobta.org/definitions.htm. [Accessed 12/6/01.]
2. Chen ML, Lin LC, Wu SC et al: The effectiveness of acupressure in improving the quality of sleep of institutionalized residents, *J Gerontol A Biol Sci Med Sci* 54A(8):M389-M394, 1999.
3. Colt GW, Hollister A: The magic of touch, *Life Mag* August:55-62, 1997.
4. Cowmeadow O: *The art of shiatsu,* Rockport, Mass, 1992, Element Books, Ltd.
5. Dibble SL, Chapman J, Mack KA et al: Acupressure for nausea: results of a pilot study, *Oncol Nurs Forum* 27(1):41-47, 2000.
6. Fan CF, Tanhui E, Joshi S et al: Acupressure treatment for prevention of postoperative nausea and vomiting, *Anesth Analg* 84(4):712-714, 821-825, 1997.
7. Felhendler D, Lisander B: Effects of non invasive stimulation of acupoints on the cardiovascular system, *Complement Ther Med* 7(4):231-234, 1999.
8. Harmon D, Gardiner J, Harrison R et al: Acupressure and the prevention of nausea and vomiting after laparoscopy [see comments], *Br J Anaesth* 82(3):387-390, 1999.
9. Harmon D, Ryan M, Kelly A et al: Acupressure and prevention of nausea and vomiting during and after spinal anaesthesia for caesarean section, *Br J Anaesth* 84(4):463-467, 2000.
10. Lundberg P: *The book of shiatsu,* New York, 1992, Simon & Schuster.
11. Maa SH, Gautheir D, Turner M: Acupressure as an adjunct to a pulmonary rehabilitation program, *J Cardiopulm Rehabil* 17:268-276, 1997.
12. Masunaga S, Ohashi W: *Zen shiatsu: how to harmonize yin and yang for better health,* New York, 1977, Japan Publications.
13. Saito K: *This is the shiatsu from Japan,* Japan Shiatsu Association of Canada. Available at www.oyayubi.com/shiatsu/story.html. [Accessed 4/01.]
14. Schlager A, Boehler M, Puhringer F: Korean hand acupressure reduces postoperative vomiting in children after strabismus surgery, *Br J Anaesth* 85(2):267-270, 2000.
15. Sergel D: *The Macrobiotic way of zen shiatsu,* New York, 1989, Japan Publications.
16. Yamamoto S, McCarty P: *Whole health shiatsu,* New York, 1993, Japan Publications.

Supplementary Readings

Kushi M: *Basic shiatsu,* Becket, Mass, 1995, One Peaceful World Press.

Liechti E: *The complete illustrated guide to shiatsu: the Japanese healing art of touch for health and fitness,* Bement, Ill, 1998, Bement Books, Ltd.

Massage Magazine. See Appendix.

Namikoshi T: *The complete book of shiatsu therapy,* Tokyo, Japan, 1994, Japan Publications.

Namikoshi T: *Shiatsu: Japanese finger-pressure therapy,* Tokyo, Japan, 1995, Japan Publications.

Ohashi W, Deangelis P: *The Ohashi bodywork book: beyond shiatsu with the Ohashiatsu method,* Tokyo, Japan, 1997, Kodansha International.

Sergel D: *The natural way of zen shiatsu,* Tokyo, Japan, 1999, Japan Publications.

Touchpoints. See Appendix.

Yamamoto S: *Barefoot shiatsu: whole-body approach to health,* New York, 1998, Putnum.

Yamamoto S, McCarty P: *The shiatsu handbook: a guide to the traditional art of shiatsu acupressure,* New York, 1996, Putnum.

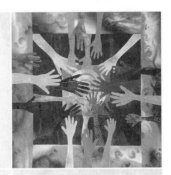

Ayurvedic Bodywork

JOHN M. MCPARTLAND

FELICIA FOSTER

HISTORY

Ayur means *life,* and *veda* means *science* or *knowledge.* *Ayurveda,* or *the science of life,* is the indigenous medical system of India. Ayurveda is reputed to be the oldest complete system of medicine. Practitioners of Chinese medicine (Chung-i) may disagree with this statement, but ancient Chinese practitioners adopted the humoral theory of Ayurveda, which suggests Ayurveda antedated Chung-i.

Brahma, the lord of creation in Hindu theology, is said to have composed a stupendous work on Ayurveda. Early Ayurvedic concepts can be found in the *Rig Veda,* dating to 2000 BC. The oldest known Ayurvedic medical textbook, the *Charaka Samhita,* was written around 320 BC. Over the past 2000 years, traditional *(Shudh)* Ayurveda has commingled with two similar systems, *Unani-Tibb* and *Siddha.* Unani-Tibb, brought to India around 1000 AD, has roots in classical Greek medicine, reworked by the Persians and Arabs. Today Unani-Tibb thrives in northwest India and Pakistan. Siddha developed at the same time as Ayurveda, and today prevails where Dravidian culture once dominated—in Tamil Nadu, Sri Lanka, Malaysia, and Singapore.

Since Indian independence, Ayurveda has enjoyed a 50-year renaissance. Before that, the British Raj suppressed Ayurveda in favor of Western medicine.[10]

Ayurveda is now becoming popular in the United States; its acceptance is on a steep growth curve, much like acupuncture 20 years ago.

PRINCIPLES AND PHILOSOPHY

Ayurveda is the art of daily living in harmony with the laws of nature. The objective of Ayurveda is to correct imbalance and maintain a continual state of balance. According to Ayurveda, balance is the evolution of prakiti, the creative principle. *Prakiti* is the basis of a person's constitutional characteristics and temperament. Prakiti is based on a person's predominant *dosha,* sometimes translated as *life force,* which is determined at the moment of conception. Prakiti is the creator of all forms in the universe (animal, vegetable, mineral, and spiritual), and we are in continual communication with all these forms. We are not separate beings with boundaries and edges, but beings participating in a cosmic dance of rhythms and vibrations. We are not static entities, but beings engaged in continual transformation and change.

In their primal states, all forms contain a perfect balance of the three *gunas,* or universal principles (*satvamaya, rajamaya,* and *tamaomaya,* described later). This state of perfect health and balance is divine, and we hold the memory of its presence within every cell of our being. While still in the womb we begin to assess and respond to the environment. We begin to perceive and interpret each moment and store these experiences in the "software" of the mind. Over time the memory of divinity and perfect health begins to fade, and life becomes linear, conditional, and materialistic.

Ayurveda moves beyond the mechanistic model and sees life as more than a series of successive cause-and-effect events. It recognizes the importance of *consciousness* and the role that consciousness plays in the process of healing. Ayurveda does not see the human body as an isolated, frozen structure, but as contextual, relational, and holistic. Each event occurring within the body is related to other events, both internally and externally. Ayurveda sees the human body as a complex metaphor, molded by its memory and perception of its entire experience of life. There is a statement in the Vedic texts, "If you want to know what your life was like in the past, look at your body now. If you want to know what your body will be like in the future, look at your life now."

Ayurvedic practitioners say that disease is the outward expression of an imbalance created by a person's inability to digest life. Our state of health and our physical bodies are a reflection of how we have chosen to live life and participate in our relationship with the universe. The daily activities of eating, breathing, metabolism, and elimination, the world of sensory experience, and the practice of wholesome living (*sadhana*) all play a part.

Allopathic medicine focuses on the systems of the physical body, such as the cardiovascular system, respiratory system, and gastrointestinal system. Ayurveda, in contrast, states that our internal healing system has supremacy over all other systems. This internal healing system is innate, divine wisdom, an eternal consciousness that is beyond the physical body and mind, a consciousness that is beyond the intellect and beyond the ego, but is always present. Thus in Ayurveda the origin of disease is believed to lie within this consciousness. Disease does not originate in its symptoms or in the mechanisms of the body.

Ayurveda teaches that our life has a purpose, and that purpose is to know or realize the Creator (cosmic consciousness) and to understand our relationship with that consciousness. Healing, according to Ayurveda, is the journey back to the self. It is about remembering our relationship with the divine and our inherent state of perfection.

Reaching and remembering this consciousness or presence is the goal of Ayurvedic treatment. Through the process of the Ayurvedic diagnosis, the person's *vikriti* (imbalance) is determined. Treatment of the person's vikriti addresses the whole life of the person and his or her relationship to the life of the universe.

AYURVEDIC DIAGNOSIS

The diagnostic process in Ayurvedic medicine begins by taking the client's history. Much of this medical history is familiar to Western practitioners, such as obtaining from the client a list of symptoms, a list of current medications, past medical and surgical history, and family history. However, Ayurvedic practitioners also obtain astrologic aspects of the client's history. The next diagnostic procedure is a visual examination of the tongue, eyes, sweat, urine, and feces. The practitioner also listens to the client's voice, auscultates the internal organs, palpates the affected

TABLE 10-1

The Tridoshas of Ayurvedic Medicine

	Vata "wind"	Pitta "bile"	Kapha "phlegm"
Elemental sources	Air and ether	Earth and fire	Earth and water
Chief characteristic	Motile, dry, cold, rough	Hot, acrid, fluid	Inertial, slow, cold, greasy, heavy
Physiology	Initiate movement, respiration	Digestion, generation of metabolism	Connective tissue, ground substance
Taste	Bitter, pungent	Sour, salty	Sweet
Proper massage oil	Sesame	Coconut	Mustard or olive (in some cases, none)

body parts (called *sparsha*), and performs an intricate form of pulse reading (*nadi vigyan* or *nadi pariksha*).

These diagnostic steps are used to determine a person's prakiti and his or her predominant dosha. Three types of doshas are recognized in Ayurveda, summarized in Table 10-1. The tridoshas are derived from environmental "elements," initially five in number (the same number as found in traditional Chinese medicine)—fire, air, water, earth, and ether. However, about 2000 years ago Indian metaphysicians dropped ether from this list.[17] Each dosha is split into subdoshas. A subdosha of vata (the "wind" dosha), for instance, is *prana*—the motile, respiratory aspect of intelligence.

Thanks to recent articles in health magazines, many people are familiar with the tridoshas listed in Table 10-1. *Trigunas* are less known but of equal importance in Ayurveda. Whereas the tridoshas manifest in a person's physical constitution, the trigunas are expressed as psychological temperament and behavior. Trigunas correlate with tridoshas: *rajamaya* correlates with *vata* in the mind as creative energy, the agitation of desires and emotions. It is active and dynamic, like Chinese *yang*. *Satvamaya* correlates with *pitta* as balanced energy, a pure luminous mind. *Tamaomaya* correlates with *kapha* in the mind as a dark, phlegmatic, forgiving yet destructive energy, like Chinese *yin*.

AYURVEDIC TREATMENT

Ayurveda's approach to healing is quite different from the Western approach of alleviating symptoms. Ayurveda's aim is to achieve balance of the four fun-

damental aspects of life: *dharma*—duty or correct action; *artha*—material success or wealth; *kama*—positive desire; and *moksha*—spiritual liberation. The foundation underlying these four aspects of life is health. Without good health we cannot perform the duties and responsibilities of daily living, we cannot create affluence and achieve success, and we cannot be creative and positive. Spiritual liberation is the result of the perfect harmony of body, mind, and consciousness or soul.

The Ayurvedic system of healing teaches that as the internal and external conditions of our lives change, we need to constantly adjust our relationship to life to maintain equilibrium. Our internal wisdom automatically initiates some of the adjusting, but conscious choice is also required. Conscious living-in-the-moment should become a way of life. Ayurveda is not a passive form of therapy; it enrolls each client as an active participant in the process of daily living and healing.

Westerners commonly equate Ayurveda with herbal medicine.[26] In fact, Ayurveda also emphasizes *pathya apathya* (dietary changes), *asanas* (yoga exercises), meditation, spiritual healing, surgery, and a highly refined variety of bodywork techniques. Ayurvedic practitioners believe that prevention is better than cure. They prescribe proper thought and behavior and timely attention to nature's needs. Even time can be conceptualized in tridosha components, so preventive measures change with the time of day and the seasons.

Ignoring prevention causes imbalance, then disease. Westerners are prone to imbalances of vata, which becomes obstructed and accumulates in weak spots, giving rise to symptoms such as headaches, nasal congestion, and heaviness in the cardiac region. Serious illness interferes with *agni* (metabolic factors), which normally transform food into *dhatus* (the seven types of body tissues) and *malas* (the three excreted wastes). Impaired *agni* results in the buildup of *ama*—unabsorbed, undigested food substances that clog intestines and blood vessels and create toxins.

Serious illness calls for serious treatment. In India, Ayurvedic practitioners are divided into a school of physicians *(Atreya sampradaya)* and a school of surgeons *(Dhanvantri sampradaya)*. Each school contains specialty branches, such as *Kayachikitsa* (*kaya* means *medicine*, *chikitsa* means *therapeutic measure;* Kayachikitsa is roughly equivalent to *internal medicine*).

Kayachikitsa has many components. Some diseases, especially vata diseases, require *Santarpana* (also called *Branhana*) or "nurturing care"—eating nourishing foods, resting, and sleeping. Pitta and kapha diseases respond better to *Apa-Tarpana* (also called *langhana*) therapeutics, which are divided into two lines of treatment:

1. *Shamana* therapeutics provide symptomatic relief; they include *kshut* (fasting), *langhana* (light diet), *trit* (restriction of fluids), *atap sevana* (sun rays), *maruta sevana* (breezes of air), *pranayama* (yogic breathing), and *vyayama* (exercises including yoga).
2. *Shodhana* therapeutics provide more than symptomatic relief; they provide a cure. Shodhana therapeutics feature the *panchakarma* (five purifications); *nasya* (nasal medications), *vamana* (emetics), *virechana* (purgatives), *basti* (enemas), and *raktamoksha* (venesection).

A person prepares for panchakarma by undergoing *purva karma* (preliminary treatment), such as *snehan* (medicated oil massages), *swedan* (sweating in herbalized saunas), and *udvartana* (anointing). Panchakarma is followed by *paschat karma* (after care), including *sansargi* (dietary restrictions) and *rasayanas* (rejuvenation with pharmacologic therapy). Rasayanas employ more than 8000 different formulations.[6] These formulations contain herbs, animal materials (e.g., cow's urine, milk, bones), minerals, and metals. Metals may be taken internally, applied to the skin, or worn as amulets.

Ayurveda also provides *daiva-vyapashraya chikitsa* (divine therapy), the treatment of diseases resulting from the curse of saints, ghosts, or other supernatural influences. This therapy makes use of divine herbs, gems, *mantras* (incantations), *mangalas* (rituals), *bali* (oblations), *upaharas* (offerings), *homas* (sacrifices), *prayaschittas* (ceremonial penitence), *upavasa* (fasting), and *gamanas* (pilgrimages).

Ayurvedic Bodywork

To focus on Ayurvedic bodywork only is somewhat artificial. Ayurveda is, after all, holistic, and asserts that anything that exists in the realm of thought or experience can influence our health. Therefore anything that can be conceptualized can be used as a healing agent. Bodywork is merely one part of our journey back to balance and harmony.

Ayurvedic healers work with an energetic concept of the body rather than a material one. This life energy or life force is conceptualized as a *dosha* in Ayurveda, but it has many synonyms around the world: *ankh* (ancient Egypt), *pneuma* or *ether* (ancient Greece), *ruach* (Judaic Hasidim), *nwyvre* (Celtic Druids), *qi* or *chi* (China), *ki* (Japan), *angin* (Malaysia), *arunquiltha* (Australian aborigines), *ha* (Hawaii), *mana* (Maori and Polynesia), *po-wa-ta* (Pueblo), *ni* (Lakota), *ton* (Dakota), *waken* or *wakonda* (Sioux), *manitou* (Algonquin), *oki* (Huron), *orenda* (Iroquois), *sila* (Inuit), *num* (!Kung bushmen), *mulungu* (Ghana tribes), *baraka* (North Africans), *m'gbe* (Pygmies), *ntu* (Bantu), *arcus energy* (Paracelcus), *animal magnetism* (Mesmer), *odic force* (von Reichenbach), *universal force* (Herder), *dynamic activity* (Bähr), *siderism* (Ritter), *vital force* (Hahnemann), *vis medicatrix naturae* (naturopathy), *innate intelligence* (chiropractic), *primary respiration* (cranial osteopathy), *orgone energy* (Reich), *radix* (Charles Kelley), *L field* (Burr), *raw power* (Iggy Pop), and *subtle energy* (the Theosophists).

Ayurvedic bodywork enhances the flow of energy through at least three types of subtle channels. *Sira* vessels carry the doshas. They are similar to Chinese meridians. There are four classes of siras; on the material plane they correspond to nerves (which carry vata), arteries and veins (which carry pitta and sometimes kapha), and lymphatic vessels (which carry kapha). *Marma* points are found along sira vessels (Figure 10-1).

Nadi channels collectively form a fine network of 72,000 subtle nerves, through which pranic and psychic energy flow. Nadi channels intersect at 360 energy centers called *chakras* (note that some clinicians count 360 acupuncture points—the number of days in the lunar year). Three primary nadi channels intertwine up the spine, running from the tailbone through the top of the head, with seven primary chakras arising along this line.

The third type of conduits, *srota* channels, are innumerable. They connect the marma points to the internal organs. They are sometimes considered lymphatic vessels, but they carry all three doshas. Srotas may be *sanga* (obstructed), *sira-granthi* (in a knotted condition), *atipravritti* (with excess flow), or *vimarga-gamana* (flowing in reverse direction).

Ayurvedic bodywork shares many common elements with osteopathic techniques used in the United States.[20] In fact, when American osteopaths began practicing in Britain, English physicians immediately compared them with Ayurvedic practitioners.[15]

Some of the aforementioned aspects of kayachikitsa, such as *asanas* (yoga exercises) and *pranayama* (yogic breathing), may be considered forms of bodywork. Asanas are a series of postures, which may be familiar to many readers. Some postures are static stretches, whereas other postures provide balanced ligamentous tension or balanced muscle tension. This form of "spontaneous release by positioning" is similar to counterstrain, an osteopathic technique.

Soft-Tissue Techniques

Ayurvedic massage enhances the flow of energy through the sira vessels (and their intersections, the marma points), nadi channels (and their intersections, the seven chakras), and srota channels. Blockage of energy flow in these channels gives rise to muscle pain and tension, and obstructed energy may solidify into boggy or knotted tissues, known to osteopaths as somatic dysfunctions and to chiropractors as subluxations.[19]

Massage is usually performed with medicated oils. Dry massage is rarely administered, but is sometimes used for afflictions of extreme kapha. To choose the correct oil, the practitioner must take into account the client's prakriti and his or her aggravated dosha. In general, aggravated vata calls for sesame oil, excess pitta requires coconut oil, and kapha needs mustard or olive oil.[12] Oils are medicated with herbal extracts or essential oils. Essential oils are volatile and provide a form of aromatherapy. The appropriateness of an essential oil can be confirmed by asking the client to inhale the oil vapor (Figure 10-2). The proper oil vapor immediately regulates the client's subtle nadi pulse.

Snehan, or medicated oil massage, prepares the client for panchakarma. The strokes used in *snehan* follow standard patterns for each aggravated dosha; they are designed to propel ama to its primary site of

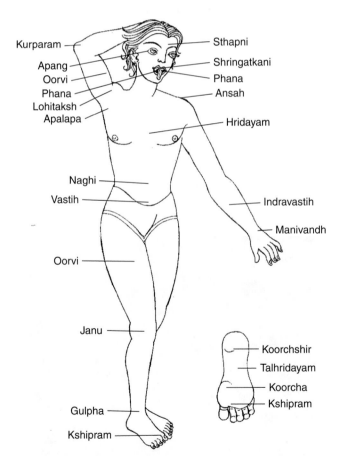

Figure 10-1 Marma points. (Modified from Johari H: Ancient Indian massage: traditional massage techniques based on the Ayurveda, New Delhi, 1984, Munshiram Manoharlal Publishers.)

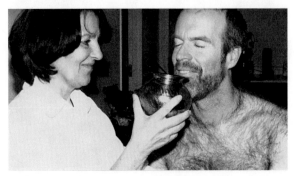

Figure 10-2 Testing the appropriateness of a medicated massage oil by inhaling its volatile vapor and checking the *nadi* pulse.

elimination, where it can be removed by panchakarma treatment (Figure 10-3).

Johari[11,12] described various types of Ayurvedic massage as follows: *jarahar,* remover of old age; *sharam har,* remover of fatigue; *vata har,* remover of the humor of wind; *drishti prasad kar,* increasing sight; *pushti kar,* making one strong; *ayu kar,* increasing longevity; *swapn kar,* inducing sleep; *twak dridh kar,* strengthening the skin; *klesh sahatwa,* providing resistance against disease and disharmony; *abhighat sahatwa,* providing resistance to injuries and power to recover quickly; *kapha vata nirodhak,* subsiding ailments caused by mucus and wind; *mrija varn bal prad,* providing strength to the skin and improving the color and texture of the skin.

These various massages use techniques similar to what Western massage therapists call *friction rubs* (localized, circular movements over muscles, tendons, and joints), *effleurage* (gliding strokes that increase blood flow), *pétrissage* (kneading or squeezing of muscles), *tapotement* (percussion that stimulates nerves and muscles), and *vibration* (an invigorating vibrato movement). The various massages differ by the amount of pressure, application of specific oils and aromas, and attention to particular body regions. For example, to improve eyesight requires gentle massage of the navel area in a clockwise direction.[12]

Some techniques of Ayurvedic massage are truly unique. A few of the techniques follow:

- *Thirummal* is used in southern India. It can be applied with the hands and the feet. English-Leuk[5] noted that thirummal can be done in a gentle, sensitive, soothing style (*satvik* massage) or a deep, intense, and often painful style (*tomasic* massage). Satvik balances the flow of energy, whereas tomasic intends to break up blocked energy.
- *Navarakizhi* massage uses rice cooked in a mixture of herbs and milk. The practitioner places the cooked jellylike mass in a small cloth sack and massages the client with it, moistening the sack from time to time by dipping it into the warm milk decoction.
- *Pizhichal* therapy uses medicated oil placed in a vessel *(dhara patram)* suspended above the supine client, positioned to direct a thin continuous stream of oil on the client's body, followed immediately by massage (Figure 10-4).
- *Spondylotherapy* is a tapotemont-like technique of rapid, light concussions applied with a hand or hammer to areas of somatic dysfunction.[20]

Ayurvedic Marma Therapy

Marma therapy treats marma points, which are comparable with Chinese acupuncture points. In the Siddha tradition practiced in Dravidian culture, marma therapy is called *varma* therapy[4] or *thanuology.*[23]

The 107 marma points manifest in 5 of the 7 dhatus. Dash and Kashyap[3] described 11 marmas in mus-

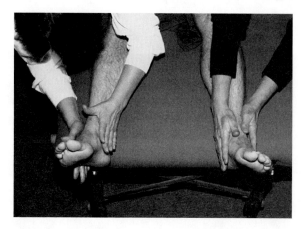

Figure 10-3 Snehan massage prepares the client for panchakarma.

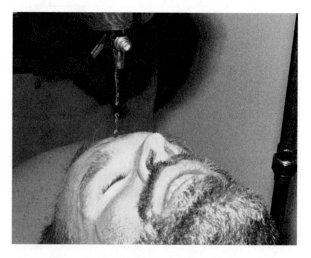

Figure 10-4 Pizhichal therapy directs a thin stream of medicated oil on the client's body.

cles, 8 in bones, 20 in joints, 27 in ligaments and nerves, and 41 in arteries and veins. They classified the marmas into those that cause instant death when damaged (located in the head, heart, and anus) and marmas that merely cause pain and deformity when damaged. Gerber[9] suggested that marmas correspond with the anatomic position of lymph nodes. As such, marma therapy is sometimes called *Ayurvedic lymphatic massage.*

Marma therapy is also called *Ayurvedic acupressure.*[21] It can be self-administered or performed by a practitioner. Although marma massage usually applies a gentle, circular motion with one finger (Figure 10-5), it may be applied more forcefully. Kurup[13] described thirummal as a marma technique. Marma therapy is used by Indian wrestlers and is considered a vital aspect of *kalarippayattu,* an Indian martial art.[9,11,12,28]

Some marma points can be needled, like acupuncture, or stimulated by a sliver of wood from the neem tree, *Azadirachta indica.*[4] Other marma points can be stimulated by yoga and pranayama. One auspicious point, *sthapni* marma (called *Thilarda varma* in the Siddha tradition, often characterized as "the third eye"), can be stimulated by simply staring at it. A trained practitioner can induce a hypnotic trance by activating this point.[4]

Sherman[25] mistakenly claimed that marma therapy was a lost art until 1987, when "the Maharishi Mahesh Yogi put Dr. John Douillard [an American chiropractor] to work at reviving it." In fact, marma therapy has remained an integral part of Ayurveda

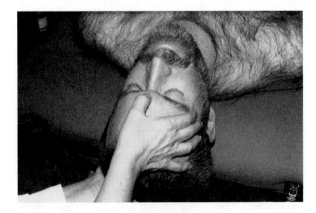

Figure 10-5 Marma massage applied to an excellent point, the *sthapni marma.*

and Siddha,[4,11] and has been popularized in the West before.[27]

Joint Articulation and Spinal Thrust

Johari[11] notes, "One who is learning about massage must learn how to put all the vertebrae in proper alignment. One should understand that massage of the spine alone can cure weak nerves and all psychic disorders."

Ayurvedic practitioners rarely use vertebral thrust techniques (the high-velocity, low-amplitude techniques used by chiropractors and osteopaths). These techniques seem to be the purview of barbers in India and Nepal, who thrust cervical vertebrae after cutting a person's hair.[19]

Cranial Work

The craniosacral mechanism is not recognized in traditional Ayurvedic medicine, although Johari[11] states, "Another important thing to remember is the role of the spinal fluid in maintaining health, vigor, vitality and virility." Gehin[8] claims that techniques akin to cranial osteopathy are practiced in Asia, but he does not elaborate on his claim.

Western Adaptations of Ayurvedic Technique

Polarity therapy was developed in the 1950s by Randolph Stone who hybridized Ayurveda with osteopathy and chiropractic. Many of Stone's techniques, such as "polar-energetics postures," are similar to Wilhelm Reich's work. Since Stone's death, Polarity therapy has diverged into several schools of thought. A satvik-oriented faction, led by Pierre Pannetier, now predominates. Many osteopathic physicians were introduced to Ayurvedic concepts through Stone, who studied with Robert Fulford, a prominent and eclectic osteopath.[7]

Arica Vortex system is an Ayurvedic hybrid developed in England. Whereas Polarity practitioners use both hands to promote a flow of energy in clients, Arica practitioners use a single pressure point to improve flow in nadi channels. Arica practitioners also use deep-tissue compression releases and deep breathing exercises.

Esoteric healing works with chakras and the etheric body. It is a form of energy healing. The phrase dates to a book of the same name written by Alice Bailey, published in 1953. Bailey was an amanuensis, influenced by Madam Blavatsky and the Theosophists. Rex Riant, a physicist from England, repopularized the study in the mid-1960s. One of Riant's protégés, Brenda Johnston, put Esoteric Healing on the map by publishing *New Age Healing* and presenting workshops around the world.

Westerners often try to box Ayurveda into the allopathic paradigm of a "diagnosis and treatment plan," and thus miss the essence of the Ayurvedic healing process. In an attempt to westernize Ayurveda, the concept of dosha and its implications are often misinterpreted and incorrectly implemented as a rigid treatment plan. Our potential for healing depends on continuous change and transformation in response to change. Ayurveda is a process of unfolding and remembering, of creating balance and harmony. Thus it complements and supports the Western modalities of healing.

Asian Adaptations: Tibetan and Thai Bodywork

Tibetan bodywork, a blend of Ayurvedic and Chinese techniques, uses massage, yogalike exercises, and acupuncture. (The Tibetans claim they invented acupuncture.) *Byugs-pa,* or Tibetan medical massage, was first described in a Tibetan medical text (the *rGyud-bzhi*) in 400 AD.

Tibetan physicians monitor energy meridians and treat imbalances with *byugs-pa.* They apply circular massage strokes to increase energy in affected areas, and linear strokes to break up energy blockages.[19] Musculoskeletal medicine is also studied in the Tibetan system, with an emphasis on osteology. In typical fashion, Tibetan osteology differs from Western approaches. Vertebrae, for instance, are numbered from the base of the neck. Hence a first vertebra in Tibetan nomenclature is our C7.[1]

Somatic dysfunctions are treated with soft-tissue techniques, including inhibitory pressure. Soft-tissue techniques also remedy arthritis and other connective tissue disorders, sinusitis, headaches, cold extremities, and psychiatric disturbances. Because most psychologic problems come from excess vata (*rLung* in the Tibetan system), selection of the correct massage oil is critical. Massage for psychologic problems focuses on the sagittal suture of the skull (along the midline of the top of the skull), first vertebra (C7, the seventh cervical vertebra in Western nomenclature),

sixth vertebra (our T5, or fifth thoracic vertebra), and the xiphisternal notch.

Tibetan physicians strive for a meditative mindset before applying treatment. They accomplish this by contemplating the Medicine Buddha, reciting mantras, and creating healing visualizations. Upon reaching a meditative state, the physician "is more sensitive to various energy blockages in the other person because he has controlled his own mind and can therefore tune into the other person mentally and physically."[1]

This meditative mindset parallels the "centering" exercises often performed by cranial osteopaths. Magoun[16] called this meditative state a "rapport in the tissues" between practitioner and client. Empathetic, meditative, centered states are known to produce strong "entrainment."[18] *Entrainment* is the harmonization of biologic oscillators. All organisms pulsate with a number of rhythms, such as diaphragmatic respiration, heart rate, heart rate variability, pulse transit time, lymph vessel oscillation, Traube-Hering modulation, brain waves, and many other fluctuations.[22] These oscillations coordinate into harmonics with each other and can be measured as a primary, fundamental rhythm. This "entrainment frequency" measured in healthy humans averages about 7.5 cycles per minute.[18]

If meditative states produce strong entrainment, centered practitioners have the ability to impose their strongly entrained rhythms onto clients.[22] Harmonization of rhythms between living things is a common phenomenon, seen in synchronously flashing fireflies, harmoniously chirping crickets, and women whose menstrual phases cycle together. Entrainment also arises between "inanimate" objects—in a room full of mechanical clocks, the "strongest" clock (the one with the heaviest pendulum) establishes the eventual overall rhythm.

Reiki, believed to be a 2500-year-old Tibetan technique, demands practice in a strongly centered meditative state. In classic Reiki technique, the practitioner places hands lightly on the client's body in a succession of twelve locations. This directs healing energy to locations roughly corresponding to chakra centers (see Chapter 12).

In Thailand, bodywork includes massage (*nûad bo ràrn*) and manipulation (*nûad càb sên*). Like the Tibetans, the Thai treat energy imbalances as well as musculoskeletal dysfunctions. Some *nûad bo ràrn* techniques resemble Chinese *Tui Na.* However, Tui Na treats 12 meridians, whereas nûad bo ràrn focuses on 72,000 sên channels (identical to the number of Ayurvedic nadi channels). Other nûad bo ràrn techniques apply vigorous traction to the extremities, with either stretch-and-hold patterns or rhythmic rocking motions. Achieving proper leverage for traction may entwine the client and practitioner in unique postures, akin to nonsexual *Kama Sutra* positions.

Another type of nûad bo ràrn approximates Chinese acupressure, but the treatment locations differ in location. Riley and colleagues[24] determined that 28% of sên points correspond to the location of Chinese acupuncture points, 8% correspond to Travell's trigger points, and 33% correspond to Chapman's reflex points.

Nûad càb sên resembles *zhong zhu,* or Chinese joint manipulation. The Thai, like the Chinese, do not recognize restrictions of spinal movement in the sagittal plane. All thrusts are directed at rotational and side-bending restrictions. Thrust forces are not localized to specific spinal segments. A Buddhist temple statue in Bangkok, reportedly 2000 years old, shows nûad càb sên manipulation of the lumbar spine. The statue was photographed by Cyriax, which is interesting because Cyriax also ignored restrictions in the sagittal plane.[2]

TRAINING AND CERTIFICATION IN AYURVEDA

India has approximately 400,000 Ayurvedic practitioners (including 40,000 Unani and 25,000 Siddha practitioners), 242 Ayurvedic hospitals, 65 Siddha hospitals, and 19 Unani hospitals.[6] There are 108 accredited undergraduate Ayurvedic colleges and 1 Ayurvedic university, 2 postgraduate institutes, and 21 postgraduate departments across India. Banaras Hindu university (BHU) uniquely supports both a faculty of Ayurveda and a faculty of Western medicine, comparable with Michigan State University (MSU), which accommodates an osteopathic college and an allopathic medical college under one roof. In 1993, BHU and MSU engaged in a scientist exchange, funded by the National Science Foundation, which initiated this study of Ayurvedic bodywork.

Training for an Ayurvedic medical degree is similar to that of the Bachelor of Medicine Bachelor of Science in the British system—the duration of undergraduate training is 5½ years after secondary schooling, and the doctorate course is another 3 years after graduation.[14]

In the United States, Ayurvedic training and certification is not regulated. No state or national licensing boards for Ayurvedic medicine currently exist. Several schools offer instruction, including the following:

- The American Institute of Vedic Studies in Santa Fe, New Mexico, offers a 250-hour correspondence course for health care professionals. The course is directed by Dr. David Frawley.
- The Ayurveda Holistic Center in Bayville, New York, offers a 2-year (750-hour) correspondence course, based on the *Ayurvedic Encyclopedia,* which was written by the center's director, Swami Sada Shiva Tirtha. A classroom course consists of 480 hours of lecture and internship instruction plus 280 hours of home study, provided by Punita Desai, BAMS.
- The Ayurvedic Institute in Albuquerque, New Mexico, offers a 4-year program (1750 classroom hours), summer-long intensive seminars, short courses, and a correspondence course. The faculty includes Dr. Vasant Lad, BAMS, MA Sc; Dr. Robert Svoboda, BAMS; Hart de Fouw (Jyotishi); Ann Harrison, LMT (yoga); Kevin Spelman, MHAHG (medical herbs); and Donald Van Howten, LMT, PIT (bodywork).
- The California College of Ayurveda in Grass Valley, California, offers a 2-year program (500 classroom hours, 250 home-study hours, and a 6-month internship), leading to certification as a Clinical Ayurvedic Specialist. The faculty includes Dr. Marc Halpern, Dr. David Frawley, Dr. Avinesh Lele, and Dr. Subhash Ranadé.
- The College of Maharishi Vedic Medicine in Fairfield, Iowa, offers a 4-year program leading to a BA degree, plus a 6-year program leading to a PhD in vedic physiology. The faculty includes Robert Schneider, MD; Vaidya H.K. Gupta, MDAy; Vaidya Manohar Palakuthi, BAMS; and Richard Averbach, MD.
- The National Institute of Ayurvedic Medicine in Brewster, New York, offers a correspon-

dence course by Scott Gerson, MD. A 3-year course being developed in collaboration with the University of Pune offers internships in India.

- The New England Institute of Ayurvedic Medicine in Cambridge, Massachusetts, offers a 1-year program of classroom and clinical instruction leading to certification. Additional programs for internship and advanced training lead to the DAy degree. The faculty includes Dr. Abbas Qutab and Dr. David Frawley.

References

1. Clifford T: *Tibetan Buddhist medicine and psychiatry,* York Beach, Me, 1984, Samuel Weiser.
2. Cyriax J: *Textbook of orthpaedic medicine,* London, 1984, Baillière Tindall.
3. Dash B, Kashyap J: *Basic principles of Ayurveda,* New Delhi, 1980, Concept Publishing.
4. Dharmalingam V, Radhink M, Balasubramanian AV: *Marma chikitsa in traditional medicine,* LSPSS Monograph No. 5, Madras, India, 1991, Lok Swaasthya Parampara Samvardhan Samithi.
5. English-Leuk JA: *Health in the new age,* Albuquerque, 1990, University of New Mexico Press.
6. Fulder S: *The handbook of complementary medicine,* ed 2, Oxford, 1988, Oxford University Press.
7. Fulford R, Stone G: *Dr. Fulford's touch of life,* New York, 1996, Pocket Books.
8. Gehin A: *Atlas of manipulative techniques for the cranium and face,* Seattle, 1985, Eastland Press.
9. Gerber ML. In Hohari H: *Ancient Indian massage: traditional massage techniques based on the Ayurveda,* New Delhi, 1984, Munshiram Manoharlal Publishers.
10. Jeffery R: *The politics of health in India,* Berkeley, 1988, University of California Press.
11. Johari H: *Ancient Indian massage: traditional massage techniques based on the Ayurveda,* New Delhi, 1984, Munshiram Manoharlal Publishers.
12. Johari H: *Ayurvedic massage: traditional Indian techniques for balancing body and mind,* Rochester, Vt, 1996, Healing Arts Press.
13. Kurup PNV: The science of life, *World Health Magazine* pp 12-15, November, 1977.
14. Kurup PNV. In Bannerman RH, Burton J, Wen-Chieh C: *Traditional medicine and health care coverage,* Geneva, 1983, World Health Organization Press.
15. Little EG: Registration of osteopaths, *BMJ* 2:815-816, 1925.
16. Magoun HI: *Osteopathy in the cranial field,* ed 3, Kirksville, Mo, 1976, The Journal Printing.
17. Mahdihassan S: Indian and Chinese cosmic elements, *Am J Chin Med* 7:316-323, 1979.
18. McCraty R, Atkinson M, Tiller WA: New electrophysiological correlates associated with intentional heart focus, *Subtle Energies* 4:251-268, 1995.
19. McPartland JM: Manual medicine at the Nepali interface, *J Manual Med* 4:25-27, 1989.
20. McPartland JM: *Ayurvedic glossary. Final report, US-India Scientist Exchange Program,* Washington, DC, 1992, National Science Foundation.
21. McPartland JM: Visit to the enchanted land: Ayurvedic medicine, as old as life, *Communique* 19(5):5, 1993.
22. McPartland JM, Mein EA: Entrainment and the cranial rhythmic impulse, *Altern Ther Health Med* 3(1):40-44, 1997.
23. Pillai SC: *Treatise on impacts to nerve centres in Varma,* Madras, India, 1991, International Institute of Thanuology.
24. Riley JN, Mitchell FL Jr, Bensky D: Thai manual medicine as represented in the Wat Pho epigraphies: preliminary comparisons, *Med Anthropol* 5(2):155-194, 1981.
25. Sherman B: *New Marma programs enliven the body's vital points* (brochure), Fairfield, Iowa, 1991, Fairfield Maharishi Ayur-Veda Center.
26. Ulrich-Merzenich G, Kraft K, Singh LM: Rheumatic diseases in Ayurveda: a historical perspective, *Arthritis Rheum* 42:1553-1554, 1999.
27. Varma D: *The human machine and its forces,* London, 1937, Health For All Publishing.
28. Zarrilli PB: Three bodies of practice in a traditional south Indian martial art, *Soc Sci Med* 28:1289-1309, 1989.

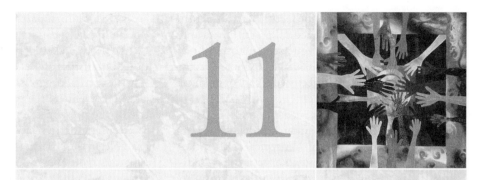

Qi Gong and Tui Na*

KEVIN V. ERGIL
MARC S. MICOZZI

CHINA'S TRADITIONAL MEDICINE

Certain considerations are important to understanding Chinese medicine. Medicine is a human endeavor and as such is shaped by the considerations of the human beings using and practicing it. These considerations sometimes have very little to do with curing disease in the most simple and efficient way and a great deal to do with economics, politics, and culture. Ideology, belief, and even simple ignorance have influenced the practice of medicine more than has ration-

ality. A medical historian or a physician might perceive medicine to be a steady march from ignorance to the light, but these are typically revisionist histories. Medicine is a human enterprise embedded in and intersected by myriad other human projects. Even the choice of how to conduct a medical procedure or what kind of health care to choose may have more to do with habit or economics than with rationality or efficacy. An example is the case of a Chinese patient choosing traditional herbal medicine to manage painful and debilitating kidney stones. Although the treatment was ultimately effective, the patient's choice was not motivated by a desire for efficacy. Had the patient opted for surgery, he or she would have been classified as an invalid and therefore barred from advancement in the workplace. Another example is a hospital that closes its doors to the prac-

*The information in this chapter was excerpted from the chapter entitled "Chinese Medicine," written by Kevin Ergil, in *Fundamentals of Complementary and Alternative Medicine*, ed 2, by Marc S. Micozzi, published by Churchill Livingstone (2001).

tice of acupuncture despite the fact that acupuncturists in the state are licensed medical practitioners and their services are routinely requested by hospital patients. In each example, considerations not directly linked to the rational and effective delivery of medical care influence medical choices.

Our own perspectives on medicine and our experience of our own medical systems provide us with ideas regarding what is normal or typical in the practice of medicine. We respond to aspects of a traditional system that correspond with our expectations. We imagine Chinese herbal medicine as a gentle therapy using nontoxic ingredients. Its use of highly toxic substances or drastic purgative therapies is easily overlooked. It is unlikely, for instance, that the traditional form of Tibetan therapeutic cautery applied with a hot iron will elicit substantial interest as a form of alternative therapy. Naturalistic and rational elements of systems intrigue us. Unfamiliar or magical diagnostic and therapeutic modes cause us concern.

We must think about medical systems as being embedded in their respective cultures. For example, the concept of neurasthenia (*sheng jin shuai ruo,* a vague fatigue thought to be caused by psychologic factors) is an important syndrome in traditional Chinese medicine and Chinese psychiatry, despite the fact that this diagnosis has fallen into disrepute among Western psychiatrists and is no longer classified as a disease entity in diagnostic manuals. Neurasthenia was an exceptionally popular diagnosis in the nineteenth century during periods of extensive medical exchange between the United States and China and Japan. The diagnosis has continued to be clinically important in China because it fits well into certain traditional medical models and responds well to cultural and political concerns about mental illness.[4] Americans and Europeans who encounter neurasthenia within the corpus of Chinese medicine sometimes find it an unusual or obscure concept despite its relevance for Chinese medical practice.

Sometimes, on encountering a new idea, we like to think about it in familiar terms. One example is the use of the word *energy* to express the idea of *qi.* An extension of this is the common practice of describing the therapeutic method of draining evil influences from channels as "sedation." Neither energy nor sedation has much to do with the concepts that underlie qi and draining; however, these terms are more familiar to us and make Chinese medicine more accessible. Unfortunately, this practice can obscure the breadth of meaning of these terms.[12]

We try to make sense of the world from our position in it, historically as well as culturally. We tend to view history as progressing, as if by design, to a specific end. Events of the past, viewed from the perspective of the present, offer tempting opportunities for reinterpretation in relation to current experience. For example, in the context of current perspectives on disease causation, Wu You Ke's statements that "miscellaneous qi" could cause epidemic disease, and his concept of "one disease, one qi,"[11] have led contemporary sources in China to suggest that such an insight, coming as it did before the invention of the microscope, is quite remarkable.[13] The implication that Wu You Ke's observation was a precursor of germ theory is attractive to Chinese practitioners who are trying to find a place for traditional practices in an increasingly biomedicalized world. In fact, the concept of miscellaneous or pestilential qi has been used extensively in adapting traditional theory to the management of human immunodeficiency virus infection. However, as Wiseman points out, this was never explored in relation to the causation of disease by microscopic organisms, nor was it ever conceived as such.

Of course, the history of Chinese medical thought includes many people who thought that they were exclusively right, but the breadth of traditional Chinese medical thought was sustained by an intellectual climate that retained all possible ideas for use and exploration. A given philosopher or clinician might reject an idea, but the idea itself would remain available for future use.

For example, during the Ming dynasty Wu You Ke (circa 1644) was the leading exponent of the "offensive precipitation sect" *(gong xia pai)* of physicians, whose tenets included a distinctive set of ideas concerning the management of epidemic disease and a wholehearted rejection of many established ideas in Chinese medicine.[14] He was subsequently viewed as a contributor to Chinese medical thought; a proponent of a divergent and uninformed theory; and finally as the intellectual antecedent of Koch, the discoverer of the tuberculosis bacillus. At no point were his ideas discarded.

Interestingly enough, in modern China, where the sheer volume of information and the nation's health care needs make it necessary to teach a standard curriculum to thousands of students each year, this tolerance for varying clinical perspectives continues. For instance, there are herbal physicians known as *Minor Bupleurum Decoction (Xiao Chai Hu Tang)* doctors because their prescriptions are organized around one formula from the *Treatise on Cold Damage (Shang Han Lun),* an early text on diagnosis and herbal therapy written during the Han dynasty (206 BC–220 AD). Some herbal physicians reject traditional formulas entirely and use contemporary perspectives on the Chinese pharmacopeia to organize their prescriptions.

There are acupuncturists whose clinical focus is dedicated almost entirely to six acupuncture points and who use computed tomography scans to plan clinical interventions. At the same time, two floors down in the same hospital physicians base their selection of acupuncture points on obscure and complex aspects of traditional calendrics and systems such as the "Magic Turtle."

HISTORY

Once it is understood that Chinese medicine is a large and varied tradition with many manifestations and philosophies, it is possible to begin its exploration. Chinese medicine has an extensive history. As is the case with most medical traditions, this history can be approached from several perspectives. One such perspective is the ancient mythology of Chinese medicine, which attributes the birth of medicine to the legendary emperors Fu Xi, Shen Nong, and Huang Di. Another is the history deduced from the careful study of available ancient texts and records. These records indicate, for example, that there is no reference to acupuncture as a therapeutic method in any Chinese text before 90 BC,[7] and that the oldest existing text to discuss medical practices that faintly resemble current Chinese medicine date from the end of the third century BC.[7] Finally, there are the more extravagant interpretations of archaeologic evidence and textual materials that seek to establish the ancient character of certain Chinese medical practices. One example of extravagant interpretation is the common assertion that the stone "needles" excavated in various parts of China were remnants of ancient acupuncture.[1,9] This assertion is based on references in texts from later periods to the ancient surgical application of sharp stones and on morphologic similarities between the excavated stones and the metal needles that were used later.

The origins of Chinese medicine are mythically linked to three legendary emperors. Fu Xi, the *Ox Tamer* (circa 2953 BC), taught people how to domesticate animals and divined the *Ba Gua,* eight symbols that became the basis for the *Yi Jing,* or *Book of Changes.* Shen Nong, the *Divine Husbandman,* is also known as the *Fire Emperor.* Shen Nong is said to have lived from 2838 to 2698 BC and is considered the founder of agriculture in China. He taught the Chinese people how to cultivate plants and raise livestock. He is also considered the originator of herbal medicine in China, having learned the therapeutic properties of herbs and substances by tasting them. Later authors attributed their work to him to indicate the antiquity and importance of their texts. The *Divine Husbandman's Classic of the Materia Medica (Shen Nong Ben Cao Jing)* is a case in point. The text was probably written in 220 AD and reconstructed in 500 AD by Tao Hong Jing. Given that all historical evidence points to the ancient character of herbal medicine in China, it is appropriate that Shen Nong is considered its originator (Figure 11-1). Huang Di, the *Yellow Emperor*

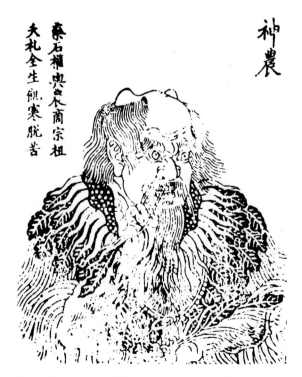

Figure 11-1 Image of Shen Nong. (From Micozzi M: *Fundamentals of complementary and alternative medicine,* ed 2. Philadelphia, 2001, Churchill Livingstone.)

(2698-2598 BC) is known as the originator of the traditional medicine of China.

QI AND THE ESSENTIAL SUBSTANCES OF THE BODY

Apart from the ideas of yin and yang and the five phases, there is no concept more crucial to Chinese medicine than qi—the idea that the body is pervaded by subtle material and mobile influences that cause most physiologic functions and maintain the health and vitality of the individual. This idea is not common to biomedical thinking about the body. Qi is commonly translated as *energy,* but this translation conceals qi's distinctly material attributes. Furthermore, although energy is defined as the capacity of a system to do work, the character of qi extends considerably further.

The Chinese character for qi is traditionally composed of two radicals (ideographs); the radical that symbolizes breath or rising vapor is placed above the radical for rice (Figure 11-2). Qi is linked with the concept of "vapors arising from food."[7] Over time this concept broadened but never lost its distinctively material aspect. Unschuld favors the use of the phrase "finest matter influences" or "influences" to translate this concept.[7] Wiseman points out that some phenomena labeled as qi do not fit conventional definitions of substance or matter, further confusing the issue.[13] Because of this confusion, many authors prefer to leave the term *qi* untranslated.

The idea of qi is extremely broad, encompassing almost every variety of natural phenomena. The body contains many different types of qi. In general, the features that distinguish each type derive from its source, location, and function. There is considerable room for debate in this area, and exploration of a wide range of materials suggests a variety of different ideas about categories of qi. In general, qi has the functions of activation, warming, defense, transformation, and containment (Table 11-1).

The qi concept is important to many aspects of Chinese medicine. Organ and channel qi are influenced by acupuncture. In fact, one characteristic feature of acupuncture treatment is the sensation of obtaining the qi or *de qi. Qi Gong* is a general term for the many systems of meditation, exercise, and therapeutics that are rooted in the concept of mobilizing and regulating the movement of qi in the body. Qi is sometimes compared with wind captured in a sail; we cannot observe the wind directly, but we can infer its pres-

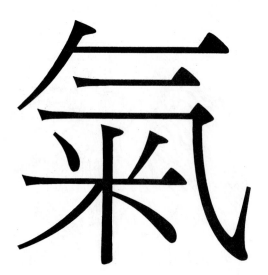

Figure 11-2 The character *qi.* (From Micozzi M: *Fundamentals of complementary and alternative medicine,* ed 2, Philadelphia, 2001, Churchill Livingstone.)

TABLE 11-1

Types of Qi

Type (Chinese)	Type (English)	Function
Ying qi	Construction qi	Supports and nourishes the body
Wei qi	Defense qi	Protects and warms the body
Jing qi	Channel qi	Flows in the channels (felt during acupuncture)
Zang qi	Organ qi	Flows in the organs (physiologic function of organs)
Zong qi	Ancestral qi	Responsible for respiration and circulation

From Micozzi M: *Fundamentals of complementary and alternative medicine,* ed 2, Philadelphia, 2001, Churchill Livingstone.

ence as it fills the sail. In a similar fashion, the movements of the body and the movement of substances within the body are all signs of the action of qi.

In relation to qi, blood and fluids constitute the yin aspects of the body. Blood is produced by the construction qi, which in turn is derived from food and water. Blood, which nourishes the body, is understood to have a slightly broader and less definite range of actions in Chinese medicine than it does in biomedicine. Qi and blood are closely linked because blood is believed to flow with qi and to be conveyed by it. This relationship often is expressed by the Chinese saying, "Qi is the commander of blood and blood is the mother of qi." It has been suggested that qi and blood are linked in the same manner as a person and his or her shadow.

Fluids are a general category of substances that serve to moisten and lubricate the body; these substances may be thin or viscous. Fluids can be conceptually separated into humor and liquid. *Humor* is thick and related to the body's organs; among its functions is the lubrication of the joints. *Liquid* is thin and is responsible for moistening the surface areas of the body, including the skin, eyes, and mouth.

CHINESE MASSAGE (TUI NA)

Tui Na, literally "pushing and pulling," refers to a system of massage, manual acupuncture point stimulation, and manipulation that is vast enough to warrant a chapter of its own. These methods have been practiced at least as long as moxibustion, if not longer, but the first Chinese massage training class was not created until 1956 in Shanghai.[8] Today, Tui Na can serve as a minor component of a traditional medical education or an area of extensive clinical specialization.

A distinct aspect of Tui Na is the extensive training of the hands necessary for clinical practice. The practitioner's hands are trained to accomplish focused and forceful movements that can be applied to various areas of the body. Techniques such as pushing, rolling, kneading, rubbing, and grasping are practiced repetitively until they become second nature. Students practice on a small bag of rice until their hands develop the necessary strength and dexterity.

Tui Na is often applied to limited areas of the body, and the techniques can be quite forceful and intense. Tui Na is applied routinely to patients with or-

thopedic and neurologic conditions. It also is applied to patients with conditions that may not be thought of as susceptible to treatment through manipulation, such as asthma, dysmenorrhea, and chronic gastritis. Tui Na is used as an adjunct to acupuncture to increase the range of motion of a joint, or instead of acupuncture when needles are uncomfortable or inappropriate, such as in pediatric applications.

As with all aspects of Chinese medicine, regional styles and family lineages of practice abound. The formal curriculum available in Chinese programs is extensive but is probably not a complete expression of the range of possibilities.

QI CULTIVATION

Qi Gong is a term that literally embraces almost every aspect of the manipulation of qi by means of exercise, breathing, and the influence of the mind. The second part of this chapter is devoted to this topic, so only a few points need to be made here. Qi Gong includes practices ranging from the meditative systems of Daoist and Buddhist practitioners to the martial arts traditions of China. Qi Gong is relevant to medicine in three specific areas. The first is to allow the practitioner to cultivate the demeanor and stamina to enable him or her to perform the strenuous activities of Tui Na, to sustain the constant demands of clinical practice, and to quiet the mind to facilitate diagnostic perception. The second involves cultivating the practitioner's ability to safely transmit qi to the patient. Practitioners may direct qi to the patient either through the needles or directly through their hands. This activity may be the main focus of treatment or an adjunctive aspect, in which case the qi paradigm is expanded to include direct interaction between the patient's qi and that of the clinician. Finally, patients may be taught to do specific Qi Gong practices that are useful for their illnesses.

Many intriguing studies of qi cultivation have been conducted in China and are beginning to be explored in the United States. Qi cultivation has been examined in relationship to an increase in immunocompetence as measured through lymphocyte profiles[5] and by changes in electroencephalography patterns. Qi cultivation has been explored as a tool for managing gastritis, and numerous Chinese studies have suggested that it may be a promising method for treating hypertension.

Unfortunately, many of the problems that have confronted acupuncture research also surround research into qi cultivation. In addition, although there is great interest in qi cultivation in the West, there has not been equivalent enthusiasm for resolving methodologic problems and beginning to establish strong research initiatives.

Research regarding the role of qi cultivation exercises in the beneficial alteration of physiologic processes is similar, in many respects, to the investigation of the effects of meditation, yoga, guided imagery, and what Benson termed the *relaxation response*. The challenge of such research is developing an effective control and ruling out other variables that may influence the results.

A researcher who attempts to examine the effects of externally transmitted qi encounters special problems. In some cases, it is believed that this phenomenon involves measurable portions of the electromagnetic spectrum. When investigators hypothesize qi as a real but presently unmeasurable phenomenon, they seek to establish the presence and effect of externally transmitted qi by examining its apparent effects on other systems that can be directly observed.

Given the extensive range of phenomena under investigation and the range of claims for the healing potential of qi cultivation, there is a certain amount of skepticism concerning the field as a whole. Even in China there is some question as to whether qi cultivation should be established as a standard method of treatment within the corpus of Chinese medicine; some observers believe that some of the practices associated with qi cultivation have the potential for abuse and charlatanism.[6]

Qi cultivation remains a challenging part of the broad fabric of China's traditional medicine. Researchers within the field hope that as time passes, it will become possible to increase the availability of well-designed studies in the field.[11]

QI GONG

Given the fundamental importance of qi to health and well being, it is not surprising that one important aspect of the practice of Chinese medicine is the systematic cultivation of qi. The methods and practices undertaken to achieve this are many. It can be said that *Qi Gong* is a term that literally embraces almost every aspect of the manipulation and development of qi by means of exercise, breathing, and creative visualization. Qi Gong can also be considered to encompass practices such as dao yin (conduction) and Tui Na (exhalation and inhalation), both of which are applied to patterning and guiding the qi in the body.

Thus the expressions *qi cultivation* or *Qi Gong* can refer to an extraordinarily broad range of practices and activities, including the meditative systems of Daoist and Buddhist practitioners, the health-giving exercises developed by ancient physicians, and the martial arts traditions of China. The unifying aspect is the intention of the practice to increase the quantity, smooth movement, and volitional control of the practitioner's qi, thus strengthening the body.

Although the practice of Daoist and Buddhist qi cultivation is aimed ultimately at spiritual realization, the practice of medical qi cultivation addresses three specific areas. The first is self-cultivation of the practitioner's health and stamina. Training to perform the strenuous activities of Tui Na, sustaining the constant demands of clinical practice, and quieting the mind to better engage in diagnosis all pertain to self-cultivation. The second area involves the cultivation of the practitioner's ability to safely transmit qi to the patient. Some practitioners believe that their qi may be directed to the patient either through needles or directly through their hands. This activity may be the main focus of treatment or an adjunctive aspect. In this case, the qi paradigm is expanded to include direct interaction between the patient's qi and that of the clinician. Finally, patients may be taught to do specific Qi Gong practices that may help treat their illness or strengthen their qi.

Qi cultivation makes extensive use of the principles of China's traditional medicine, and its history is intertwined with that of famous physicians. The history of qi cultivation practices is believed to extend back into antiquity and to point to an early recognition of the importance of exercise to health. In Lu's *Spring and Autumn* annals, a famous aphorism relates the importance of movement to the maintenance of health and function: "Flowing water will never turn stale, the hinge of the door will never be eaten by worms. They never rest in their activity: that's why."[3] In this text Lu described the role of dance and movement in correcting the movement of qi and yin within the body and benefiting the muscles.[15]

Descriptions of qi cultivation practices and exercises are attributed to the early Daoist masters. Zhuang Zi, writing in the fourth century BC, reveals the role of breathing and physical exercise in promoting longevity and describes a sage intent on extending his life.[2] "To pant, to puff, to hail, to sip, to spit out the old breath and draw in the new, practicing bear hangings and bird-stretches, longevity his only concern."[10]

Among the texts recovered at Ma Huang Dui are a series of illustrated guides to the practice of conduction *(dao yin)* that provide guidance to the physical postures and therapeutic properties of this form of qi cultivation.[2] The famous physician of the second century, China Hua Tou, is credited with the creation of a series of exercises. Based on the movements of the tiger, the deer, the bear, the monkey, and the bird, these exercises were to be practiced to ward off disease. Zhang Zhong Jing in his *Golden Cabinet Prescriptions* recommended the practices of *dao yin* or conduction and Tui Na or exhalation and inhalation to treat disease.

A wide variety of qi cultivation forms were developed over the centuries, and many have achieved great popularity. From the 1950s on, Qi Gong training programs were implemented and sanatoria were built, specializing in the therapeutic application of Qi Gong to the treatment of disease.

FUNDAMENTAL CONCEPTS

Qi cultivation rests on several fundamental principles intended to support activity to enhance the movement of qi and to increase health. Most discussions of qi cultivation address relaxation of the body, regulation or control of breathing, and calming of the mind. Qi cultivation generally is performed in a relaxed standing, sitting, or lying posture. Once the correct position is achieved, the practitioner begins to regulate breathing in concert with specific mental and physical exercises.

For example, one form of Qi Gong involves visualizing the internal and external pathways of the channels and imagining the movement of the qi along these channels in concert with the breath. As the practice develops, the practitioner begins to experience the sensation of qi traveling along the channel pathways. Traditionally, it is believed that the mind guides the qi to a specific area of the body and that

the qi then guides the blood there as well, improving circulation in the area. From this point of view, this particular exercise trains the qi and blood to move freely along the channel pathways, leading to good health.

Another exercise involves the use of breath, visualization, and simple physical exercises to benefit the qi of the lungs. This therapeutic exercise is recommended for bronchitis, emphysema, and bronchial asthma. It is begun by assuming a relaxed posture, whether sitting, lying, or standing. The exercise is begun by breathing naturally and allowing the mind to become calm. The upper and lower teeth are then clicked together by closing the mouth gently 36 times. As saliva is produced it is retained in the mouth, swirled with the tongue, and then swallowed in three parts while the client imagines that it is flowing into the middle of the chest and then to an area about three fingerbreadths below the navel (the *dan tian,* or cinnabar field). At this point, the client imagines that he or she is sitting in front of a reservoir of white qi that enters the mouth on inhalation and is transmitted through the body as the client exhales, first to the lungs, then to the *dan tian,* and finally out to the skin and body hair. This process of visualization is repeated 18 times.

This process uses the relationship between the mind and qi to strengthen the function of the lungs and to pattern areas of the body associated with the area in which the lung and respiration qi is stored. This area is associated with the acupuncture point *dan zhong,* or chest center (ren 17), which is located in the middle of the chest. (*Ren* are acupuncture points.) Next the qi is directed to the cinnabar field, which is associated with another location on the ren channel *qi hai,* or sea of qi (ren 6), just below the umbilicus. This area is considered important in the production and storage of the body's qi and to the lungs on exhalation.

This exercise typifies the aspect of a Qi Gong exercise described previously; it induces relaxation through mental concentration, because focusing on breathing and visualization help remove distracting thoughts from the mind, and patterning the breath with visualization controls and regulates the breathing.

It should be stressed that although many forms of Qi Gong exist, they share general principles of application and a relationship to Chinese medicine concepts.

References

1. Chuang Y: *The historical development of acupuncture,* Los Angeles, 1982, Oriental Healing Arts Institute.
2. Despeux C: Gymnastics: the ancient tradition. In Kohn L, editor: *Taoist meditation and longevity techniques,* Ann Arbor, Mich, 1989, Center for Chinese Studies, The University of Michigan.
3. Engelhardt U: Qi for life: longevity in the Tang. In Kohn L, editor: *Taoist meditation and longevity techniques,* Ann Arbor, Mich, 1989, Center for Chinese Studies, The University of Michigan.
4. Kleinman A: *Social origins of distress and disease: depression, neurasthenia, and pain in modern China,* New Haven, Conn, 1986, Yale University Press.
5. Ryu H, Jun CD, Lee BS et al: Effect of qigong training on proportions of T lymphocyte subsets in human peripheral blood, *Am J Chin Med* 23:27-36, 1995.
6. Tang KC: Qigong therapy—its effectiveness and regulation, *Am J Chin Med* 22:235-242, 1994.
7. Unschuld P: *Medicine in China: a history of ideas,* Berkeley, Calif, 1985, University of California.
8. Wang G, Fan Y, Guan Z: Chinese massage. In Zhang E, editor, WenPing Y, translator: *A practical English-Chinese library of traditional Chinese medicine,* Shanghai, 1990, Publishing House of Shanghai College of Traditional Chinese Medicine.
9. Wang X: Research on the origin and development of Chinese acupuncture and moxibustion. In Xiangtong Z, editor: *Research on acupuncture, moxibustion and acupuncture anesthesia,* New York, 1986, Springer-Verlag.
10. Watson B: *The complete works of Chuang-tzu,* New York, 1968, Columbia University Press.
11. Wiseman N: *A list of Chinese formulas,* Taiwan, 1993, unpublished paper.
12. Wiseman N, Boss K: *Glossary of Chinese medical terms and acupuncture points,* Brookline, Mass, 1990, Paradigm Publications.
13. Wiseman N, Ellis A, Zmiewski P et al. In Wiseman N, Ellis A, translators: *Fundamentals of Chinese medicine,* Brookline, Mass, 1995, Paradigm Publications.
14. Wong CK, Wu TL: *History of Chinese medicine: being a chronicle of medical happenings in China from ancient times to the present period,* Taipei, Taiwan, 1985, Southern Materials Center.
15. Zhang E: Clinic of traditional Chinese medicine. In Zhang E, editor, Zou J, translator: *A practical English-Chinese library of traditional Chinese medicine,* Shanghai, 1990, Publishing House of Shanghai College of Traditional Chinese Medicine.

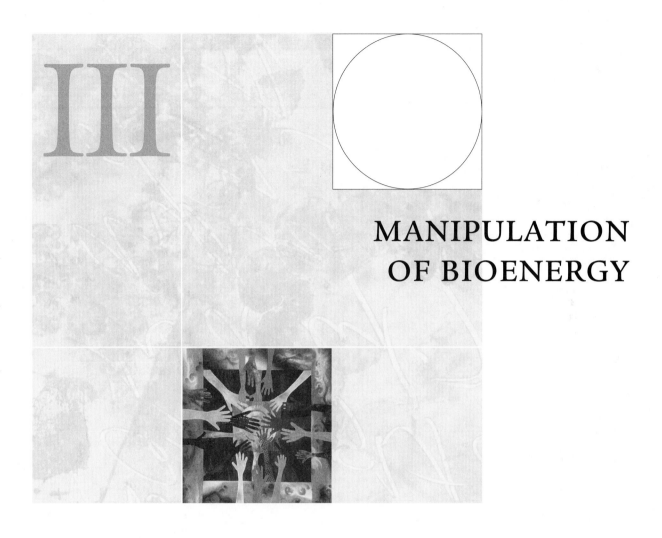

III

MANIPULATION
OF BIOENERGY

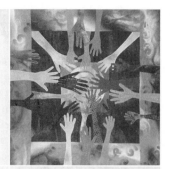

Reiki
The Usui System of Natural Healing

EARLENE GLEISNER

Spiritual Precepts of Reiki
Just for Today . . . Do Not Anger
Just for Today . . . Do Not Worry
Honor your parents, teachers, and elders
Earn your living honestly
Show gratitude to all living things

eiki, which is translated from Japanese as *universal life energy,*[2] is the intrinsic power used in the Usui System of Natural Healing. This power is channeled through practitioners to wherever it is needed in a person, plant, or animal, and even, as one anecdote suggests, to a weak car battery. Handed down from Master to student, the Usui System is an oral tradition. This method of hands-on heal-ing has become popular all over the world. Many dif-ferent schools, or *streams* as they are described in the present day Japanese view,[20] have developed from the original teachings of Mikao Usui in the early 1920s.

Reiki requires no particular religious orientation, no physiologic or anatomic knowledge, and no train-ing in body manipulation techniques such as mas-sage.[6,12,13] Because it is so simple, it easily accompanies other allopathic and holistic therapies, but can stand alone as a single therapy to promote healing.

Because Reiki actually stimulates the body's own healing abilities, it can be used in all manner of preoperative and postoperative treatments, oncologic regimens, stress management modalities, and chronic disease and pain management.[1,3,9] The beauty of the system is that it can be learned by doctors and clients so that both are joined in the effort to attain the client's highest level of balanced wellness.

HISTORY

The roots of the Usui System of Natural Healing have been traced to Shinto, the earliest religion of the indigenous Japanese peoples. However, the system is also known to rely on Buddhist tradition in some of its practices.[20] Shintoism, as practiced in its earliest form (200 BC), included a belief in spirit beings and the resultant energy of every living thing, as well as entities the Western mind finds difficult to believe as alive, such as stones and waterfalls.[19] Hence Reiki, or universal life energy, can be better understood in its fullest capacity when linked with a Shinto world view, which recognizes and honors spiritual forces and energy, rather than the Buddhist view,[4] which regards the world and its elements as transient.

As told in the origination myth of the Usui System of Natural Healing, Dr. Mikao Usui was searching for concrete ways in which Jesus and the Buddha were able to heal with the laying on of hands. All documented oral histories agree that the point of origin for this system occurred when Dr. Usui undertook a lengthy meditation and fast on Mount Kuiyama outside Kyoto, Japan, and received information, guidance, and initiation into this healing modality.[2,5,12,18]

Dr. Usui began teaching this method in 1920; a year later he opened a Reiki practice in Harajuko, Tokyo, close to the Meiji Jinju.[20] Dr. Usui developed and taught the Five Precepts, or Five Spiritual Precepts, as guidelines for everyday living and foci for personal meditation. Followers disagree about the basis of these precepts. Some believe they are based on the Meiji Emperor's Five Rules of Life. Others believe these writings were developed as positive reflections of the Five Hindrances to spiritual enlightenment presented by the Buddha.

Several Reiki lineages have grown out of the original teachings of Dr. Usui. It is universally recognized that a Hawaiian-born, Japanese-American woman, Hawayo Takata, began teaching Reiki to the Western World in the 1970s. Her story is widely known because it has been chronicled in many books and retold at almost every First Degree Class throughout the world.[2,5,11,12]

In the United States, many schools have developed. These schools have varying requirements in training, but all of them hold one thing as true: the transfer of this energy, Reiki, from a human being to any other living being is real. It is relaxing, healing, and responsible for a growing mass of anecdotal evidence regarding the rebalancing of mind, body, and spirit and the release of disease or pain.

Research is beginning to document this system as a valid therapy, the results of which can be replicated.[15] The Usui System of Natural Healing is being taught to nurses in hospitals and in nursing schools. Doctors, dentists, psychologists, and other health care providers are learning this technique to add a dimension of calming, healing touch to their practices.[7]

Like Shintoism, which had no formal organization until it was used as a political tool to enhance the lineage of the Meiji Emperors,[19] Reiki had no textbook or written instructions until very recently. Now there are manuals and written treatises, even cassettes and videos, discussing a wide array of personal interpretations of this system. Techniques of application have been diverse; they depended on the oral teachings of each Master as he or she initiated and instructed students. Not until the Usui System faced competition from other emerging Reiki schools and styles was there any attempt by a professional organization to establish a systematic application. In 1993 the Reiki Alliance, which was originally formed to support the teachings of Hawayo Takata through her granddaughter Phyllis Furumoto,[18] began to define the qualifications for and ethical behavior of a Reiki practitioner. Several organizations have subsequently developed their own criteria to promote wider acceptance by the medical community (see Reiki Organizations in the Appendix).

PRINCIPLES, PHILOSOPHY, AND DIAGNOSIS

Most Reiki practitioners are not concerned with a client's diagnosis unless they are coordinating with a doctor or other medical provider. This is because

Reiki has a unique relationship with disease and pain—it supports healing only of what needs to be healed rather than what the practitioner intends to be healed. For this reason, Reiki practitioners generally do not promise any specific symptom improvement or "cure."[10]

What is promised is a relaxing moment in time. Sometimes only one session is needed and sometimes multiple sessions are needed for the clients to begin to realize they are experiencing shifts in their perspectives of life, disease, attitudes, and the nature of the symptoms that brought them to the treatment room in the first place.[2,23,24]

Touch

Because the Usui System of Natural Healing teaches a system of touching, part of its effectiveness can be attributed to the body's response to gentle, appropriate contact between practitioner and client.[7] The practitioner gains permission to touch the client, then places his or her hands in a prescribed pattern on the client's body. The client is clothed and may be standing, sitting, or reclining on a bed, massage table, or the floor. Several nursing studies[8,14,16,17] have shown that this gentle act of appropriate touch can help a person make a profound shift, from the tense response of the fight-or-flight pattern of the sympathetic autonomic nervous system to the healing response of the relaxation pattern of the parasympathetic autonomic nervous system (Table 12-1).[22]

When a client's anxiety is relieved, symptoms are reduced.[21] Occasionally the opposite sequence is observed—symptoms abate and then anxiety is relieved. In either case, at this degree of deep relaxation the natural healing ability of the body is supported and enhanced. By the second or third hand position on the head, most clients are asleep. Thus on this very basic level of touch, much is accomplished toward individualized healing.

Energy

In her early diary, documented in the *Reiki Alliance Student Handbook* (or *Blue Book*),[18] Hawayo Takata, the energetic woman who brought the teaching and use of the Usui System out of Japan, stated that "this power [Reiki] is unfathomable, immeasurable, and

TABLE 12-1

Effects of Autonomic Nervous System Stimulation

Sympathetic	Parasympathetic
Increased alertness	
Increased heart rate, force, and contraction	Decreased heart rate
Dilation of vessels in the coronary arteries, pulmonary arteries, and skeletal muscles	Relaxation of vessels of gastrointestinal tract and skin
Constriction of vessels of the gastrointestinal tract and skin	Increased lacrimal, salivary, bronchial secretions; increased skin temperature
Dilation of bronchioles	Constriction of bronchioles
Decreased gastrointestinal motility and secretions	Increased gastrointestinal motility and secretions
Dilation of pupils	Constriction of pupils
Sweating	
Relaxation of the bladder detrusor muscle	Contraction of internal urethral sphincter
Contraction of bladder detrusor muscle	Relaxation of internal urethral sphincter
Glycogenolysis, lipolysis	Glycogenesis, lipogenesis

being a universal life force, it is incomprehensible to man. Yet, every living being is receiving its blessings daily, awake and asleep."

Many compare the feeling of receiving Reiki to the sensation felt when praying, meditating, singing, walking in the woods, or in any other way actively seeking God. The physical sensations associated with these activities are so similar that many Reiki practitioners believe they are the physical responses to making a connection with a power greater than themselves. Skepticism of this connection is a culturally held belief, especially in our hurry-up, stress-filled world. Our society reinforces the belief that none of us are connected to any kind of greater source or higher power. In the First Degree Class of this system, students are assisted in becoming aware (again) of the Universal Energy—that it is a life force that abounds in everything and that human beings benefit when they remain open to it.[2,3]

The body automatically directs healing energy to wounds, strain, tension, and other ailments. It is believed that the receiver of Reiki draws this energy through the hands of the practitioner, who is open to its universal availability. It is the need for healing energy that invites Reiki to be drawn through the practitioners hands.[3] This is why practitioners can offer Reiki to themselves. The hands are simply placed over an area of pain or infection or tension and the mind is opened and energy is allowed to flow. There is no manipulation of muscles or of the "electromagnetic field" of a client. The only method is to apply touch to a client's body in the prescribed hand positions or to be guided by an intuitive force. Some schools of Reiki do not allow the practitioner's hands to touch the client's body. The origin of this practice is not clear; traditional practitioners use this "hands-off" technique only when treating open or fresh wounds caused by accident or surgery. Some schools of Reiki teach that the practitioner's hands should remain in place for a period of 3 to 5 minutes. The traditional practitioner leaves the hands in position until the flow of energy is no longer felt.

For any condition, the basic routine is to offer a complete treatment session and then return to the sites of the original pain, stress, or tension. However, case reports indicate that after applying the full body treatment, a practitioner has no need to return to the original areas of complaint because the problem has been resolved.[2,3]

Principles

Although many research projects regarding the efficacy of Reiki are being developed, the collected experiences of Reiki practitioners are the most definitive validation of the system at this time. The following clinical observations describe the effectiveness of the practice of The Usui System of Natural Healing.

When a practitioner places hands on a client, both the practitioner and the client observe sensory changes around or under the hands of the practitioner.[2,9] These changes include the sensations of warmth, tingling, cold, extra fullness, and electrical charge. These sensations can change from one day to the next, from one client to the next, and can be experienced differently by the practitioner and the client. These sensory changes indicate that something is passing between the practitioner and the client. When the sensation dissipates after a time of holding the hands in one position, it signals the practitioner to change hand positions; in other words, to move on.

There is no conscious effort needed on the part of a practitioner to "turn Reiki on." When the body is in pain, has sustained a wound, or is beset by an unbalanced glandular, metabolic, or enzymatic process, it gives out an electromagnetic, neural, atomic, or vibrational alarm to stimulate a healing response from the rest of the body. How else does the body's immune system send its cells to determine the form of an intruding bacteria, or platelets to a wound to help stop bleeding? If we could record this signal with sensitive diagnostic equipment, we would understand the call of the body for internal or external energy. The fact that the sensation of Reiki energy flow dissipates after a time tells us that the particular need has been satisfied for the time being.[2,7,9] The time frame for this shift may be as little as a few seconds or as long as 45 minutes, or until the practitioner tires of holding the position.

The phenomenon of energy exchange can also explain the intuitive experience of many practitioners who find their hands drawn to a particular part of the client's body. Very often the recipient asks, "How did you know I had tension there?" The practitioner has no conscious knowledge of where the client is holding tension. It has been explained that the energy itself, meaning Reiki, feels the call of the body and is pulled to the need.

In the recent proliferation of anecdotes in books and on the Internet, no harmful effects of Reiki have been reported. One of the issues frequently discussed is the role of the intent of the practitioner. It is most often agreed that the only necessary intent is to be *available* to channel the energy rather than the intent "to heal" a certain symptom or condition. Clients are often healed in unexpected ways.[2,3] For this reason, traditional Reiki practitioners make no promises regarding the efficacy of treatment. Many practitioners, seeking to avoid any promise of therapeutic value, refer to the hour-long applications of energy simply as "sessions" or "therapy appointments."

The many anecdotal testimonies show Reiki to support the natural healing process of the body to such an extent that it can stimulate what is called a *healing crisis* (e.g., bringing a boil to a head, thus allowing the wound to be cleaned, or causing a quick rise in temperature in someone with an infection, followed by a gradual return to normal).[3,21] Some practitioners have reported that cuts, surgical wounds, and broken bones healed faster than expected after application of Reiki. There is also anecdotal evidence of Reiki resulting in a reduction of the side effects of chemotherapy and radiation treatment.

Reiki is often described as working on the root cause of a disease or imbalance. If a mental, emotional, or spiritual disturbance is a major factor in a physical impairment, the client often recognizes the disturbance during a Reiki session. How to deal with a painful relationship or a financial problem can be revealed during a session. As stated earlier, healing can come in many forms.[2,3]

When practitioners or others who have been attuned to Reiki regularly apply this energy to themselves they experience a dramatic reduction in day to day stress levels. When energy application is coupled with focused attention, through "processing work," or meditation, on the Five Precepts, personal understanding and an increase in compassion and openness to life can also occur.[7]

People who have attended classes describe personal experiences that defy logical explanation. These experiences are designated as mystical, synchronistic, or cosmic. Because they are often very personal, these experiences are not referred to in medically oriented classes so as not to put off clinicians who require concrete explanations.

PRACTICES, TECHNIQUES, AND TREATMENT

The practitioner's hands are held with fingers and thumb together then cupped slightly. They are placed in this preferred position in a relaxed manner on a person's clothed body.[2,3] The practitioner begins the treatment sitting at the head of the bed or massage table.

As taught in most schools, a full session of Reiki application begins with three hand positions on the head while the client is lying comfortably on his or her back. Every effort is made to ensure the comfort of the client and to prevent any stress in cases of diminished heart or lung capacity. If the client cannot recline on a bed, these hand positions are accomplished in the best possible manner. The first position (Figure 12-1) is over the eyes and sinuses, the second (Figure 12-2) is over the ears, including the temporomandibular joint, and the third (Figure 12-3) is the cradling of the head in the palms of the hands with fingertips at the client's occipital ridge.

After the three hand positions have been applied to the head, the practitioner remains seated at the head of the massage table and continues. The fourth position (Figure 12-4) is around the neck, thumbs to the back of the neck and fingertips overlapping the thyroid gland. The hands often cover the cervical lymph nodes. In the fifth position (Figure 12-5) the hands cover the bronchial tree, sternum, and thymus gland.

When applying hands to the front of the body, the practitioner stands on the client's right side and begins a new series of hand positions. The first position is with both hands on the right lung area. Precise

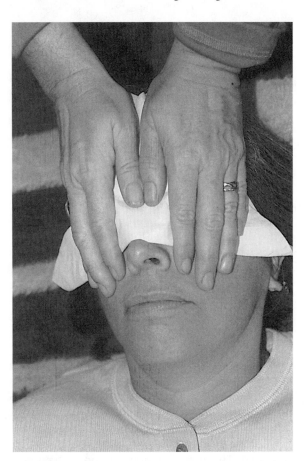

Figure 12-1 First head position.

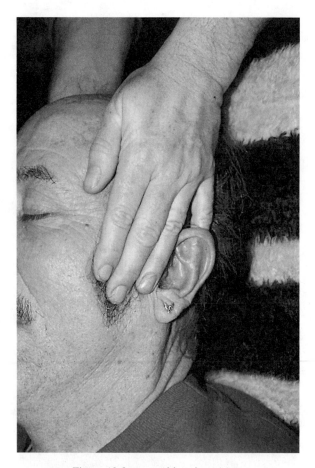

Figure 12-2 Second head position.

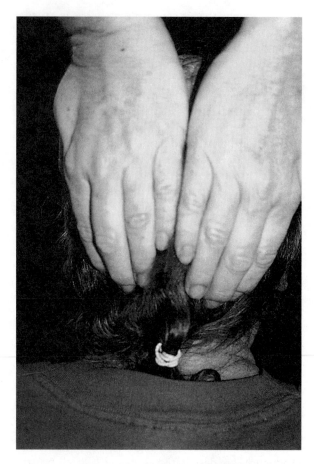

Figure 12-3 Third head position.

placement puts the middle finger of the upper hand at the bottom level of the sternum. The second position is directly over the left lung area. The third position is with the hands separated and parallel across the diaphragm, stomach, and upper liver area. This position also covers the gall bladder and spleen. The fourth position is below the belt line, between the ischial tuberosities of the pelvic girdle. A fifth position is often marked at the area over the uterus of a woman or the prostate of a man.

Many schools continue the treatment with a hand position that treats the inguinal area of both males and females. Often included are "knee sandwiches" in which one hand is palming the underside of the knee and the other is palming the patella. This position is held until both hand sensations are equalized. This same palming method is often used on each foot.

While the client is on his or her stomach, the back is offered Reiki with four main hand positions. Standing on the same side of the client as when working on the front, the practitioner palpates the lower margin of the scapula, then places the hands side by side over the left lung and heart area (Figure 12-6). The second position is with hands side by side over the right lung area. The third position is above the belt line or waist over the kidneys. The fourth is below the waist at the lumbar-sacral curve.

A fifth position is often called the "T-hold" (Figure 12-7). One hand is placed with the fingertips just touching the coccyx and the palm of the hand covering the rectal area. The other hand is held across the fingertips of the first hand, which cross the longer part of the sacrum. The practitioner must stand in a comfortable position to accomplish this application. It serves the rectum, the back of the uterus or

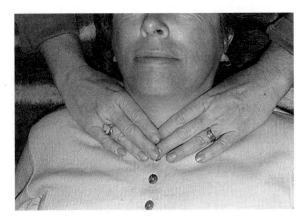

Figure 12-4 Neck position.

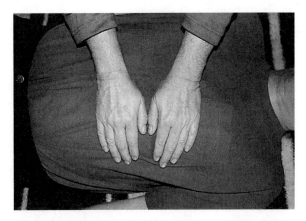

Figure 12-5 Second chest position.

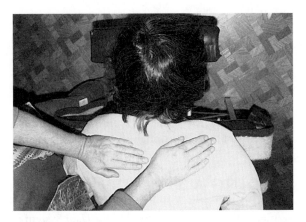

Figure 12-6 Optional shoulder position done before beginning hand positions on back.

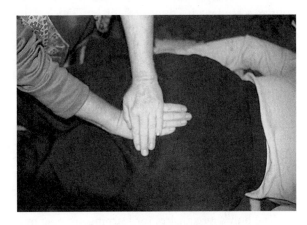

Figure 12-7 "T-hold" position.

prostate, and the back of the bladder, and has been reported to relieve impotency. An optional balancing position is one hand at the base of the neck, and the other hand over the sacrum (Figure 12-8).

European treatment styles differ from those taught in American schools. Some teach more hand positions and often offer the application of Reiki to clients who are covered with only a sheet or blanket. Other styles of Reiki applications are not described in relationship to body organs as has been done here. One school of Reiki designates a series of hand positions in relation to chakras, energy centers in line from the pubic bone to the top of the head. This chakra system is derived from Hindu philosophy and was not in the original teachings of the Usui System.

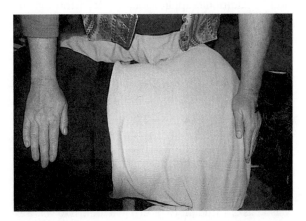

Figure 12-8 Optional balancing position: one hand at base of neck; other hand over sacrum.

The Levels of Reiki

Traditionally there have been three levels or degrees in the Usui System of Natural Healing.[2,9]

First Degree (Reiki I) is often erroneously referred to as Beginning Reiki. This creates a misunderstanding in that it can lead a person to believe that he or she has to take the next levels to have a complete understanding of Reiki or to be able to completely use the Usui System of Natural Healing. In the traditional system, Reiki I is sufficient to become a Reiki practitioner or to offer Reiki to oneself and family members for health maintenance and stress prevention.

This class is taught in three 4-hour sessions and includes four initiations or "attunements," which are the methods of connecting an individual with the source of energy, Reiki. Once connected to that source, a student is connected for life. During this class, students are taught the history of Reiki, observe the hand positions, and are invited to give and experience a full body application. Discussion of the Five Precepts is encouraged. Students are also encouraged to experience self-treatment and to investigate the application of Reiki in emergency situations, in hospices or hospitals, and to clients with acute or chronic conditions. Many case studies are reviewed and the dynamic potential of having access to this energy is outlined. Often students experience changes in their health, their relationships, or other human conditions during this training.

The only prerequisites for learning are openness, a desire to learn, and a commitment to use Reiki regularly.[5]

Second Degree (Reiki II) Class in some schools is referred to as Advanced Training. It involves instruction in additional applications of Reiki through the use of symbols or energy patterns. These additional applications include being able to offer Reiki to a person who is not in the room. This person can be next door or on the other side of the globe. The technique is called *Sending Reiki* or *Distant Reiki* and is akin to distant healing. Another application is that of mental rebalancing, which involves a specific hand position and techniques to help relieve addictions and habits and also to improve mental clarity. A third application is the ability to focus Reiki into a laser-like beam or to intensify its concentration. This class is taught over 2 days, or a minimum of two sessions. Often a Reiki Master asks a student to return in a month to share experiences regarding practice at this level of application.

In the traditional school of the Usui System of Natural Healing, the third level is referred to as Reiki III,

Third Degree Reiki, or Master Training, and may last as long as a year. Other schools have divided this training into two levels, Third Degree and Master Teacher Training, and others have consolidated this training into a 1-day experience. Many agree that this level of training can be taxing on the person who wishes to pursue this plateau of commitment to the Usui System. According to the Reiki Alliance, a student of Reiki should have been actively working with Reiki for 3 to 10 years before moving into this level of training.

A person who completes this training has the knowledge and technique with which to educate and open others to Reiki. How to initiate others into all three degrees is only one part of this mastery. Several organizations have developed teaching protocols for all levels of training. Each Master may add his or her own requirements.

All three levels are taught by a Master who has fulfilled all training requirements. They are known as Reiki Masters, not because they have mastered the energy, but because they have made a commitment to stand in the light of Reiki and allow their lives to exemplify the qualities described in the Five Precepts. This commitment is made on many levels, including financial, political, emotional, and spiritual.

FINDING A TEACHER

So many changes have occurred in the Usui System of Natural Healing since Hawayo Takata initiated her 22 Masters before her death in 1980. Some of these changes have occurred through the vision or ego of a particular Master. If a person seeks to learn Reiki, one of the questions to ask a potential Master is how his or her lineage is traced to Takata.[9] A Master's lineage demonstrates his or her proximity to the original teachings. A Master who knows and shares his or her lineage honors that lineage, an important element of the Usui System. There are other important questions to ask of a Master, including the following:

1. For how many years did you practice the Usui System of Natural Healing or Reiki Healing before seeking to be trained as a Master?
2. How do you see your role in practicing Reiki Healing, both in private practice and in serving the community at large?
3. Over what period of time was your Master training completed?
4. May I contact some former students of your classes?

5. Is there practice time during the training (whether for First or Second Degree)?
6. Can I receive a treatment from you before committing to the class?

Most traditional Masters also teach the history of Reiki, specifically how Dr. Usui received and applied his knowledge and vision. This story is the point of origin and the moment in time when energy became named as Reiki and the Usui System became manifest.[2,5,9,12,18] As with any other origination story, it offers its own teachings relevant to the system. The importance of this history gives rise to additional questions to ask a Master, including questions regarding the importance of the Five Precepts, the value of the teachings, and the continued availability of the Master to the student.

Most traditional Masters agree that, because Reiki can do no harm, any way in which a person may be drawn into the essence of this energy will prove beneficial. To gain a deeper understanding of the original teachings, a student needs to be aware of these important questions to ask a potential teacher so as to test the integrity and responsibility that the Master brings to the teachings. Choosing a Master can be the beginning of a lifelong relationship.[9]

References

1. Alandydy P, Alandydy K: Using Reiki to support surgical patients, *J Nurs Care Qual* 13(4):89-91, 1999.
2. Baginsky B, Sharamon S: *Reiki: universal life energy,* Mendocino, Calif, 1989, LifeRhythm.
3. Barnett L, Chambers M: *Reiki energy medicine,* Rochester, NY, 1996, Healing Arts Press.
4. Boorstein S: *It's easier than you think,* San Francisco, Calif, 1995, HarperCollins
5. Brown F: *Living Reiki: Takata's teachings,* Mendocino, Calif, 1992, LifeRhythm.
6. Brown F: *Reiki, the Usui system of natural healing.* Paper presented to Paranormal Research proceedings for the International Conference for Paranormal Research, Colorado, 1988.
7. Eos N: *Reiki & medicine,* Laytonville, Calif, 1994, White Feather Press.
8. Fakouri C, Jones P: Relaxation Rx: slow stroke back rub, *J Gerontol Nurs* 13:32-35, 1987.
9. Gleisner E: *Reiki as a complementary therapy: scientific and practical evidence of the value of touch and universal life energy,* Laytonville, Calif, 1997, White Feather Press.
10. Gleisner E: *Reiki in everyday living: how universal energy is a natural part of life, medicine, and personal growth,* Laytonville, Calif, 1992, White Feather Press.
11. Graham V: Mrs. Takata opens minds to Reiki, *San Mateo Times,* May 17, 1975.
12. Haberle H: *Hawayo Takata's story,* Olney, Md, 1990, Archedigm Publications.
13. Hammond S: *We are all healers,* New York, 1973, Ballantine Books.
14. Lynch J, Flaherty L, Emrich C et al: Effects of human contact on the heart activity of curarized patients in a shock trauma unit, *Am Heart J* 88:160-169, 1974.
15. Mansour AA, Beuche M, Laing G et al: Nurse J: A study to test the effectiveness of placebo Reiki standardization procedures developed for a planned Reiki efficacy study, *J Altern Complement Med* 5(2):53-64, 1999.
16. Melzak R, Wall PD: Pain mechanisms: a new theory, *Science* 150:971-979, 1965.
17. Mills M, Thomas SA, Lynch JJ et al: Effect of pulse palpitation on cardiac arrhythmia in coronary care patients, *Nurs Res* 25:378-382, 1976.
18. Mitchell P: *The Usui system of natural healing,* Cataldo, Idaho, 1985, Reiki Alliance.
19. Ono S: *Shinto, the kami way,* Tokyo, 1962, Charles E. Tuttle Company.
20. Petter FA: *Reiki: The legacy of Dr. Usui,* Twin Lakes, Wis, 1998, Lotus Press.
21. Sawyer J: The first Reiki practitioner in our OR, *AORN J* 67(3):674-677, 1998.
22. Tattam A: Reiki—healing and dealing, *Aust Nurs J* 2(23):52, 1994.
23. Tovar K, Cassneyer V: Touch, *AORN J* 49(5):1356-61, 1989.
24. van Sell SL: Reiki: an ancient touch therapy, *RN* 59(2):57-59, 1996.

Supplementary Readings

Bullock M: Reiki: a complementary therapy for life, *Am J Hosp Palliat Care* 14(1):31-33, 1997.

Kelner M, Wellman B: Who seeks alternative health care? A profile of the users of five modes of treatment, *J Altern Complement Med* 3(2):127-140, 1997.

Kelner M, Wellman B: Health care and consumer choice: medical and alternative therapies, *Soc Sci Med* 45(2):203-212, 1997.

Wirth DP, Barrett MJ: Complementary healing therapies, *Int J Psychosom* 41:61-67, 1994.

Wirth DP, Richardson JT, Eidelman WS: Wound healing and complementary therapies: a review, *J Altern Complement Med* 2(4):493-502, 1996.

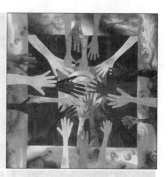

Healing Touch and Therapeutic Touch

DIANE WIND WARDELL

Although Healing Touch (HT) and Therapeutic Touch (TT) are different approaches to healing with touch or the hands, both methods were developed and promoted within the nursing profession. As such, most of the individuals who practice HT and TT are nurses. HT and TT are often used in settings in which traditional medical care is offered, such as hospitals and clinics. However, this type of healing can be done anywhere. Although both modalities use the word *touch* in their name, actual physical touch is not required in the application of either modality. HT and TT are considered *energy-based* or *biofield* therapies.

HT and TT are contemporary interpretations of ancient healing practices. HT uses physical touch to influence the human energy system, thus affecting physical, emotional, mental, and spiritual health. TT is defined as "an intentionally directed process of energy exchange during which the practitioner uses the hands as a focus for facilitating healing."[18]

The view of the client or patient in these modalities is that he or she consists of physical, emotional, mental, and spiritual aspects, each of which can be influenced to assist the person's capacity to self-heal. This is the foundation of HT and TT practice. Both methods promote healing for the individual's "highest good," meaning that the cure is not necessarily the focus; the focus is the individual facilitating his or her own growth or undergoing "self-healing."[30] Each method is believed to be useful in a variety of ways, including reducing pain, decreasing anxiety, and accelerating self-healing. It is important to realize, however, that the response to these healing methods is individualized.

HT and TT are often used to augment traditional or "routine" medical care, which currently is considered the "standard of care." Such use has been referred to as *integrative,* which implies that these techniques or systems have been outside the biomedical model and are now being integrated into the commonly accepted system of health care. In the future, it may be that other systems of care based on holistic methods that consider a patient's physical, emotional, mental, and spiritual aspects may serve as the standard of care, and that biomedical techniques will be integrated into that system.

HISTORY

The art of healing is a basic human practice found across cultures and time. Modern medicine is relatively new in contrast to these ancient forms of healing that involve energy or biofield therapies. Energy-based therapies were described as early as 2500 to 5000 years ago in the writing of *Huang Ti Ching Su Wen* of China, the source of basic concepts in Chinese medical theory.[11] In addition, ancient carvings from the Egyptian Third Dynasty depict the use of the hands to heal.[24]

Healing Touch

The Healing Touch Program developed from the energy-based healing practice of a nurse, Janet Mentgen, in the early 1980s.[29] Mentgen's introduction to healing came when she attended a beginning lecture on TT presented at a conference near Denver. She later met the instructor and was invited to the advanced class in TT the next day. After this exposure, she took a TT course at a local hospital in the Denver area, where she realized that she had the ability to facilitate others' healing, see auras, and develop her intuition. She left her nursing job to develop a healing practice full time and taught continuing education classes on healing in nursing at the local community college in Red Rocks, Colorado. To expand her clinical skills and her understanding of energy-based therapies, she continued to study with a number of therapists and lay healers in different alternative therapies, and gained extensive training in biofeedback. She integrated what she learned into the college classes she was teaching, and began to offer different classes and levels of training over several semesters. Although her foundation was TT, she realized what she was teaching included other techniques as well. Therefore the term *healing touch* was eventually coined to describe her method.

In 1988 a group of nurses who had been teaching a variety of healing techniques came together at the request of the American Holistic Nurses Association to bring a healing program forward as a certificate program of the organization. Because HT had already been taught as a series of courses, the group decided to support this program. It was first offered as a pilot project as a weekend or intensive course at the University of Tennessee and in Gainesville, Florida, in 1989, and became a certificate program of the American Holistic Nurses Association in 1990. During its first year, 25 programs were offered across the United States. By 1997, there were more than 500 programs available. More than 55,000 people have taken at least the first level of the course, and there are almost 2000 certified practitioners of HT as of this writing. In addition to the United States, courses have been taught in Canada, New Zealand, Australia, South Africa, Peru, Great Britain, Finland, Netherlands, Germany, France, Romania, and Trinidad-Tobago. As its popularity continues to spread, HT is being brought to areas where medical care is limited and the need is great, such as South America and Africa.

Janet Mentgen continues to be an active teacher of the program and its instructors today. Throughout her work she supports the program's vision to take HT to all people who affect health care. She believes that "we are teaching how to do the work and nobody owns the work. It is a collective."[18]

In 1996 Healing Touch International, Inc. (HTI), was formed as a nonprofit education corporation to administer the HT certification process for practitioners and instructors. HTI is also responsible for the International Standards of Practice and Code of Ethics for HT practitioners worldwide.

Therapeutic Touch

TT was developed by Dolores Krieger in the early 1970s. Krieger's interest in touch evolved from her research interest in healers and her interactions with Dora Kunz, a clairvoyant and noted healer. She tells her story in the book *The Therapeutic Touch: How to Use Your Hands to Heal.*[13] Krieger said that Dora Kunz, who was able to see the subtle energy patterns (auras) around individuals, studied with Charles Leadbeater, a twentieth-century "seer," since the time she was a child. With this training and ability, she worked throughout her life to use her hands as instruments of healing with noted doctors and scientists. When Krieger first met her, Kunz was studying the processes of different healers, including Oskar Estebany.

Mr. Estebany had been a colonel in the Hungarian cavalry. When his horse became ill, instead of putting the animal to sleep as advised, he worked all night massaging, caressing, talking to, and praying for her. In the morning, much to his and others' surprise, the horse was well. After that incident, others brought their animals to him. A desperate father once asked Estebany to heal his child. Although he declined at first, Estebany relented and worked on the child, who recovered. Estebany eventually came to Canada and became part of a research study that Krieger was observing. A subsequent study allowed Krieger to work more closely with Estebany. Although she found his technique quite simple, she was unable to capture his "intense interior experience." Estebany did not believe that people could be taught a method that would allow them to do what he did, because what he did was the result of a "gift" imparted at birth. Dora Kunz thought differently and agreed to teach others, including Dolores Krieger. That was the beginning of their life-long relationship.

Krieger went on to offer a class called "Frontiers in Nursing: The Actualization of Potential for Therapeutic Human Field Interaction," within the master's degree program at New York University. TT is now taught around the world to nurses and others in continuing education programs offered through universities and professional organizations.

The Nurse Healers Professional Associates International, Inc., is the official organization of TT. It was developed in 1979 as a "body of professional persons in the health field who are interested in healing."[15] The form of TT associated with this organization is referred to as the *Krieger/Kunz model* of TT.

Healing Work Today

A recent study found that 13% more individuals are using complementary therapies than 5 years ago, and that energy healing is one of the forms of therapy that has increased to the greatest degree.[6] HT and TT con-

tinue to rise in popularity as complementary therapies are offered in hospitals. Some hospices for example, encourage HT and TT training for all nursing staff. At Wilcox Hospital in Kauai, Hawaii, 95% of the doctors have given blanket permission for nurses to use HT on their patients. Even State Boards of Nursing (e.g., Nevada) are suggesting that Healing Touch be considered standard nursing care.

PRINCIPLES, PHILOSOPHY, AND DIAGNOSIS

HT promotes self-healing for the individual's highest good, meaning that "cure" is not the focus; the focus is the facilitation of self-healing and growth. This is accomplished by restoring balance and harmony in the human energy system, which can benefit clients with any number of physical ailments, from specific problems to systemic imbalances.[9] TT also accomplishes these goals. It is administered with the "intent of enabling the person to repattern their energy in the direction of health." TT works *with* the individual and facilitates healing.

The foundations of HT and TT are similar. The body is seen as an internal energy system that interacts with the external world, and the healing force is thought to come from another source such as the universe.[1] Human beings (and all living things) are connected through the unity of creation. Consequently, even a small amount of interference in the pattern of energy affects the entire structure of the universe simultaneously.[8]

The interconnectedness of the body and mind is one way to understand the basis for these techniques. Many people are now aware of this interconnectedness, in part because of the effect that stress and other consequences of contemporary life have on the body, especially the immune system, resulting in increased incidence of heart disease, cancer, depression, asthma, and arthritis. If a person is stressed and anxious, the body becomes tight and conditions such as sore muscles, tension headache, and hyperventilation may develop. A person who is aware of what is happening to his or her body during stressful periods is able to consciously work to alter these symptoms. Conversely, if no action is taken, this stressed state can eventually lead to disease.

The body's molecular structure is actually a complex network of interwoven energy fields, and is nourished by subtle energy systems affected by our emotions, level of spiritual balance, nutrition, and environment.[8] We are all a part of and contributors to this subtle energy field.[25] Although recent research has led some to state that the energy field does in fact exist and can be measured,[22] our understanding of how these techniques actually work is still theoretic.

It is known that every unit of matter can be broken down into smaller and smaller parts until what remains is a signature vibration. When two objects have similar natural frequencies, they can interact without touching and their vibrations can become entrained and can resonate. This is one of the theories that supports touch therapies, because the therapist and client entrain and seek a higher vibration that affects the healing process.[3]

Modern interpretation of the human energy field or the designation of the field is extrapolated from ancient systems. The meridian system found in traditional Chinese medicine can be traced back thousands of years, as can the chakra system found in the texts of ancient India. The chakra system is the energy system that is identified and manipulated within HT and TT. *Chakra*, a Sanskrit word used by the Hindus, means *wheel of light*.[5] Seven chakras constitute the major energy centers of the body, and minor chakras are found over the joints and throughout the body (Figure 13-1). These centers are not static; their motion in a healthy individual has been described as "beautifully balanced, symmetrical and organic with all the parts flowing together in a rhythmic pattern. Their motion is, in fact, harmonic or musical in character, with rhythms which vary according to individual, constitutional and temperamental differences."[12]

According to Bruyere,[5] each of the seven major chakras has a physical, emotional, creative (or mental), and spiritual (or celestial) component. The endocrine system is believed to be closely associated with the functions of the chakras.[2] In addition, each chakra has a purpose or *body*. The body for the first chakra, which deals with survival and physical sensation, is the physical body. The body for the second chakra is the emotional body, related to the people with whom we share our feelings (e.g., spouse, children). The body for the third chakra is the mental body, which has to do with thoughts, opinions, and will. The body for the fourth chakra is the heart center or astral body, which bridges between the material and spirit. The body for the fifth chakra, the etheric body, is the template for the perfect body, "light

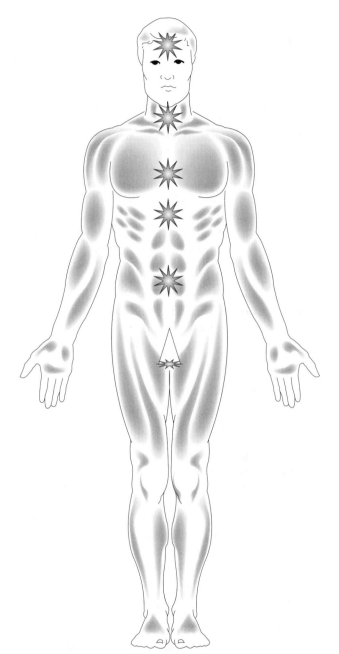

Figure 13-1 The seven major chakras.

body," or higher potential and is about speaking our truth. The body of the sixth chakra is often called the "third eye," and is about "sight" (involving intuition and insight). The body of the seventh or "crown" chakra is related to the spiritual realm and our spiritual life. Each of the seven chakras is also associated with a color.

The human aura is viewed as the totality of the human being; what we actually see is only part of this physical manifestation. Dora Kunz was noted for her ability to see and interpret human energy fields.[16] She saw them as concentric spheres that are part of the universal field of the entire earth. Auras are like a "moving picture . . . in an ongoing process of living."[16] They are usually ovoid, with many colors depicting the emotional energy. Auras can vary in size without a "true" norm. They can be about 12 to 18 inches and can expand or shrink considerably. The chakras, as energy centers, are believed to function as both transmitters and transformers of energy from field to field, acting to synchronize the emotional, mental, and etheric energies.[12]

The ability to see or detect an aura is not a requirement for the provider of HT or TT treatment. Nor is it necessary for clients receiving the healing to have knowledge of or belief in the theory or explanatory rationale.

Three modern nursing theorists, Rogers, Watson, and Newman, have been influential in the development of HT and TT. Rogers' theory of the Science of the Unitary Human Being has formed the basis for much of the research that has been conducted on TT as a healing modality.[27] The theory posits the four meta-paradigms of man: health, environment, and nursing in interaction with a dynamic health-patterning model that actualizes potential. What are the four things? They are the study of "unitary, irreducible, indivisible human and environmental fields: people and their worlds."[28] Margaret Newman was a student of Rogers and has explored the mutuality of the interaction between nurse and client, the uniqueness and wholeness in the pattern of the interaction, and movement to a higher consciousness.[19] The founder of nursing, Florence Nightingale (1820-1910), described nursing as developing the ability to put patients in the best condition for nature to act upon them.[20] She recognized the healing properties of the environment, including fresh air, sunlight, and warmth, and saw people as complex beings inseparable from their environment.

Jean Watson's postmodern framework of transpersonal care has proposed that modalities that involve touch flow from a spiritual path of human development and form the foundation for transpersonal practice.[31] HT provides a way to articulate this process. Watson's work in the transpersonal-healing-caring framework provides more explicit application of energy therapies to the holistic health care needs of clients.[31] Some of the premises of this model include being vulnerable; cultivating the ability to ground, energize, and center the self and the other; using focused intentionality to potentiate wholeness, harmony, and healing; and being mindfully present. The model also encourages connecting with the deeper self, cultivating an awe of the unknown, and conveying caring and acceptance for others.

Diagnosis

No medical diagnosis is made with HT or TT. HT and TT help a person to self-heal, promoting the client's health and well being by maintaining balance within the energy field.

If the person offering the healing session is a nurse, a nursing diagnosis may be used. The terminology of nursing diagnoses has been developed through The North American Nursing Diagnosis Association. The nursing diagnosis for working with the body's energy system is: "Energy field disturbance: a condition in which a disturbance of the human energy field manifests a disharmony in the human-environmental energy field mutual process."[17] If the practitioner/healer is not a nurse, he or she will use other terminology to describe this imbalance.

Many of the words that have been used to describe energy imbalance are associated with the senses. Words associated with sense of touch or feeling, for example, include *congestion, spikes, heat,* and *cold.* A description based on sight may use words that describe color, such as *gray* or *brown,* or shade, such as *dark* or *light.* The visual sense might also include terms such as *murky* or *thick.* Descriptions based on the auditory senses might include words like *buzzing* or *hum.* The olfactory sense might assign a *smoky* or *pungent* odor. The intuitive sense can also be developed. Although the practitioner watches for these changes in the energy field of the patient, it is not necessary to be able to detect them to conduct a healing session. Although many beginning practitioners and even some advanced practitioners have not yet learned to trust their senses, the healing work still can be done effectively. However, it should always be remembered that the client directs the session. Belief in the system is not necessary, although it is usually considered helpful. Clients identify their goals for the work in discussion with the practitioner and a mutual goal set is established. For example, if a client desires freedom from pain, a mutual goal for the session may be to work for that person's highest good in reducing his or her pain.

Practitioners of HT and TT follow the basic guidelines established within the curriculum of study for their respective modalities. Each curriculum teaches the healer to follow the nursing process. This involves a step-by-step protocol, which includes an energy-based interview, energy field assessment, plan and intervention using one or more of the HT techniques or TT, and evaluation. Again, the client remains the central focus. The healer is there to facilitate the client's healing.

PRACTICES, TECHNIQUES, AND TREATMENT

Touch can benefit clients with any number of physical ailments, specific problems as well as systemic imbalances. It can assist with pain reduction, wound healing, postoperative recovery, spiritual growth, and relief of symptoms.

Interaction of the Client and Practitioner

The interaction of the client and practitioner may include a formal or informal contract. The client has the ultimate responsibility for his or her healing, whereas the practitioner is obligated to provide the client with information about what is being performed and the expected outcome. No false promises of a "cure" should be made, because this is not the focus of treatment.

Certain information should be provided before a session. An example is the information that has recently been mandated by the state of Minnesota in the Minnesota Uniform Health Care Act (HF No. 3839). According to this Act, which is referred to as the Complementary and Alternative Health Care Client Bill of Rights, the following information must be provided before a healing session from an alternative provider begins:

- The degrees, training, experience, or other qualifications of the practitioner

- The name of the practitioner's supervisor, if any
- The fees charged for the service and how they may be paid
- A brief summary of the theoretic approach used
- Information concerning the assessment and recommended service, including the duration of services
- A promise of courteous treatment
- Assurances that records are confidential and will be made available to the client
- A statement that other services may be available and where information regarding such services may be found
- A declaration of the patient's right to choose and/or change providers
- A statement regarding the client's right to refuse treatment

Constraints of the Practitioner

Anyone can do HT and TT, regardless of age, physical condition, or education. The healing work can be provided by nonprofessionals for family members and friends. It may also be incorporated into the routine care provided by professionals such as nurses or massage therapists. For example, a nurse may smooth the energy field above a patient's arm before and after inserting an intravenous line, with the intent to ease insertion, decrease discomfort, and repattern the energy field. A massage therapist may perform a technique such as *mind clearing* (from the HT lexicon) to promote relaxation before beginning the massage. The techniques can also be helpful for managing the practitioner's own health and well being.

Practitioners who have pursued the healing work to a more advanced level with extensive study may elect to offer the service to others in a more comprehensive way. One way to do this is as part of an existing professional practice. For example, an HT or TT practitioner may be employed by an institution (e.g., hospital, hospice, or wellness center) to provide treatment to clients who request it or for whom it is recommended. This service may or may not be part of routine care at the facility. Another way to provide a more comprehensive service is to establish a private practice in which the client can individually contract for the treatment.

A practitioner who has a physical limitation may practice in any of the ways described, although this may require making adjustments regarding time, setting, and techniques used. Many of the techniques can be practiced without physically touching the body and may be provided even from a distance.

Practitioners develop confidence with time and, more importantly, with practice. The HT program includes many different techniques for beginning and advanced practitioners. Although the TT method is relatively simple to master, it takes time to become proficient. The healer's comfort level with using either of these therapeutic modalities varies with experience and training. Attributes of an effective healer include the ability to set intention to the highest good of the client, the motivation to help another, an open mind, an open heart able to provide unconditional love and acceptance, and the ability to let go of expectations.

Mutual interaction is inherent in the healing process. Therefore a person who is engaged in healing is also engaged in self-healing. It is important to recognize this mutuality. During training, healers must commit to being aware of personal qualities that need to be refocused or redirected to health and healing.

Indications and Contraindications

There are no contraindications for using HT or TT. Because HT and TT are noninvasive techniques that do not present any documented risks, they can be used for all conditions. This does not mean to imply that they are the only treatment modalities for illness or emotional distress. They should be used in conjunction with traditional medical care. Ideally, there should be interaction among all health care professionals involved in assisting a client to manage his or her health.

It has been noted that 33% of clients do not inform their physicians that they are engaged in complementary therapies.[6] Physicians may not understand the risks and benefits of different complementary therapies, which may cause confusion and discord. However, primary care providers and others involved in patient care should be aware of the various therapies being used (a cogent argument for curriculum development in medical schools and schools of allied health professions). For example, when the HT technique of *magnetic unruffling* is used it may alter postoperative recovery. It is postulated that this technique helps to remove accumulated debris or congestion (in this case, the anesthetic residue) from the energy field, allowing the person to awaken sooner and with fewer side effects.[9]

HT and TT can be used to promote health and well being. The focus on maintaining balance within the energy field is a preventive strategy. HT and TT also have the potential to beneficially affect individuals with a variety of conditions—they may be used to decrease pain and bleeding; relieve headache pain; help break up congestion; aid in the healing of fractured bones, tendonitis, and tumors; and promote relaxation and improve mental focus.[9,14] In addition, preoperative and postoperative energy work can help prepare patients for surgery through relaxation and energy balancing, thus improving the rate of recovery. Evidence also suggests that TT has beneficial effects for pregnant women and people suffering from psychiatric disorders.

There are some constraints on the application of HT and TT techniques. For example, with the very young or old and the very frail it is best to work for short periods of time. However, the amount or intensity of the energy is less important than the ability of the therapist to "integrate the healee's energies into a synchronous flow."[14] In HT it is believed that no harm can be done during a session if the intent of the provider is applied to the client's highest good and follows the direction of his or her energy. Working within this framework, only the energy that is needed is available to the client. During the interaction, there should be dialogue between the practitioner and client so that if problems do arise they can be addressed. If a situation or problem arises that was not present before the session it "most likely has an energetic component and will dissipate if you work through it."

There is a somewhat different view in TT practice. The Policy and Procedure for Health Professionals states that TT "does not usually exceed 30 minutes." It has been suggested that a treatment session should not exceed 20 to 25 minutes because it is believed possible to "overdose on energy."[14]

The response to HT and TT may be immediate or may take several hours or days. There may be a sense of general relaxation, comfort, or increased sense of well being. There may also be tension release that may manifest as crying, slowing of breathing, and decrease in heart rate, blood pressure, perspiration, and other bodily sensations.

Techniques

Healing Touch

In HT the practitioner first interviews the client regarding treatment goals and then assesses the energy field. Depending on the length of time available for a session, techniques that best meet the client's needs at the time are selected. The client is usually asked to lie on a massage table, but treatment can be given in any position or in any setting (e.g., hospital bed, chair, home, or office). The client remains fully clothed; a blanket or light covering may be placed over the client for comfort. The practitioner may use light touch on certain areas (e.g., the joints, chakras, or problem area) of the body after confirming that the client is amenable to touch. All techniques can also be done without touching, and certain techniques are routinely performed this way.

The treatment session varies depending on the setting and on the health condition, age, need, and desire of the client. HT sessions can take from a few minutes to an hour. The healer first centers himself or herself before discussing the client's concerns. This communication requires a relaxed body, a clear mind, and a sense of spiritual calm. The healer focuses on the client's highest good without imposing his or her own wishes or desires for the outcome of the session. The discussion may reveal the reason for the visit, description of the problem, and the client's goals. The client then lies prone or sits in a chair. The practitioner then assesses the energy field surrounding the client by sweeping the hands several inches over the client and noting any changes in the energy field, which can be felt as tingling, warmth, and coolness, among other sensations. A pendulum can also be used as an assessment device to indicate whether the major energy centers or chakras are open and functioning.

A nursing diagnosis may be made based on these findings. The planned intervention then uses one or more of the HT techniques to provide balance in the energy system. If a full session is being offered, it usually begins with an opening technique or full body technique that balances the entire system, such as chakra connection, spiral opening, and full-body connection. Table 13-1 presents the goals, indications, and a brief description of the major HT full-body techniques. If any imbalances are noticed while the initial technique is applied, or if the client has identi-

fied a particular area of concern, additional techniques are used. For example, local techniques include the pain drain for pain relief; "ultrasound" to break up congestion; and modulation of energy to aid in the healing of fractured bones.[9] Other localized techniques can be used to promote relaxation and increase focus. Full-body HT techniques such as the lymphatic drain and chelation are used for systemic imbalances and transitions, and usually take more time to complete. The full-body techniques promote complete balancing of the entire energy field and usually have more sustained effect.

While providing treatment, the healer may place his or her hands directly on the clothed body, or may choose to situate them a few inches above the body if this is more comfortable for the client. During the session the client may experience a variety of responses, including falling asleep, visual or sensory experiences, or a sense of peace. After the session the healer evaluates the outcome by performing another energy assessment to determine whether balance has been achieved and eliciting feedback from the client about his or her experiences. This information is documented on the client's record.

Additional techniques are taught in Advanced Practice classes, which are delivered solely by Janet Mentgen, the founder of HT. These advanced techniques are not included in the standard program of study for certification. They are used for balancing the system at multiple levels, deeper spiritual healing, healing of chronic pain from traumatic events, and aligning the energy centers. The practitioner's voice may also be used to promote relaxation.

Therapeutic Touch

TT was first described as a five-step procedure of centering, assessment, unruffling, directing, and modulating the transfer of energy, and recognizing the time to stop.[13] This five-step procedure is now referred to as the *Krieger/Kunz method*. *Centering* involves "bringing body, mind, and emotions to a quiet, focused state of consciousness."[21] *Assessment* of the energy field around the client involves the basic principle of symmetry. The field should feel the same on both sides; dissimilarities have often been described as areas of congestion, prickling, heat, or coolness. *Unruffling* or clearing involves movement of the hands outward toward the periphery of the field so that there is a gentle sweeping of the pressure or congested areas

TABLE 13-1

Selected Healing Touch Techniques

Full-body techniques	Goals	Indications	Brief description
Chakra connection	Open and balance the energy centers.	Systemic or chronic disease, trauma, anxiety.	Practitioner places the hands lightly on the body or off the body, starting at the feet, and holds each position for about 1 minute. The hands gradually move up the body over the joints of the legs and arms and the major centers on the trunk and head.
Magnetic unruffle	Cleanse and clear the body or remove congested energy and emotional debris.	Postanesthesia, smoking (current or past), chronic pain, trauma, medication or drug use, systemic disease, and emotional clearing.	With hands above the body at all times, the practitioner starts at the head and moves slowly down to and off (above) the feet. Repeated on each side of the body until the practitioner feels the field is clear, usually approximately 15 minutes, more or less.
Chakra spread	Open chakras and promote deep healing.	Transitions: to ease dying, severe pain, severe stress, and spiritual growth.	Practitioner holds each foot and then each hand, then works above the body, starting at the head with hands together and gently opening each chakra down the body. Practitioner ends by holding the client's hand and placing other hand over the heart.
"Ultrasound"	Provide deep penetration to facilitate healing by breaking up congestion, patterns, and blocks.	Pain (e.g., arthritic joints), decreasing bleeding, sealing lacerations, ear or eye problems, fractures and joint injuries.	Practitioner directs the finger at the area above the body. The hand moves. Can be done for a few minutes or more.
Pain drain	Remove pain or congestion.	Acute and chronic pain from injury, surgical incisions, and disease process.	Practitioner places one hand on or above the painful area until a change is felt and then places the other hand on or above the area. Usually takes 5-10 minutes.
Wound sealing	Repair field from incisions, trauma, or childbirth.	New wounds and old wounds that have remained painful or create discomfort.	With the palms down, practitioner moves hands back and forth slightly above the injured area for a short time, gathering energy, and then holds palm directly over area for 1 minute.
Unruffling and pain ridge	Remove congestion.	Pain (acute), anxiety, stress, nausea and vomiting.	Calm and rhythmic movements of the hands, palms facing the body at a distance of 1-6 inches, brushing down and away from above to below.

in the energy field. *Directing and modulating energy* involves transferring or channeling energy to the client and also modulating it so that part of the field may be energized and another calmed.

TT treatment is individualized and is usually done with the fully-clothed client sitting in a chair or reclining, whichever is more comfortable. The practitioner's hands, held approximately 2 to 4 inches above the client's skin, are passed from the head to the toe, both front and back, to assess the field. The therapist may then use rhythmic, sweeping motions of the hands, perhaps touching the client. The hands may then be placed gently on or slightly off the body over an area that was felt to be dissimilar or a place the client identified as having a problem. When the practitioner believes the session is complete, he or she rechecks the field.

Differences

HT and TT are very similar disciplines, yet there are differences between them are minor. HT uses a greater variety of techniques for specific purposes than TT. The hands may be placed on or over the body more often in HT. TT sessions are usually shorter, although they may last as long or longer than an HT session, depending on the circumstances in which they are offered. The training programs are different. (See the following.)

TRAINING AND CERTIFICATION

The programs of study in HT and TT were originally offered only to nurses, but are now available to others interested in healing. "Any man or woman—given real interest and prompted by the incentive to serve—who thinks and loves can be a healer."[2] The focus is on a "heart-centered" approach in which peace and calm provide the foundation for the interaction between client and practitioner.[10] It is important that practitioners be present in the moment so they can listen to the clients fully.

Healing Touch

There are several levels of training in the course of study for HT practitioners. Self-care is stressed throughout the HT program because it is the basis for transferring the focused, intentional energy that is needed to perform HT with others.[9] The learning process is life-long, and requires commitment to self-healing and spiritual discipline through adequate rest, a healthy diet, and striving for emotional balance.[7]

The Code of Ethics developed by HTI in 1996 is based on the premise that HT helps the client to self-heal and is based on a heart-centered, caring relationship. The client is not judged and his or her humanness is respected because he or she is considered whole and holy. The client is seen as part of a unity and individual rights are upheld. Respect for coping mechanisms is always maintained. The client's health care choices are honored and interventions are based on energetic assessments, which are documented. Information is provided according to expressed need, context, and personal situation. The confidentiality of the client is respected. Adhering to the principle of "do no harm," no energy is given beyond the person's capacity to receive it. Appropriate health care referral is made whenever necessary. Practitioners practice within the scope of their background and training and meet their obligations accordingly. Supervision and consultation are sought when needed.

There are eight standards of practice, which describe facets of what the HT practitioner must do or be. These standards follow:

1. Integrates HT within the scope of his or her background, and clearly represents background to the client and public
2. Is a resource within the community for information regarding the practice of HT
3. Has a good grasp of the theoretic base of HT and maintains a commitment to continual learning
4. Obtains health information and energy assessment from the client
5. Assesses the energy system of the client
6. Facilitates the healing process but allows the client to guide the pacing, openness, and intensity of HT at all times
7. Respects the client's spiritual beliefs and practices by operating from a broad, universal concept of spirituality
8. Explains the treatment fully, allowing the client to be a knowledgeable participant in the healing process, based on his or her ability

Training

A person can take as few as one or as many as all of the available courses to become a practitioner of HT. It is a multilevel continuing education program of 120 hours of standardized curriculum. Each level includes both didactic and experiential learning (e.g., lecture, practice of techniques, and exercises to enhance learning). The program is sequenced in five levels of instruction: Level I, Level IIA, Level IIB, Level IIIA, and Level IIIB. An additional level is for instructor training.

Level of Practice

The level of practice a practitioner may establish is based on his or her training. The "Student of Healing Touch" has completed the Level I course taught by a certified instructor and is actively participating in the HT educational program. The "Healing Touch Practitioner Apprentice" has completed the Level IIIA course (the fourth course) and is participating in a minimum 1-year mentorship process. The "Healing Touch Practitioner" has completed 120 contact hours of course work within Levels 1 through IIIB and has received a Certificate of Completion from the Healing Touch Program Director. The "Certified Healing Touch Practitioner" is an HT practitioner who, in addition to completing the program of study, has met the certification criteria established by HTI and has been reviewed and approved by the HTI Certification Board.

Program Description, Objectives, and Content

The program includes four levels from beginner to instructor. The second and third levels are divided into two separate courses.

- **Level I** usually consists of 20 hours of instruction. The content includes the basics of the chakra and energy systems and the concepts of the human energy field as it relates to modern scientific principles. The student learns how to assess the energy field with hand scanning and the pendulum. Centering techniques are developed and the student is introduced to therapeutic touch. Intervention techniques for stress, pain, and balancing are taught, including magnetic unruffling, chakra connection, ultrasound, laser, chakra spread, and headache techniques. A discussion of how to apply HT in personal and professional practice is provided. Principles of self-healing and personal development are explored.

- **Level II** includes 30 or more hours divided into two training sessions. The person learns healing sequences for specific client needs (e.g., back pain) and also develops therapeutic interaction skills.
  - In **Level IIA** the content includes development of assessment, interview, and documentation techniques. Specific techniques for working with the back and neck, sequencing, wound closure, pain management, and spiral meditation are presented. A 1-hour healing sequence for specific client problems is conducted.
  - In **Level IIB** the content includes self-care techniques that support the process of becoming a healer. The philosophies of noted healers such as Brennan, Bruyere, and Bailey are reviewed. The student learns Hara alignment meditation and advanced techniques such as etheric unruffling, lymphatic drain, chelation, and spinal cleansing. Instruction is provided on advanced studies of the human energy system, including chakra function, aura perception, layers, and energy blocks. The perceptual tools of the student are developed. The student views healing from the standpoints of practitioner, client, and observer or coach and performs a complete treatment session.

- **Level III** includes two educational sessions with a 6-month to 1-year course of study in between. The focus is on case studies, mentoring, ethics, client-practitioner relationships, practice establishment, and integration of community. There are specific requirements for practice, education, and service for successful completion of this level of study. A certificate of completion is awarded. After completing Level III, students can apply for certification as an HT practitioner.

- An additional level is for certified practitioners who are interested in teaching HT. Instructor training involves additional course work and a minimum of seven supervised teaching experiences.

Certified Practitioner

An HT practitioner obtains certification from HTI by submitting an application documenting that he or she has met the criteria established. The application must provide the following information and documentation:

- Evidence of completion of all course work
- Professional resume
- Summary of experience with healing modalities and a 1-year mentorship and mentorship approval (approval of the preceptor by the HTI)
- A description of educational experiences, including books read and conferences attended
- A case study of in-depth work with one client over a minimum of three to five sessions and documentation of the use of HT curriculum techniques
- A description of self-study, including a statement of purpose regarding personal development, growth, and practice as an HT practitioner

Therapeutic Touch

Nurse Healers-Professional Associates, Inc. (NH-PA), is the approved provider of continuing education offerings for TT. NH-PA facilitates the exchange of research findings, teaching strategies, and new developments in the area of healing. It also maintains a *Statement of Ethics and Conduct for Practice of Therapeutic Touch.* This document explicitly states that the practitioner is to provide the treatment process as taught, with integrity, and based on the client's needs, while respecting the client's rights and responsibilities. The statement also identifies the principles of obtaining permission; fee notification; nonexploitiveness; maintaining confidentiality and personal boundaries; and making a commitment to strengthen abilities.

Training

TT classes are taught in universities and other venues around the world. There are different classes for beginning, intermediate, and advanced students. According to the *Curriculum and Guidelines for Teaching Krieger/Kunz Therapeutic Touch,* the characteristics and expectations of the student in the different classes are as follows:

- The beginner class prepares students to understand the history, assumptions, concepts, and research associated with the practice of TT. Students learn to center and do the phases of TT. They learn the importance of applying

ethical principles and proper conduct, and the need for self-healing and personal growth. Students are taught the importance of giving and receiving ongoing TT sessions with peer review.
- Intermediate students recognize the effects of TT on outcomes and perform all phases of TT. They understand the use of imagery, color, and modulation, and apply and demonstrate ethical principles. They participate in a program of self-healing. They appreciate the value of giving and receiving sessions with peer review.
- Advanced students acknowledge TT as a unique and effective healing modality. They understand how TT affects the emotional field, the endocrine system, and the autonomic nervous system. They learn to adapt TT as a nonlinear application and to adhere to ethical principles and conduct. In addition, advanced students recognize a need to maintain a program of self-healing and personal growth. They accept responsibility for giving and receiving sessions on an ongoing basis.

Practitioner

According to NH-PAI 2000, the criteria for health care professionals who use TT in a medical setting are that they should have completed a minimum 12 contact hour, Basic Level workshop taught by a qualified TT practitioner. In addition, they are required to have a 1-year mentorship, during which time they may practice at the discretion and under supervision of their mentors. A further requirement is the completion of a 14 contact hour, Intermediate Level course.

RESEARCH

TT has been the subject of most of the research on energy-based therapies in nursing. Numerous studies have related the effects of TT on stress, wound healing, and relief of symptoms. A recent metaanalysis indicated that most studies support the efficacy of TT, although several studies had mixed or negative results.[36] Another metaanalysis examined physiologic and psychologic variables in nine studies.[26] A medium effect was demonstrated, but not enough information was available to calculate the weighted mean. Further analysis indicated that a stronger probability for effectiveness was present within the physiologic variables than in psychologic distress variables. Individual studies indicated that TT was effective in increasing periods of abstinence in individuals with drug addiction[8a] and altering time perception, decreasing stress, and many other positive indicators.[6a]

There are more than 35 completed studies of HT. Preliminary evidence indicates HT may decrease depression and lost workdays from back injury.[4,23] Other studies have examined the effect of HT in decreasing chronic pain and as an intervention in improving spasticity in children. It has been postulated that because energy enhances normal function, there is no inherent harm that can be done by HT.

Anything that is done to or around us affects us in some way; some effects are just more obvious than others. Subtle effects may be short term or long lasting; long-lasting effects clearly have greater ability to facilitate change over time. Research that has been done with TT and HT is contradictory; improvement is demonstrated in some studies and not in others. This may be because our methods of study are not sophisticated enough to measure the actual changes that are occurring; and it is possible that when the intent is set for a person's highest good, paradoxical results may occur.

Case Study Example

The following was an unsolicited response sent by e-mail to one of the participants in an HT Level I class.

In Sunday's class you worked on my nose. I don't remember all that I had told you about my nose. The septum started dissolving slowly about 25 years ago. It has been raw and bloody inside every day for all those years. Not once has it ever healed over. The doctors have never been able to figure out why and even did a biopsy to check for cancer.

It was negative. I had to have corrective surgery about 12 years ago to build back up the area just up from the top lip because my nose was sagging. Sounds kinda horrible doesn't it!? I just wanted you to know what the past has been like so you can understand what a miracle you did for me. That evening when you worked on my nose it felt red hot deep inside where it is always raw and like something heavy was sitting inside my sinuses. That evening [I could tell] right away the swelling was down because I could breathe a little easier. But the best was yet to

come! A few days later I noticed no blood was dripping out and I blew my nose just to see if there was any blood and just a slight amount was there. Now, today, there isn't any raw bloody tissue anymore anywhere inside my nose! I checked it out with a Q-tip and not one spot of blood showed up. It only took about a week and a half to finally heal after you worked on me. You accomplished something in minutes that no doctor in over 20 years could do. I will be forever grateful to you! Take care of those hands of yours. They are worth more than all the gold in the world.

References

1. *Alternative medicine: expanding medical horizons. A report to the National Institutes of Health on alternative medical systems and practices in the US.* Chantilly, Va, Sept 14-16, 1992, Workshop on Alternative Medicine.
2. Bailey AA: *Esoteric healing,* NY, 1953, Lucis.
3. Braden G: *Awakening to zero point: the collective initiation,* Bellevue, Wash, 1994, LL Productions.
4. Bradway C: The effects of healing touch on depression, *Colorado Center for Healing Touch Newsletter: Research Edition* 8(3):2, 1998.
5. Bruyere R: *Wheels of light,* New York, 1994, Simon & Schuster.
6. Eisenberg DM, Davis RB, Ehner SL et al: Trends in alternative medicine use in the US, 1990-1997, *JAMA* 280(18):1569-1575, 1998.
6a. Engle V, Graney M: Biobehavioral effects of Therapeutic Touch, *J Nurs Schol* 32(30):287-293, 2000.
7. Etheridge CE: *Right rhythmic living,* Sacramento, Calif, 1996, Stovall-Hinkle.
8. Gerber R: *Vibrational medicine: new choices for healing ourselves,* Sante Fe, N Mex, 1996, Bear & Company.
8a. Hagemaster J: Use of Therapeutic Touch in treatment of drug addictions, *Holist Nurs Pract* 14(3):14-20, 2000.
9. Hover-Kramer D, Mentgen J, Scnadrett-Hibdon S: *Healing touch: resource for health care professionals,* Albany, NY, 1996, Delmar Publishers.
10. Joy WB: *Joy's Way,* Los Angeles, 1979, JP Tarcher.
11. Kaptchuk TJ: *The web that has no weaver: understanding Chinese medicine,* New York, 1983, Congdon and Weed.
12. Karagulla S, Kunz D: *The chakras and the human energy fields,* Wheaton, Ill, 1989, Quest Books.
13. Krieger D: *The therapeutic touch. How to use your hands to heal,* Englewood Cliffs, NJ, 1979, Prentice-Hall.
14. Krieger D: *Accepting your power to heal,* Sante Fe, N Mex, 1993, Bear & Company.
15. Krieger D: Letter in my point of view, *Coop Connec* 21(4):1-12, 2000.
16. Kunz D: *The personal aura,* Wheaton, Ill, 1991, Quest Books.

17. McFarland GK, McFarland EA: *Nursing diagnosis and intervention: planning for patient care,* ed 3, St Louis, 1997, Mosby.
18. Mentgen J, Bulbrook MJ: *Healing Touch level I notebook,* Carrboro, NC, 1994, North Carolina Center for Healing Touch.
19. Newman M: *Health as expanding consciousness,* New York, 1994, National League for Nursing.
20. Nightingale F: *Notes on nursing,* New York, 1969, Dover Publications.
21. Nurse Healers-Professional Associates: *Therapeutic touch teaching guidelines: beginners level Krieger/Kunz method,* Allison Park, Pa, 1992, Nurse Healers-Professional Associates, Inc.
22. Oschman JL: *Energy medicine: the scientific basis,* New York, 2000, Churchill Livingstone.
23. Osterlund H, Davids D, Gima A et al: HeToBa study at the Queen's Medical Center, *Healing Touch Newsletter: Research Edition* 8(3):16, 1998.
24. Pavek R: *Manual healing methods: physical and biofield* (Report), Washington DC, 1993, National Institutes of Health, Office of Alternative Medicine.
25. Pearsell P: *The heart's code: tapping the wisdom and power of our heart energy,* New York, 1998, Broadway Books.
26. Peters RM: The effectiveness of therapeutic touch: a meta-analytic review, *NSQ* 12(1):52-61, 1999.
27. Rogers ME: *An introduction to the theoretical basis of nursing,* Philadelphia, 1970, FA Davis.
28. Rogers ME: Nursing: science of unitary, irreducible, human beings: Update 1990. In Barrett EA, editor: *Visions of Rogers' science-based nursing,* New York, 1990, National League for Nursing.
29. Wardell DW: *White shadow: walking with Janet Mentgen,* Lakewood, Colo, 2001, Colorado Center for Healing Touch.
30. Wardell DW, Mentgen J: Healing Touch: an energy-based approach to healing, *Imprint* 46(2):34-35, 51, 1999.
31. Watson J: *Postmodern nursing and beyond,* New York, 1999, Churchill Livingstone.
32. Winstead-Fry P: An integrative review of meta-analysis of therapeutic touch research, *Altern Ther Health Med* 5(6):58-67, 1999.

APPENDIX

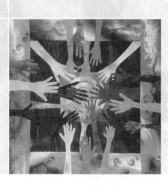

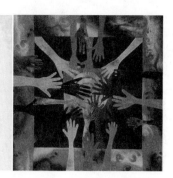

Resources and Contacts (Professional Organizations and Referral Services)

CHAPTER 1: OSTEOPATHIC MEDICINE

Associations

American Osteopathic Association
142 East Ontario Street, Chicago, IL 60611
Phone: (800) 621-1773
Fax: (312) 202-8200
Website: www.aoa-net.org

American Association of Colleges of Osteopathic
    Medicine (AACOM)
5550 Friendship Boulevard, Suite 310
Chevy Chase, MD 20815-7231
Phone: (301) 968-4100
Fax: (301) 968-4101
Website: www.aacom.org

American Academy of Osteopathy
3500 DePaw Boulevard, Suite 1080
Indianapolis, IN 46268
Phone: (317) 879-1881
Fax: (317) 879-0563
Website: www.academyofosteopathy.org

CHAPTER 2: CHIROPRACTIC

Associations

American Chiropractic Association
1701 Clarendon Boulevard
Arlington, VA 22209
Phone: (800) 986-4636
Email: AmerChiro@aol.com
Website: www.amerchiro.org

World Federation of Chiropractic
3080 Yonge Street, Suite 5065
Toronto, Ontario, M4N3N1, Canada
Phone: (416) 484-9978
Email: worldfed@sympatico.ca
Website: www.wfc.org

International Chiropractors Association
1110 North Glebe Road, Suite 1000
Arlington, VA 22201
Phone: (800) 423-4690
Email: chiro@erols.com
Website: www.chiropractic.org

Canadian Chiropractic Association
1396 Eglinton Avenue West
Toronto, Ontario, M6C2E4
Canada
Phone: (416) 781-5656
Website: www.ccachiro.org

Foundation for Chiropractic Education
    and Research
704 East Fourth Street
Des Moines, Iowa 50309
Phone: (515) 282-7118
Email: fcernow@aol.com
Website: www.fcer.org

National Board of Chiropractic Examiners
901 54th Avenue
Greeley, CO 80634
Phone: (970) 356-9100
Email: nbce@nbce.org

Council on Chiropractic Education
8049 N. 85th Way
Scottsdale, AZ 85258
Phone: (602) 443-8877
Email: cce@adata.com

Additional Links

www.chiroweb.com
www.chiro.org

CHAPTER 3: MASSAGE THERAPY: TOUCHABILITIES™

Professional Organizations

There are many professional organizations for massage and bodywork. They provide support, status, education, camaraderie, leadership opportunities, buying power, lobbying power, and networking to practitioners. Two professional organizations that cater to the broadest spectrum of bodyworkers and massage therapists are the American Massage Therapy Association (AMTA), which is focused on but not limited to Western techniques, and the American Organization for Bodywork Therapies of Asia (AOBTA), which is focused on Eastern techniques. Many individual modalities have established organizations that represent their specialized interests. To reference these groups, refer to the listing in every issue of *Massage Magazine*.

American Massage Therapy Association
820 Davis Street, Suite 100
Evanston, IL 60201
Phone: (847) 864-0123
Website: www.amtamassage.org

American Organization for Bodywork Therapies
    of Asia
1010 Haddonfield-Berlin Road, Suite 408
Voorhees, NJ 08043
Phone: (856) 782-1616
Website: www.aobta.org

Publications

The following periodicals feature editorials and articles on research, modalities, and trends in the field. Some may include product and seminar advertising, listings of conventions, articles on business development, practice management, and legislative updates. They discuss the issues facing the profession and present personal stories and experiences. All are available by subscription, and most are available at newsstands and in bookstores.

Massage Magazine
1636 West First Avenue, #100
Spokane, WA 99204
Phone: (800) 872-1282 or (509) 324-8117
Website: www.massagemagazine.com
    Massage Magazine includes a regular listing of the associations for the various modalities, reports the latest guidelines for licensure in the states that regulate massage, and provides a resource directory of schools.

Massage Therapy Journal
820 Davis Street, Suite 100
Evanston, IL 60201
Phone: (847) 864-0123, ext. 113
Website: www.amtamassage.org
    Massage Therapy Journal is the publication of the AMTA and can be subscribed to independent of membership. It features listings of schools that are accredited by the Commission on Massage Training Accreditation (COMTA).

Journal of Bodywork and Movement Therapies
Harcourt Publishers Ltd.
Foots Cray, Sidcup
Kent, England DA145HP
United Kingdom
U.S. toll-free phone number: (877) 839-7126
Website: www.churchill.com/journals.html
    The *Journal of Bodywork and Movement Therapies* is the only academic peer-reviewed publication for the bodywork and movement professions. It has no advertisement other than for its own yearly conference; it features editorials, peer-reviewed articles, technique papers, and strategies for working with practical issues in musculoskeletal function, treatment, and rehabilitation. This is available through subscription only.

Massage and Bodywork
c/o ABMP 1271 Sugarbush Drive
Evergreen, CO 80439
Phone: (800) 458-2267
Website: www.abmp.com

Massage and Bodywork magazine is a publication of the Associated Bodywork and Massage Professionals, a private, for-profit group that offers insurance and networking opportunities for massage therapists.

Books

Ford C: *Where healing waters meet: touching the mind and emotions through the body,* New York, 1992, Talman Company (out of print).
Goldman J: *Healing sounds: the power of harmonics,* London, 1996, Harper Collins.
Hugh M: *Heart of listening: a visionary approach to craniosacral work: anatomy, technique, transcendence,* Berkeley, Calif, 1998, North Atlantic Books.
Knaster M: *Discovering the body's wisdom,* New York, 1986, Bantam Books.
Oschman J: *Energy medicine: the scientific basis,* Kent, England, 2000, Churchill-Livingstone.
Smith FF: *Inner bridges: a guide to energy movement and body structure,* Atlanta, 1986, Humanics Pub Group.

Regulatory Agencies

Commission on Massage Training Accreditation (COMTA)
820 Davis Street, Suite 100
Evanston, IL 60201
Phone: (847) 864-0123
Website: www.amtamassage.org

COMTA is the accrediting agency for schools of massage and bodywork. As a regulating organization, its purpose is to set entry-level standards for massage education and ensure that a school accredited by them meets specific criteria. To become accredited, each school must comply with a stringent set of standards aligned with the guidelines of the U.S. Department of Education. The Commission is composed of nine elected members. They meet twice a year to consider new applicants and oversee and review issues that pertain to currently accredited schools. COMTA status provides assurance for the prospective student that these schools can deliver the training and skills necessary to provide high-quality education.

National Certification Board of Therapeutic Massage and Bodywork (NCBTMB)
8201 Greensboro Drive, Suite 300
McClean, VA 22102
Phone: (800) 296-0664 or (703) 610-9015
Website: www.ncbtmb.com

NCBTMB is the certifying agency for individual therapists. It is the board that sets minimum competency standards for the practice of professional massage therapy. To become certified, a therapist must complete approved educational programs and pass a national exam. NCBTMB certification status supports the therapist because it signifies professionalism and credibility. It also assures the public by identifying those practitioners who have acquired the education and skills necessary to provide high-quality care.

CHAPTER 4: MODERN NEUROMUSCULAR TECHNIQUES

Publications

Chaitow L, *Modern neuromuscular techniques,* ed 2, Edinburgh, 2002, Churchill Livingstone.
Chaitow L, DeLany J: *Clinical application of neuromuscular techniques,* vol 1, the upper body and vol 2, the lower body, Edinburgh, 2000 and 2002, respectively, Churchill Livingstone.

These two, highly illustrated, strongly referenced texts, written by the authors of this chapter to offer step-by-step protocols of neuromuscular techniques as well as foundational anatomy, supporting modalities and information pertinent to the practice of NMT. Although the text does not replace the need for hands-on, supervised training, it does move the training of NMT into a new realm, supported by study guides and computer-interactive programs. In addition, trainees may study the text before taking an NMT class, thereby entering the class with a stronger foundation of understanding, and then review the text after the class to help solidify comprehension.

Journal of Bodywork and Movement Therapies,
Harcourt Health Sciences.
Neuromuscular therapy approaches are often included in articles published in *Journal of Bodywork and Movement Therapies.* This peer-reviewed, highly referenced journal incorporates multiple disciplines of

manual therapies and offers practical, clinically relevant material for integrative health care. Sample journal articles and subscription information are available at the following website:
www.harcourt-international.com/journals/jbmt/

Organizations with NMT Seminar Training

American Version NMT
NMT Center, Judith DeLany, Director
900 14th Avenue North
St. Petersburg, FL 33705
Phone: (727) 821-7167
Email: nmtcenter@aol.com

St. John Method NMT
St. John Seminars, Paul St. John, Director
10710 Seminole Boulevard, Suite 1
Largo, FL 33778
Phone: (727) 397-5525
Email: info@stjohnnmtseminars.com

Schools with American Version NMT Curriculum Training

Colorado Institute of Massage Therapy, Roger
    Patrizio, Director
2601 East St. Vrain
Colorado Springs, CO 80909
Phone: (719) 634-7347
Email: coimt@excelonline.com

Rising Spirit Institute of Natural Health (formerly
    New Life Institute)
Drs. Bruce & Martha Costello, Directors
4330 Georgetown Square II, #500
Atlanta, GA 30338
Phone: (770) 457-2021
Email: drbruce@mindspring.com

Tennessee Institute of Healing Arts, Alan Jordan,
    Executive Director
7010 Lee Highway, Suite 712
Chattanooga, TN 37421
Phone: (423) 892-9882
Email: TIHA@aol.com

Schools with European Version NMT Curriculum Training

School of Integrative Health, University
    of Westminster
115 New Cavendish Street
London, W1M8JS, United Kingdom
Phone: 44-7911-5000, ext. 3699
NCBTMB Phone: (703) 610-9015

CHAPTER 5: CULTIVATING THE VERTICAL: THE ROLF METHOD OF STRUCTURAL INTEGRATION

The Rolf Institute
205 Canyon Boulevard
Boulder, CO 80302
Phone: (800) 530-8875
Colorado residents: (303) 449-5903
Fax: (303) 449-5978
Website: www.rolf.org

CHAPTER 6: APPLIED KINESIOLOGY

Associations

International College of Applied Kinesiology (ICAK)
    The website offers papers written by ICAK members (updated monthly), information on seminars, professional links, and news.
International College of Applied Kinesiology Executive Offices
Phone: (913) 384-5336
Email: icak@usa.net
Website: www.icak.com

International College of Applied Kinesiology—USA
    Chapter
    The website includes information for professionals, in-depth information about Applied Kinesiology, research papers, the ICAK status statement, AK classes (for professionals who are licensed to diagnose), and links to other sites, as well as general information about AK and a listing of AK doctors.

The ICAK-USA Central Office
6405 Metcalf Avenue, Suite 503
Shawnee Mission, KS 66202-3929
Phone: (913) 384-5336
Website: www.icakusa.com

Additional Links

Applied Kinesiology Seminars
   This site provides Applied Kinesiology training courses, books, articles, charts, information, and links (in English and German). Free membership is offered to those who translate AK articles from German into English.
   Website: www.akse.de

Kinesiology Net
   This site provides a listing of 17 Internet domain names dedicated to specific methods of Kinesiology and the official websites of specific methods.
   Website: www.kinesiology.net

Books

Barrett S: Applied Kinesiology: muscle-testing for "allergies" and "nutrient deficiencies," *Quackwatch* May, 1998. Available online: www.quackwatch.com.
Burton Goldberg Group, editors: *Alternative medicine: the definitive guide,* Puyallup, Wash, 1994, Future Medicine Publishing.
Zwicky JF: *Reader's guide to alternative health methods,* Chicago, 1993, American Medical Association.

CHAPTER 7: THE TRAGER® APPROACH

Association

Trager International
3800 Park East Drive
Suite 100, Room 1
Beachwood, OH 44122
Phone: (216) 896-9383
Email in the United States: trager@trager.com
International Email: admin@trager.com
Website: www.trager.com

For additional information about The Trager Approach:
1. *Trager Mentastics: Movement as a Way to Agelessness*
   Milton Trager, MD, with Cathy Guadagno, 1987
   Station Hill Press, Barrytown, NY 12507
2. *Movement as a Way to Agelessness: A Guide to Trager Mentastics*
   Milton Trager, MD, and Cathy Hammond, 1995
   Station Hill Press, Barrrytown, NY 12507
3. *Moving Medicine, the Life and Work of Milton Trager, MD*
   Jack Liskin, 1996
   Statin Hill Press, Barrytown, NY 12507

CHAPTER 8: FELDENKRAIS METHOD

Associations

Feldenkrais Guild of North America
   The Feldenkrais Guild was established in 1977 by Moshe Feldenkrais, DSc, to be the professional organization of practitioners and teachers of the Feldenkrais Method. In 1997 the name was changed to Feldenkrais Guild of North America (FGNA). FGNA is a nonprofit, tax exempt, professional organization concerned with increasing public awareness of the Feldenkrais Method of Somatic Education, the certification and continuing education of practitioners, the protection of the quality of the Feldenkrais work, and research in the Method's effectiveness. Only people personally trained by Dr. Feldenkrais or graduates of Guild-Accredited Training Programs are eligible to be certified, to become members of FGNA, and to use its service-marked terms (see p. 119). There are additional national Feldenkrais guilds in at least 14 other countries.
   The FGNA website includes a worldwide directory of certified Feldenkrais practitioners; explanations of the Feldenkrais Method; the Feldenkrais Standards of Practice; sample lessons of *Awareness Through Movement;* an extensive bibliography of books, chapters, and articles by and about Moshe Feldenkrais and the Feldenkrais Method; a list of current Feldenkrais Professional Training Programs; and a reference list of all research articles to date.

Feldenkrais Guild of North America
3611 SW Hood Avenue, Suite 100
Portland, OR 97201
Phone: (503) 221-6612
Fax: (503) 221-6616
Email: guild@feldenkrais.com
Website: www.feldenkrais-method.org
International Feldenkrais Federation

The International Feldenkrais Federation (IFF) was founded and incorporated in Paris in 1992 and is the coordinating organization of most Feldenkrais professional organizations worldwide. An enormous archive of previously unpublished original materials from the life and work of Moshe Feldenkrais has been cataloged and maintained through the IFF. This includes the hundreds of *Awareness Through Movement* lessons taught and tape recorded by Feldenkrais during the years he taught his public classes on Alexander Yanai Street in Tel Aviv, Israel. This voluminous resource is being painstakingly translated from the original Hebrew and transcribed to expand the learning of Feldenkrais practitioners worldwide. The website includes a biography of Feldenkrais, extensive explanations of the method, the standards of practice, and links to the general and research bibliographies.
International Feldenkrais Federation
30, rue Monsieur le Prince
75006 Paris, France
Phone/Fax: 33.1.43.74.15.19
Email: iff@peak.org
Website: www.feldenkrais-method.org

Publications

Many of the books listed in the bibliography are available through FGNA and a private company called Feldenkrais Resources, which is owned and operated by two Feldenkrais trainers.
Feldenkrais Resources
830 Bancroft Way, Suite 112
Berkeley, CA 94710
Phone: (800) 765-1907 or (510) 540-7600
Fax: (510) 540-7683
Email: feldenres@aol.com

The Feldenkrais Method is also recommended in the books of Andrew Weil, MD, and his website is linked to the website of the FGNA.
Website: www.drweil.com

CHAPTER 9: SHIATSU

Kerry Palanjian, MBA, CMT
Nationally Certified Massage Therapist
Shiatsu Therapy & Owner, Shiatsu On-Site
Corporate and Private Practice
More than just Massage-in-a-chair
Greater Philadelphia
300 Horsham, E-8
Phone: 215-674-3086
Fax: 215-674-3138
Email: sosbykp@aol.com

Associations

American Organization for Bodywork Therapies of Asia (AOBTA)
1010 Haddonfield-Berlin Road, Suite 408
Voorhees, NJ 08043
Phone: (856) 782-1616
Fax: (856) 782-1653
Email: aobta@prodigy.net
Website: www.aobta.org

The American Organization for Bodywork Therapies of Asia is a national not-for-profit professional association of practitioners of Bodywork Therapies of Asia. All forms that are recognized by AOBTA originally had their roots in China. Over the centuries China, Japan, Thailand, Korea, and more recently, North America and Europe have changed and evolved these forms into separate and distinct modalities. The AOBTA recognizes 12 forms of Asian Bodywork Therapy. The AOBTA was formed in 1989 with the coming together of a number of associations, which represented individual disciplines of Asian Bodywork Therapy. AOBTA currently has 1400 active members in the United States and abroad.

Associated Bodywork & Massage Professionals (ABMP)
1271 Sugarbush Drive
Evergreen, CO 80439
Phone: (800) 458-2267 or (303) 674-8478
Fax: (303) 674-0859 or (800) 667-8260
Email: expectmore@abmp.com
Website: www.abmp.com

Associated Bodywork and Massage Professionals (ABMP) is a membership organization serving the massage, bodywork, somatic, and esthetic professions. ABMP competes effectively for members by providing the best value and most responsive, knowledgeable service. Our business philosophy is summed up by our credo: "Expect more."

The American Massage Therapy Association (AMTA)
820 Davis Street, Suite 100
Evanston, IL 60201-4444
Phone: (888) 843-2682 or (847) 864-0123
Fax: (847) 864-1178
Website: www.amtamassage.org/about/about.htm

British Columbia Acupressure Therapists'
    Association
Email: bcata@islandnet.com
Website: www.islandnet.com/~bcata/

Commission on Massage Therapy Accreditation
820 Davis Street, Suite 100
Evanston, IL 60201-4444
Phone: (847) 869-5039
Email: cellisamtamassage.org
Website: www.info@comta.org

European-Shiatsu-Association (ESI)
German Shiatsu Association
Email: GSDshiatsu@aol.com
Website: www.shiatsu-gsd.de/

The International Macrobiotic Shiatsu Society

The International Macrobiotic Shiatsu Society (IMSS) is a forum for friends interested in the healing arts of macrobiotics and Shiatsu. This dynamic combination is based on the teaching of Shizuko Yamamoto. Macrobiotics is a natural approach to living that includes a whole foods diet. Shiatsu is a touch technique based on traditional Asian medicine. Shiatsu literally means finger pressure. It is similar to acupuncture but without needles. In the United States it is sometimes called acupressure. The Yamamoto macrobiotic style is also known as Barefoot Shiatsu. IMSS is a membership organization. All are welcome to join.

Founded in 1986, after almost five decades of experience by Shiatsu Master Shizuko Yamamoto, the IMSS promotes a natural approach to living. Macrobiotic Shiatsu uniquely combines the power of natural foods in the macrobiotic diet with the traditional Asian healing techniques of Shiatsu. As all things be-

long to nature, it is natural to be healthy and happy. When imbalances arise, simple techniques can help to correct them. In a practical manner, macrobiotic Shiatsu unifies body, mind, and spirit.
International Macrobiotic Shiatsu Society (IMSS)
2807 Wright Avenue
Winter Park, FL 32789
Email: mbshiatsu@aol.com
Website: www.imss.macrobiotic.net

AOBTA-Approved Schools

Arizona

Desert Institute of the Healing Arts
Margaret Avery-Moon, Director
639 North Sixth Avenue
Tucson, AZ 85705
Phone: (520) 882-0899
Fax: (520) 624-2996
Email: info@diha.org
Website: www.desertinstitute.org

California

Acupressure Institute of America
Michael Reed Gach, Founder
1533 Shattuck Avenue
Berkeley, CA 94709
Phone: (510) 845-1059
Fax: (510) 845-1496
Website: www.acupressure.com
Email: info@acupressure.com

Heartwood Institute
Chela Burger, Director
220 Harmony Lane
Garberville, CA 95542
Phone: (707) 923-5000
Fax: (707) 923-5010
Website: www.heartwoodinstitute.com
Email: hello@heartwoodinstitute.com

International Professional School of Bodywork
    (IPSB)
Barbara Clark, Director
1366 Hornblend Street
San Diego, CA 92109
Phone: (800) 748-6497
Fax: (619) 272-4772
Email: beingipsb@aol.com

Mueller College of Holistic Studies
Penny Youngberg, Director of Administration
4607 Park Boulevard
San Diego, CA 92116
Phone: (619) 291-9811 or (800) 245-1976
Fax: (619) 543-1113
Email: info@MuellerCollege.com
Website: www.MuellerCollege.com

Pacific College of Oriental Medicine
Jack Miller, President
7445 Mission Valley Road, Suite 105
San Diego, CA 92108
Phone: (619) 574-6909
Fax: (619) 574-6641
Website: www.ormed.edu

Jin Shin Do Foundation for Bodymind Acupressure
Iona Marsaa Teeguarden, MA, Director
P.O. Box 416
Idyllwild, CA 92549
Phone: (831) 763-7702
Fax: (909) 659-5707
Website: www.jinshindo.org

Louisiana

Blue Cliff School of Therapeutic Massage
Richard Denney, Director
3501 Severn Avenue, Suite 20
Metairie, LA 70002
Phone: (504) 456-3140
Fax: (504) 466-8514
Vernon Smith: smithyne@aol.com
Richard Denney: massage@ametro.net

Massachusetts

Acupressure Therapy Institute
Barbara Blanchard, Director and President
355 Turnpike Street
Canton, MA 02021
Phone: (617) 497-1477

Boston Shiatsu School
Kiku Zutrau Miyazaki, Director
1972 Massachusetts Avenue
Cambridge, MA 02140
Phone: (617) 876-4048
Fax: (617) 497-4892
Website: www.bostonshiatsu.org
Email: eastwestinst@mindspring.com

Minnesota

Center Point
Cari Johnson Pelava, Founder
1313 5th Street SE, #336
Minneapolis, MN 55414
Phone: (612) 617-9090
Fax: (612) 617-9292
Email: nlsmt@pro-ns.net

New Jersey

Associates for Creative Wellness School of Asian
    Healing Arts
Ruth Dalphin, Director
Suite G-38
1930 East Marlton Park
Cherry Hill, NJ 08034
Phone: (856) 985-8320
Email: acwsaha@bellatlantic.net

New York

Swedish Institute School of Massage Therapy &
    Acupuncture, Inc.
Paula J. Eckardt, Director
226 West 26th Street, 5th Floor
New York, NY 10001
Phone: (212) 924-5900
Fax: (212) 924-7600
Email: Admission@swedishinstitute.com

The New York College for Wholistic Health,
    Education, and Research
Steven Schenkman, President
6801 Jericho Turnpike, Suite 300
Syosset, NY 11791
Phone: (516) 364-0808
Fax: (516) 364-0989
Email: info@nycollege.edu

Pennsylvania

International School of Shiatsu
Saul Goodman, Director
10 South Clinton Street, Suite 300
Doylestown, PA 18901
Phone: (215) 340-9918
Fax: (215) 340-9181
Email: info@shiatsubo.com

Meridian Institute
Carolee Parker, Director
998 Old Eagle School Road, Suite 1212
Wayne, PA 19087
Phone: (610) 293-4030
Fax: (610) 971-9860

Texas
Academy of Oriental Medicine
Stuart Watts, President
Pamela Ferguson, Dean of Asian Bodywork
2700 West Anderson Lane, Suite 204
Austin, TX 78757
Phone: (512) 454-1188
Fax: (512) 454-7001
Email: acuaoma@aol.com

Additional Educational Institutions and Links

Acupuncture/Acupressure Internet Resources
Website:
  www.holisticmed.com/www/acupuncture.html

American Association of Asian Medicine
Website: www.aaom.org/

Living Earth School of Natural Therapies
401 Richmond Street West, Studio 1
Toronto, Ontario M5V 3A8, Canada
Phone: (415) 691-0400
Fax: (905) 303-8724
Website: www.livingearthschool.com

The Ohashi Institute (Ohashiatsu)
  The Ohashi Institute is a nationally respected and internationally recognized nonprofit educational organization dedicated to the promotion and understanding of the Asian healing arts. Their stated mission is to serve the planet by bringing excellence to the art of healing and serenity to the art of living. Their motto is "Touch for peace."
147 West 25th Street, 8th Floor
New York, NY 10001
Phone: (800) 810-4190 or (646) 486-1187
Fax: (646) 486-1409
Website: www.ohashi.com/
Email: ohashiinst@aol.com

Natural Healers.com
  This is an excellent link for detailed information on finding a school.
Website: www.naturalhealers.com/find.shtml

School of Shiatsu and Massage at Harbin Hot Springs
P.O. Box 570
21208 Calistoga Street, Suite A
Middletown, CA 95461
Phone: (800) 693-3296
Fax: (707) 987-9638
Website: www.schoolofshiatsuandmassage.com

The British School of Shiatsu Do
3 Farnham Park Drive
Upper Hale, Farnham, Surrey
GU9 0HS, England
United Kingdom
Phone: +44 (0) 1252 724059
Email: registrar@farnham.shiatsu-do.co.uk
Website: www.shiatsu-do.co.uk
David M Winter, Principal (Farnham)
Phone/Fax: 01252-724059

Worldwide Aquatic Bodywork Association (Watsu)
Website: www.waba.edu

Jin Shin Do Foundation for Bodymind Acupressure
P.O. Box 416
Idyllwild, CA 92549
Fax: (909) 659-5707
Website: www.jinshindo.org

Touch Research Institutes (TRI), University of Miami School of Medicine

Considered the pioneer of and premium research institute for massage therapy, the first Touch Research Institute was formally established in 1992 by Director Tiffany Field, PhD, at the University of Miami School of Medicine via a start-up grant from Johnson & Johnson. The TRI was the first center in the world devoted solely to the study of touch and its application in science and medicine. The TRI's distinguished team of researchers, representing Duke, Harvard, Maryland, and other universities, has successfully improved the definition of touch as it promotes health and contributes to the treatment of disease. Research efforts that began in 1982 and continue today have shown that touch therapy has numerous beneficial effects on health and well-being. A second TRI is located in the Philippines. A group of neonatologists there have replicated earlier studies showing that preterm infants' weight gain can be facilitated by massage therapy. A third TRI is located at the University of Paris and studies the role of touch in perception, learning, and psychopathology. A fourth TRI is located at the UCLA Medical School Pediatric Pain Center and is focused on the use of touch therapies with children's pain syndromes.

P.O. Box 016820
Miami, FL 33101
Phone: (305) 243-6781
Fax: (305) 243-6488
Email: tfield@med.miami.edu
Website: www.miami.edu/touch-research/

National Certification Board for Therapeutic
    Massage and Bodywork (NCBTMB)
8201 Greensboro Drive, Suite 300
McLean, VA 22102
Phone: (800) 296-0664 or (703) 610-9015
Fax: (703) 610-9005
Email: info@ncbtmb.com
Website: www.ncbtmb.com

Massage Magazine
    Massage Magazine covers the massage trade with articles on technique, research, and laws; profiles; and industry news. In publication since 1985, it is circulated internationally, bimonthly.
Massage Magazine
1636 West First Avenue
Spokane, WA 99204
Phone: (800) 872-1282 or (509) 324-8117
Website: www.massagemagazine.com

The Shiatsu Society (UK)—United Kingdom

The Shiatsu Society is a nonprofit umbrella organization for all types and styles of Shiatsu.

The society sets standards in training that are implemented by registered teachers through its assessment subcommittee. The society maintains a register of qualified practitioners who have passed the society's assessment. The society was set up in 1981 to facilitate communication within the field of Shiatsu and to inform the public of the benefits of this form of natural healing. Since that time, the society has grown to form a network linking interested individuals, students, and teachers and to fulfill the role of Professional Association for Shiatsu Practitioners.

The Shiatsu Society
Eastlands Court, St. Peters Road
Rugby CV21 3QP
United Kingdom
Tel: 01788 555051
Fax: 01788 555052
Email: admin@shiatsu.org
Website: www.shiatsu.org

Shiatsu Therapy Association of Ontario (STAO)

The STAO is a nonprofit organization that represents professionally trained Certified Shiatsu Therapists (CSTs) in Ontario, throughout Canada, and internationally. The association is a self-regulatory body mandated to protect the interests of the public by setting the highest standards of training and practice in North America.

Email: info@shiatsuassociation.com
Phone (Toronto, Canada): (416) 923-7826 (STAO)
Toll-free Phone (Canada & U.S.): (877) 923-7826
    (STAO)

Other Links

www.psychotherapiepraxis.at/shiatsu1.htm—Great site for numerous links to Shiatsu and related information

www.abmp.com/home.html—Associated Bodywork Massage Professionals referral source for practitioners

gehon.ir.miami.edu/touch-research/index.html— Touch Research Institute home page

www.shiatsu.8m.com/workshops.htm—Shiatsu information pages, numerous links

www.rianvisser.nl/shiatsu/e_index.htm—Shiatsu links, The Netherlands

www.kushiinstitute.com—Kushi Institute Macrobiotic educational link www.copernic.com/index.html—Excellent free search engine for Shiatsu links; first download it, and then enter *Shiatsu* or *Shiatsu Research;* it searches multiple search engines and provides all links

findwhat.com—Good search engine; simply enter *Shiatsu*

Additional Reading

Kushi M, et al: *Basic Shiatsu,* Becket, Mass, 1995, One Peaceful World Press.

Liechti E: *The complete illustrated guide to Shiatsu: the Japanese healing art of touch for health and fitness,* Bement, Ill, 1998, Bement Books.

Namikoshi T: *The complete book of Shiatsu therapy,* Tokyo, Japan, 1994, Japan Publications.

Namikoshi T: *Shiatsu: Japanese finger-pressure therapy,* Tokyo, Japan, 1995, Japan Publications.

Ohashi W, Deangelis P: *The Ohashi bodywork book: beyond Shiatsu with the Ohashiatsu method,* Tokyo, Japan, 1997, Kodansha International.

Sergel D: *The natural way of Zen,* Tokyo, Japan, 1999, Japan Publications.

Yamamoto S, McCarty P: *The Shiatsu handbook: a guide to the traditional art of Shiatsu acupressure,* New York, 1996, Putnam.

Yamamoto S, et al: *Barefoot Shiatsu,* New York, 1998, Putnam.

Massage Magazine, see Contacts section.

Touchpoints—Newsletter published quarterly by Touch Research Institute, see Contacts section.

Additional Book Sources

Website:
    www.omega23.com/books/med/shiatsu.html

CHAPTER 10: AYURVEDIC BODYWORK

Resources

The American Institute of Vedic
    Studies
P.O. Box 8357
Santa Fe, NM 87504-8357
Phone: (505) 983-9385
Fax: (505) 982-5807
Website: www.vedanet.com

The Ayurveda Holistic Center
82A Bayville Avenue
Bayville, NY 11709
Phone: (800) 452-1798
Website: ayurvedahc.com

The Ayurvedic Institute
11311 Menaul Boulevard NE
Albuquerque, NM 87112
Phone: (505) 291-9698
Fax: (505) 294-7572
Email: info@ayurveda.com
Website: www.ayurveda.com

The California College of Ayurveda
1117-A East Main Street
Grass Valley, CA 95945
Phone: (530) 274-9100
Website: www.ayurvedacollege.com

The College of Maharishi Vedic Medicine
Maharishi University of Management
Fairfield, IA 52557
Phone: (641) 472-4600
Website: www.mum.edu/CMVM/index.html

The National Institute of Ayurvedic Medicine
584 Milltown Road
Brewster, NY 10509
Phone: (845) 278-8700
Website: http://niam.com

The New England Institute of Ayurvedic Medicine
1815 Massachusetts Avenue
Cambridge, MA 02140
Phone: (508) 755-3744
Email: ayurveda@hotmail.com

CHAPTER 11: QI GONG AND TUI NA

Publication

Cassidy CM: *Contemporary Chinese medicine and acupuncture,* Philadelphia, 2002, Elsevier Science.

Links

CHI-LEL™ Qi Gong

This site provides access to workshops and retreats, books and tapes, the certification program, and a directory of teachers.
Website: www.chilel-qigong.com

National Qigong (Chi Kung) Association—USA

The National Qigong Association (NQA) is the umbrella organization that embraces and supports equally all schools, traditions, teaching styles, and philosophies of Qigong and Tai Chi.
Website: www.nqa.org

Natural Health Web

This site provides links to additional websites and articles online.
Website:
    www.naturalhealthweb.com/topics/subtopics/
    qi_gong.html

Talamasca

This site provides a list of recommended books and additional Qi Gong–related websites.
Website: www.talamasca.org/avatar/qigong.html

QI: The Journal of Traditional Health and Fitness

This magazine and website target consumer-level Qi Gong enthusiasts. The website includes an extensive list of Qi Gong teachers and practitioners.
Website: qi-journal.com

American College of Acupuncture & Oriental Medicine

The college offers a master's of science program in acupuncture and herbal medicine.
Website: www.acaom.edu

Qigong Association of America

This site provides access to books, CDs, message boards, and teachers.
Website: www.qi.org

Qigong Institute

This site contains a directory of teachers, lectures and workshops, databases, videos, books, and scientific papers.
Website: www.qigonginstitute.org

The Taoist Sanctuary of San Diego

The sanctuary is a nonprofit organization involved in the teaching of Taijiquan, Qi Gong and Taoist meditation, Taoist philosophy, and traditional Chinese healing methods. The school was founded in 1975.
Website: www.taoistsanctuary.org

Qi Medicine

This fledgling site features a few good images and some history regarding Qi Gong in its variety of forms and applications.
www.qi-medicine.co.uk

Other Links

www.allmasters.com
www.acupuncture.com
www.wujiproductions.com

CHAPTER 12: REIKI: THE USUI SYSTEM OF NATURAL HEALING

Reiki Organizations and Websites

The Reiki Alliance
P.O. Box 41
Cataldo, ID 83810
Phone: (208) 783-3535
Website: www.reikialliance.com
Email: internationaloffice@reikialliance.org

Reiki Alliance—Europe
Honthorstraat 40 111 1071 DG
Amsterdam, The Netherlands
Phone: 31-20-6719276
Fax: 31-20-6711736
Phyllis Lei Furumoto, Grand Master
Email: phyllis@furumoto.org

American Reiki Master Association
Omega Dawn Sanctuary of the Healing Arts
P.O. Box 130
Lake City, FL 32056-0130
Phone/Fax: (904) 755-9638
Email: arma@atlantic.net
Website: www.atlantic.net/~arma/
Dr. Arthur L. Robertson, Reiki Master

The Reiki Do Institute
Windpferd Verlag
Friesenrieder Straße 45
Aitrang 97648, Germany

Reiki Outreach International
P.O. Box 191156
San Diego, CA 92159-1156
Website: www.annieo.com/reikioutreach/
Mary A. McFadyen, Founder

The Reiki Touch
P.O. Box 571785
Houston, TX 77057
Judy-Carol Stewart, Reiki Master

The International Center for Reiki
    Training
21421 Hilltop Street, #28
Southfield, MI 48034-1023
Phone: (248) 948-8112 or (800) 332-8112
Fax: (248) 948-9534
Email: center@reiki.org
Website: www.reiki.org
William Rand, Reiki Master

Sacred Earth Center
6255 East Avon Lima Road
Avon, NY 14414
Phone: (716) 226-8233
Email: wddancer@yahoo.com
Website: members.tripod.com/~jwinddancer
S. Jeanne Gunn, Reiki Master

Reiki Plus® Institute
707 Barcelona Road
Key Largo, FL 33037
Phone: (305) 451-9881
Email: reikiplus@mindspring.com
Website: www.reikiplus.com
David Jarrell, Reiki Master

The Reiki Healing Connection
633 Isaac Frye Highway
Wilton, NH 03086
Phone: (603) 654-2787 or (888) REIKI-4-U
Fax: (603) 654-2771
Email: reiki@reikienergy.com
Website: www.reikienergy.com/
Libby Barnett, Reiki Master
Maggie Chambers, Reiki Master

The Healing Source
P.O. Box 31907
Phoenix, AZ 85046
Phone: (602) 265-9096
S.S. Sangeet Khalsa, Reiki Master

The Reiki Training Centre of Canada
P.O. Box 3294
Sherwood Park, Alberta
Canada, T8A 2A6
Phone: (780) 448-0817
Fax: (780) 922-1147
Email: anny@success-and-more.com
Anny Slegten, Reiki Master

Centre for the Traditional Healing Methods
10000 Zagreb
Veslaeka 27, Croatia
Phone/Fax: +3851/324-325

Reiki Kyokai Usui Shiki Ryoho
Secretary
218 Osborne Road
Jesmond, Newcastle upon Tyne
NE2 3LB, United Kingdom
Phone/Fax: +44 (0) 191 281 7442
Email: 106622.1776@compuserve.com
Website: ourworld.compuserve.com/homepages/

Healing Touch
UK Ottawa Area Reiki Centre
3428 Woodroffe Avenue
Nepean, Ontario, K3J4G5 Canada
Phone: (613) 823-7113

The Reiki Foundation™
P.O. Box 362
Brewster, NY 10509-0362
Phone: (845) 278-3038
Fax: (845) 279-5260
Email: asunam@msn.com
Websites: www.asunam.com/
www.asunam.com/reiki_foundation.htm

International Association of Reiki
Lesni 14, 46001 Liberec 1
Czech Republic
Phone/Fax: (420) 48 424-629
Email: reiki@pvtnet.cz
Website: www.wisechoices.holowww.com/
Mari Hall, Reiki Master

The Awareness Institute
110 Smith Street, Suite A
Mount Shasta, CA 96067-2636
Phone: (530) 926-0260
Fax: (530) 926-0981
Email: awarinst@gate.net
Website: www.awarinst.com
Dr. Charles A. Thomas, Reiki Master

Reiki Center for Healing Arts
1764 Hamlet Street
San Mateo, CA 94403
Phone: (413) 345-7666
Rev. Fran Brown, Reiki Master

Reiki Healing Institute
449 Sante Fe Drive, #303
Encinitas, CA 92024
Phone: (619) 436-6875
Marsha Burack, Reiki Master

Traditional Japanese Reiki Association
c/o Aurora Holistic Centre
4556 - 99 Street
Edmonton, Alberta, T6E 5H5, Canada
Phone: (403) 437-5481
Email: tjreiki@connect.ab.ca
Website: www.reikilinks.com/home/tjreiki/
Dave King or Adrienne Bouchard

The International Reiki Healing Association
2261 Market Street, Suite 238
San Francisco, CA 94114
Phone: (415) 771-4991
Cheryl Coleman and Claudia McGregor, Reiki
    Masters

Northwest Reiki Institute
P.O. Box 342
Langley, WA 98260
Phone: (360) 221-6143
Fax: (360) 221-6961
Gordon Rosenberg, Reiki Master

Institute for the Study and Propagation of Men
    Chhos Rei Kei
38548 Redwood Highway (199), 8A
O'Brien, OR 97534
Lama Yeshe Drugpa Thrinley Odzer, Founder

The RN Reiki Connection
1248 Hunt Club Lane
Media, PA 19063
Phone: (610) 566-5669
Email: bhceres@optononline.net
Website: members.aol.com/KarunaRN
Marion Yaglinski, RN, Reiki Master

Reiki New Zealand Inc.
P.O. Box 60-226
Titirangi, Auckland, New Zealand
Email: info@reiki.org.nz

Reiki Healer's Association
5462 Noyestar Road
East Hardwick, VT 05836-9826
Phone: (802) 533-2527
Email: pemadolk@plainfield.bypass.com
Website: www.inc.com/users/ReikiHealers.html
Mari Cordes, Reiki Master

European Reiki Association (ERA)
Viale S. Antonio, 59
21100 Varese VA, Italy
Phone: (IT) 0332-966064
Fax: (IT) 0347-4180414
Email: erava@innocent.com and caocis@tin.it
Prof. Dr. Stefano Maria Rattazzi, Founder
Dr. Giacomo Motta, Manager

International Association of Reiki Professionals
P.O. Box 104
Harrisville, NH 03450
Phone: (603) 827-3290
Fax: (603) 827-3737
Email: info@iarp.org
Website: www.iarp.org/

Atlantic Usui Reiki Association
RR #2 Stewiacke
Nova Scotia, Canada B0N 2J0
Email: jsettle@atcon.com

CHAPTER 13: HEALING TOUCH AND THERAPEUTIC TOUCH

Contacts

American Holistic Nurses Association
P.O. Box 2130
Flagstaff, AZ 86003-3120
Phone: (800) 278-AHNA
Email: AHNA-Flag@flaglink.com
Website: www.ahna.org

Colorado Center for Healing Touch, Inc.
12477 West Cedar Drive, Suite 206
Lakewood, CO 80228
Phone: (303) 989-0581
Email: ccheal@aol.com

The Canadian Therapeutic Touch Network
P.O. Box 85551
1048 Eglinton Avenue West
Toronto, Ontario M6C 2C5, Canada
Website: www.therapeutictouchnetwork.com

Healing Touch International, Inc.
12477 West Cedar Drive, Suite 202
Lakewood, CO. 80228
Phone: (303) 989-7982
Email: HTIheal@aol.com
Website: www.healingtouch.net

Nurse Healers-Professional Associates, Inc.
3760 South Highland Drive, Suite #429
Salt Lake City, Utah 84106
Phone: (801) 273-3399
Website: www.therapeutic-touch.org

INDEX

Page numbers followed by f indicate figures; t, tables; b, boxes.

A
Abhighat sahatwa, 160
Act-ure, 126
Acupressure
  Ayurveda, 161
  shiatsu, 151-152
Acupuncture points, 144
Acupuncture *versus* shiatsu, 144-145, 145t
Agni, 158
AK. *See* Applied kinesiology (AK).
Apa-Tarpana therapeutics, 158
Applied kinesiology (AK), 100-101
  acupuncture meridian system, 106
  cerebrospinal fluid, 106
  chemical health, 104
  International College of Applied Kinesiology, 108
  logo, 102, 102f
  manual muscle tests, 101-102, 101f
    interpretation of, 107-108
  mental/spiritual health, 104-105
  muscle-organ/gland association, 106
  nervous system, 105
  neurolymphatic reflexes, 105-106
  neurovascular reflexes, 106
  research, 108-109
  structural health, 103-104
    evaluation of, 102-103
  therapy localization, 107
  training, 109
  treatment factors, 105
    acupuncture meridian system, 106
    cerebrospinal fluid, 106
    nerve, 105
    neurolymphatic reflexes, 105-106
    neurovascular reflexes, 106

Applied kinesiology (AK)—cont'd
  triad of health, 102, 103
    chemical factors, 104
    interplay within, 104f, 105
    mental/spiritual factors, 104-105
    structural factors, 103-104
Arica Vortex system, 161
Artha, 157
Asanas, 157, 159
ATM. *See* Awareness Through Movement (ATM).
Atreya sampradaya, 158
Attachment trigger points (ATrPs), 81-82
Auras, 188
Awareness Through Movement (ATM), 127
  lesson excerpts, 127-131
  practice strategies, 131-132, 133f, 135f
Ayu kar, 160
Ayurveda, 155-156
  Arica Vortex system, 161
  bodywork, 158-159
    marma therapy, 160-161
    soft-tissue techniques, 161-163
    Thai, 162-163
    Tibetan, 162
    western adaptations, 161-162
  cranial work, 161
  diagnosis, 156-157
  esoteric healing, 161-162
  joint articulation and spinal thrust, 161
  marma points, 158, 159f, 161
  marma therapy, 160-161
  philosophy and principles, 156
  polarity therapy, 161
  shamana therapeutics, 158
  shodhana therapeutics, 158
  soft-tissue techniques, 159-160
  Thai bodywork, 162-163
  Tibetan bodywork, 162
  training and certification, 163-164

Ayurveda—cont'd
    treatment, 157-153
    western adaptations, 161-162
Azadirachta indica, 161

B
Bali, 158
Barnes, John, 8
Barral, Jean-Pierre, 16
Bindegewebsmassage, 76
Bone-out-of-place theory, 32
Bo-shin, 147
Branhana, 158
British osteopathic practitioners, 20
Bun-shin, 147
Butterfly effect, 13

C
Cassidy, J.R., 36
CCCR (Consortial Center for Chiropractic Research), 27
Central trigger points (CTrPs), 80-81
Chakras, 144, 158, 187-188
Chapman's reflexes, 106
Chila, Anthony, 15
Chinese massage, 163, 169
Chinese traditional medicine, 165-167
    history of, 167-168
    qi, 168-169, 168f, 168t,
        cultivation, 169-170
    Qi Gong, 168, 169-171
Chiropractic, 26-27
    bone-out-of-place theory, 32
    clinical settings, 36
    contention and controversy, 28-30
    core principles, 31
    diagnostic logic, 36-37
    future health care systems, in, 46-47
    high-velocity, low-amplitude thrust adjustment, 34, 36
    infantile colic research, 43-44
    intellectual foundations, 30
    interprofessional cooperation, 30
    low back cases with leg pain, 42
    low back pain manual adjustment, 40-42
    manual therapies used by, 34, 36. *See also* Spinal manual
        therapy (SMT).
    modernist approach, 31
    motion theory, 32-33
    musculoskeletal disorders research, 39, 43
        early research, 39
        headaches, 42-43
        low back pain manual adjustment, 40-42
        low back pain with leg pain, 40-42
        University of Colorado project, 39
    natural healing precepts, 30-31

Chiropractic—cont'd
    "one cause-one cure" philosophy, 27-28
    osteopathy, as offshoot of, 8
    pain, approach to, 37, 38
    referrals to allopathic physicians, 38
    research, 38-46
    segmental dysfunction, 32-33, 34, 35f
    segmental facilitation, 34
    traditionalist approach, 31
    visceral disorders research, 39, 44
        infantile colic, 43-44
        methodological challenges, 44-46
    Western precursors, 27
Colleges and schools
    Ayurveda instruction, 163
    chiropractic, 27
    International College of Applied Kinesiology, 108
    osteopathy. *See* Osteopathy: medical schools/colleges.
    Reiki, 176
    shiatsu, 152
Consortial Center for Chiropractic Research (CCCR), 27
Cranial osteopathy, 16
Craniosacral therapy, as offshoot of osteopathy, 8
CTrPs (central trigger points), 80-81

D
Daiva-vyapashraya chikitsa, 158
De Jarnette, Major Bertrand, 39
Dhanvantri sampradaya, 158
Dharma, 157
Dhatus, 158
Direct treatment, defined, 14
Doshas, 157, 158
Dysponesis, 102-103

E
Effleurage, 150, 160
Esoteric healing, 161-162

F
Fascia, defined, 51
Feldenkrais, Moshe, 122-126, 120f
Feldenkrais Method (FM), 119-120
    act-ure as biologic necessity, 126
    attention and discrimination, 125
    Awareness Through Movement, 127
        lesson excerpts, 127-131
        practice strategies, 131, 133f, 135f
    brain created by experience, 123
    certification in, 134
    differentiation and integration, 125
    experience, role of, 123

Feldenkrais Method (FM)—cont'd
    Functional Integration, 127
        lesson excerpts, 127-131
        practice strategies, 131
    historical development, 120-121
    homunculus, individuality of, 124
    images and habits, 123
    infant learning model, 124-125
    Jiu-Jitsu, 121f
    lesson excerpts, 127-131
    movement patterns, individuality of, 124
    nervous reorganization, 122-123
    organic learning, 123-124
    practice strategies, 131
    research, 134
        dynamic systems theory, 136
        effectiveness, 137, 136t
        functional performance and motor control, 135
        pain management, 134-135
        psychological effects of method, 135-136
        quality of life improvements, 136
    risk and safety, 133
    self-image, 124
    self-improvement through movement, 125
    skeletal conductivity of movement, 126
    skeletal support and the mobilization of muscle
        tension, 126
    spontaneity, 123
    Training Accreditation Board, 133-134
    training programs, 133, 134f
FI. See Functional Integration (FI).
Fight or flight arousal, 125
Five element shiatsu, 152
Five factors of intervertebral foramen, 105-106
Fixation subluxations, 32
FM. See Feldenkrais Method (FM).
French osteopathic practitioners, 20
Functional Integration (FI), 127
    lesson excerpts, 127-131, 127f
    practice strategies, 131,

G
Gamanas, 158
Gillet, Henri, 39
Gonstead, Clarence, 39
Goodheart, George J., Jr., 100-101
Grammar of spontaneity, 123
Gunas, 156

H
Headaches, chiropractic research on, 42-43
Healing touch (HT), 184-185
    case study, 96
    client-practitioner interaction, 189

Healing touch (HT)—cont'd
    current use, 186
    diagnosis, 188-189
    history of, 185
    indications, 190
    philosophy and principles, 186-188
    practitioner constraints, 189-190
    research, 195-196
    techniques, 191, 192t
    therapeutic touch, distinguished, 193
    training and certification, 193-195
High-velocity, low-amplitude (HVLA) thrust
    chiropractic adjustment, 34, 36
    osteopathy, 15
Homas, 158
Homeostasis, 52, 59
    mechanisms, self-sufficiency of, 13
Homunculus, individuality of, 124
Hook up state, 113-114
HT. See Healing touch (HT).
HVLA thrust. See High-velocity, low-amplitude (HVLA)
        thrust.
Hyperalgesic skin zone, 76

I
Illi, Fred, 39
Indirect treatment, defined, 14
Infantile colic chiropractic research, 43-44
Integrated neuromuscular inhibition technique (INIT),
        85-86
International College of Applied Kinesiology (ICAK), 108
International osteopathic practitioners, 20
International Rolf Institute, 91-92
Internships for osteopaths, 21

J
Janse, Joseph, 39
Japanese shiatsu, 152
Jarahar, 160
Jing, 143
Jitsu, 146
Joint hypermobility, 33
Jones, Lawrence, 15

K
Kama, 157
Kapha vata nirodhak, 160
Kayachikitsa, 158
Kieraku, 143
Kinesiology. See Applied kinesiology (AK).
Klesh sahatwa, 160
Korr, Irvin, 24
Krieger, Dolores, 185-186
Kyo, 146

L

Langhana therapeutics, 158
Ling, Per Henrik, 52
Littlejohn, J. Martin, 19
Lymphatic treatment
    marma therapy, 161
    osteopathy, 15

M

Macrobiotics and shiatsu, 146, 152
Malas, 158
Mangalas, 158
Mantras, 158
Marma points, 158, 159t, 161
Marma therapy, 160-161
Massage therapy, 50-51
    body views, 51
        convergent view, 52
        energetic view, 51-52
        functional view, 51
        movement view, 51
        structural view, 51
    Chinese massage, 169
    licensure, 66
    modalities, 52-54
        creation of, 51
        touch abilities. *See* TouchAbilities.
    relaxation paradigm, 92
    shiatsu. *See* Shiatsu.
    training, 66
Mead, Margaret, 122f
Meade, T.W., 40
Medical schools. *See* Osteopathy.
Mentastics, 114f, 115-116
Mentgen, Janet, 185
Meridians or channels, 143
    internal organs, relationship to, 145
Mitchell, Fred, Sr., 15
Moksha, 157
Mon-shin, 147
Mrija varn bal prad, 160
Musculoskeletal disorders
    chiropractic research, 39, 43
        early research, 39
        headaches, 42-43
        low back pain, manual adjustment for, 40-42
        low back pain with leg pain, 40-42
        University of Colorado project, 39
    neuromuscular therapy techniques. *See* Neuromuscular
        therapy (NMT).
    neuromusculoskeletal medicine osteopathy, 19
    Trager Approach, use of, 116
Myofascial release, 15-16
    osteopathy, as offshoot of, 8

N

Nadi channels, 158-159
Nadi pariksha, 157
Nadi vigyan, 157
Navarakizhi massage, 160
Neuromuscular therapy (NMT), 72
    American NMT, 82-84
        assessment protocols, 83b
        training and certification, 87
        treatment framework, 86-87
    assessment, 70-72
        American NMT protocols, 83b
        to treatment, 79
    attachment trigger points, 81-82
    biochemical factors, 71
    central trigger points, 80-81
    certification, 87
    compression techniques, 78
    contraindications, 73
    discomfort scale, use of, 75-76
    European NMT, 84
        Lief's finger techniques, 85, 85f, 86f
        thumb techniques, 84-85, 85f
        training and certification, 87
        treatment framework, 86-87
    flat compression, 78, 78f
    flat palpation, 77-78
    historical development, 69-70
    indications, 72-73
    lubricants, use of, 79-80
    nutritional factors, 71-72
    palpation techniques, 75
        discomfort scale, use of, 75-76
        flat palpation, 77-78, 77f
        panniculosis, 76-77
        snapping palpation, 78-79, 79f
        trigger points, 80
    panniculosis, 76-77
    pincer compression, 78, 78f
    postural and use factors, 71
    protocols sequencing, 74-75
    psychosocial factors, 72
    snapping palpation, 78-79, 79f
    Trager Approach, use of, 116
    training, 87
    trigger points, palpation of, 80
    trigger points, treatment of, 80
        attachment, 81-82
        central, 80-81
        considerations, 82
        European INIT protocol, 85-86
        palpating, 80
Neuromusculoskeletal medicine osteopathy, 19
NMT. *See* Neuromuscular therapy (NMT).
Northup, George W., 11

O

OCF. *See* Osteopathy in the cranial field (OCF). 16
Organic learning, 123-124
Osteopathic manipulative technique (OMT). *See* Osteopathy: manipulation.
Osteopathy
  articulatory technique, 15
  biofeedback, validation of, 12
  chaos mathematics, use of, 13
  classical osteopathy
    philosophy, 9
    practice of, 19
  contemporary philosophy, 12-13
    ""Our Platform,"" differences from, 10b-11b
  counterstrain technique, 15
  cranial field, 16
  craniosacral therapy, 16
  diagnosis, 16-17
    case examples, 17
  drugs, use of, 9-12, 18
  exercise needs, 12, 13
  facilitated positional release, 15
  fractal analysis, use of, 13
  genetics, promise of, 12
  high-velocity, low-amplitude thrust, 15
  history of, 3-8
  lymphatic treatment, 15
  macroscopic level of manipulation, 18
  manipulation, 18
    practitioners, levels of, 19
    surgery patients, 10
    techniques, 14-16
  medical schools/colleges, 21, 24, 22t-23t
    historical development, 5-6
    interviews, 21
    matriculation requirements, 21
    postgraduate education, 21, 24
    research, 24
  medicines, use of, 9-12, 18
  microscopic level of manipulation, 18
  mind/body approaches, 12
  muscle energy treatment, 15
  myofascial release, 15-16
    osteopathy, as offshoot of, 8
  nutrition, importance of, 12, 13
  "Our Platform," 6, 10b
    contemporary differences, 10b-11b
  philosophy and principles, 8-9, 10b-11b
    classical, 9
    contemporary, 12-13
    current principles, 13-14
    evolution of, 9-12
    implementation, levels of, 18-20
  primary care specialties, 19

Osteopathy—cont'd
  profession of
    history of, 3-8
    internationally, 19-20
    internships, 21
    levels of practice, 18-20
    offshoots of, 8
    practice rights, 20
  psychological counseling, use of, 12
  reductionist manipulative specialists, 19
  relaxation response, validation of, 12
  soft tissue treatment, 15
  solar radiation, dangers of, 12
  surgery
    OMT for patients, 10
    use of, 18
  techniques/treatment, 14-16
    articulatory technique, 15
    case examples, 17
    counterstrain technique, 15
    direct treatment, defined, 14
    high-velocity, low-amplitude thrust, 15
    indirect treatment, defined, 14
    lymphatic treatment, 15
    muscle energy treatment, 15
    myofascial release, 8, 15-16
    osteopathy in the cranial field, 16
    soft tissue treatment, 15
    visceral techniques, 16
  wellness and illness, 13
Osteopathy in the cranial field (OCF), 16

P

Pain
  chiropractic
    approaches to pain, 37, 38
    low back cases with leg pain, 42
    low back pain manual adjustment, 40-42
  Feldenkrais Method research, 134
  medical approaches to, 37
Palmer, B.J., 39
Palmer, Daniel David, 8, 27-29, 28f
Panniculosis, 76-77
Paschat karma, 158
Pathya apathya, 157
Peckham, John, 15
Pétrissage, 160
Physical therapy, as offshoot of osteopathy, 8
Pincer compression, 78, 78f
Pizhichal therapy, 160
Polarity therapy, 161
Prakiti, 156
Pranayama, 159
Prasad kar, 160

Prayaschittas, 158
Purva karma, 158
Pushti kar, 160

Q
Qi, 168-169, 168f, 168t
    cultivation, 169-170
Qi Gong, 168, 169-171

R
Rajamaya, 156, 157
Rasayanas, 158
Reiki, 175-176
    diagnosis, 176-177
    energy, 177-178
    European treatment styles, 181
    hand positions, 179
        on back, 180, 181f
        balancing position, 181, 181f
        on chest, 179, 181f
        on head, 179, 179f, 180
        inguinal area, 180
        around neck, 179, 181
        "T-hold" position, 180-181, 181f
    history, 176
    instruction, 182-183
    levels of, 182
    Masters, 182-283
    philosophy and principles, 177, 178-179
    schools, 176
    touch, 177
Research
    applied kinesiology, 108-109
    chiropractic
        musculoskeletal disorders research. See Chiropractic.
        visceral disorders research. See Chiropractic.
    Feldenkrais Method. See Feldenkrais Method (FM).
    healing touch, 196
    osteopathic institutions, 24
    Rolf Method of Structural Integration, 98
    shiatsu. See Shiatsu.
    therapeutic touch, 195-196
    Trager Approach, 117
Rogers, M.E., 188
Rolf, Ida, 8, 89-92
Rolf Method of Structural Integration, 89
    adaptability principle, 94
    biologic organization and morphology, 96-97
    closure principle, 95
    continuity principle, 94-95
    corrective paradigm, 92
    goals of, 92-93
    historical development, 89-91
    holistic paradigm, holistic principles of intervention, 94-96

Rolf Method of Structural Integration—cont'd
    integration in gravity, 92-93
    less invasive/less painful techniques, 96
    logo, 91-92, 91f, 93
    new developments, 93-96
    normality, 93, 94
    osteopathy, as offshoot of, 8
    palintonic principle, 95
    professional organizations, 98
    relaxation paradigm, 92
    research, 98
    somatic idealism and formulism, 92-94
    "structure determines function" principle, 90
    support principle, 94
    10-session protocol ("The Recipe"), 90, 92, 97
    training, 97-98
    typical session, 97

S
Sadhana, 156
Sansargi, 158
Santarpana, 158
Satvamaya, 156, 157
Schools. See Colleges and schools.
Segmental dysfunction (SDF), 32-33
    diagnosis, 34, 35f
Segmental facilitation, 34
Sensitive dependence on initial conditions, 13
Set su-shin, 147
Shamana therapeutics, 158
Sharam har, 160
Shiatsu, 141
    acupressure, 151-152
    acupuncture, distinguished, 144-145, 145t
    Anma Therapy, 152
    chakras, 144
    diagnosis, 147-149, 150
    energy principle, 143
    five element shiatsu, 152
    history of, 141-143
    Japanese, 152
    jitsu, 146
    kyo, 146
    macrobiotics and, 146, 152
    meridians or channels, 143
        internal organs, relationship to, 145
    philosophy and principles, 143-147
    practice of, 149
    preparation for, 149
    research, 153
        cardiovascular, 153
        nausea and vomiting, 153-154
        nausea with breast cancer chemotherapy, 153
    techniques, 149-152

Shiatsu—cont'd
   training and certification, 147, 152-153
   Tsubos, 144
      internal organs, relationship to, 145
   typical session, 150
   yin and yang, 145
   Zen, 152
Shiatsu Anma Therapy, 152
Shintoism, 176
Shodhana therapeutics, 158
Sira vessels, 158, 159f
SMT. *See* Spinal manual therapy (SMT).
Snapping palpation, 78-79, 79f
Snehan, 158, 159-160
Sparsha, 157
Spinal manual therapy (SMT), 27. *See also* Chiropractic.
   AHCPR guidelines endorsement, 30
   headaches research, 42-43
   indications and contraindications, 34, 35f
   infantile colic research, 43-44
   low back pain research
      acute *versus* chronic pain, 40
      chronic cases, evidence for manual methods in, 41
      chronic cases, preventing acute cases from becoming, 41-42
      low back cases with leg pain, 42
      manual adjustment for pain, 40-42
   techniques, 34, 36
   Western precursors, 27
Spondylotherapy, 150
Srota channels, 159
Sthapni marma, 161
Still, Andrew Taylor, 3, 4-6, 4f, 8, 24
Still technique, 15
Sutherland, William G., 16
Swapn kar, 160
Swedan, 158

T
Takata, Hawayo, 177
Tamaomaya, 156, 157
Tapotement, 160
TART diagnosis, 16
Thai bodywork, 162-163
Thanulogy, 160-161
Therapeutic touch (TT), 184-185
   client-practitioner interaction, 189
   current use, 186
   diagnosis, 188-189
   healing touch, distinguished, 193
   history of, 185-186
   indications, 190
   philosophy and principles, 186-188
   practitioner constraints, 189-190

Therapeutic touch (TT)—cont'd
   research, 195-196
   techniques, 191, 193
   training and certification, 195
Thirummal, 160
Tibetan bodywork, 162
TouchAbilities, 53-54
   breathing component, 54
      BodyWays using techniques, 55b
      directing, 55
      observing, 54
      synchronizing, 55
   compression component, 59
      BodyWays using techniques, 60b
      pressing and pushing, 59-60
      squeezing and pinching, 60
      twisting and wringing, 60
   energetic component, 58-59
      balancing, 59
      BodyWays using techniques, 59b
      intuiting, 58
      sensing, 58
   expansion component, 60-61
      BodyWays using techniques, 61b
      lifting, 61
      pulling, 61
      rolling, 61
   gliding component, 65
      BodyWays using techniques, 66b
      rubbing, 65
      stroking, 65
   kinetic component, 61-62
      BodyWays using techniques, 63b
      holding and supporting, 62
      letting go and dropping, 62-63
      mobilizing, 62
      stabilizing, 63
   mental component, 55
      BodyWays using techniques, 57b
      focusing, 57
      inquiring, 56
      intending, 56-57
      transmitting, 57
      visualizing, 56
   oscillation component, 63
      BodyWays using techniques, 64b
      collective intentions, 64-65
      shaking, 64
      striking, 64
      vibrating, 64
Traditional Chinese medicine (TCM). *See* Chinese traditional medicine.
Trager, Milton, 110-111, 113f, 114f

Trager Approach, 111-112
  contraindications, 117
  deep relaxation state, 112-113
  diagnostic approach, 112, 114
  goals of, 114-115
  history of, 110-111
  hook up state, 113-114
  indications, 116-117
  mentastics, 114f, 115-116
  philosophy and principles, 111-115
  reflex-response, 116
  research, 117
  table work, 115
  training and certification, 117
Triano, John, 36
Tridoshas, 157
Trigger points (TrPs). *See* Neuromuscular therapy (NMT).
Trigunas, 157
TrPs (trigger points). *See* Neuromuscular therapy (NMT).
Tsubos, 144
  internal organs, relationship to, 145
TT. *See* Therapeutic touch (TT).
Tui Na, 153, 169
Twak dridh kar, 160

U
Udvartana, 158
University of Colorado chiropractic research project, 39

Upaharas, 158
Upavasa, 158
Upledger, John, 8
Usui, Mikao, 175, 176
Usui System of Natural Healing. *See* Reiki.

V
Varma therapy, 160-161
Vata har, 160
Vibration
  Ayurvedic massage, 160
  TouchAbilities, 64
Visceral disorders
  chiropractic research, 39, 44
    infantile colic, 43-44
    methodological challenges, 44-46
  osteopathic techniques, 16

W
Ward, Robert, 15
Watson, Jean, 188

Y
Yin and yang, 145

Z
Zen shiatsu, 152